Current Concepts in Sports Medicine

Editor

LAWRENCE M. OLOFF

CLINICS IN PODIATRIC MEDICINE AND SURGERY

www.podiatric.theclinics.com

Consulting Editor
THOMAS J. CHANG

January 2023 • Volume 40 • Number 1

ELSEVIER

1600 John F. Kennedy Boulevard • Suite 1800 • Philadelphia, Pennsylvania, 19103-2899

http://www.theclinics.com

CLINICS IN PODIATRIC MEDICINE AND SURGERY Volume 40, Number 1
January 2023 ISSN 0891-8422, ISBN-13: 978-0-323-98693-9

Editor: Megan Ashdown
Developmental Editor: Diana Grace Ang

Clinics in Podiatric Medicine and Surgery (ISSN 0891-8422) is published quarterly by Elsevier Inc., 360 Park Avenue South, New York, NY 10010-1710. Months of issue are January, April, July, and October. Business and Editorial Offices: 1600 John F. Kennedy Blvd., Ste. 1800, Philadelphia, PA 19103-2899. Customer Service Office: 3251 Riverport Lane, Maryland Heights, MO 63043. Periodicals postage paid at New York, NY and additional mailing offices. Subscription prices are $329.00 per year for US individuals, $625.00 per year for US institutions, $100.00 per year for US students and residents, $405.00 per year for Canadian individuals, $754.00 for Canadian institutions, $490.00 for international individuals, $754.00 per year for international institutions, $100.00 per year for Canadian students/residents, and $220.00 per year for foreign students/residents. To receive student/resident rate, orders must be accompanied by name of affiliated institution, date of term, and the *signature* of program/residency coordinator on institution letterhead. Orders will be billed at individual rate until proof of status is received. Foreign air speed delivery is included in all *Clinics* subscription prices. All prices are subject to change without notice. POSTMASTER: Send address changes to *Clinics in Podiatric Medicine and Surgery*, Elsevier Health Sciences Division, Subscription Customer Service, 3251 Riverport Lane, Maryland Heights, MO 63043. **Customer Service: 1-800-654-2452 (US). From outside of the US, call 314-447-8871. Fax: 314-447-8029. E-mail: JournalsCustomerService-usa@elsevier.com (for print support); JournalsOnlineSupport-usa@elsevier.com (for online support).**

Reprints. For copies of 100 or more of articles in this publication, please contact the Commercial Reprints Department, Elsevier Inc., 360 Park Avenue South, New York, NY 10010-1710. Tel.: 212-633-3874; Fax: 212-633-3820; E-mail: reprints@elsevier.com.

Clinics in Podiatric Medicine and Surgery is covered in *MEDLINE/PubMed (Index Medicus) and EMBASE/Excerpta Medica.*

Contributors

CONSULTING EDITOR

THOMAS J. CHANG, DPM
Clinical Professor and Past Chairman, Department of Podiatric Surgery, California College of Podiatric Medicine, Faculty, The Podiatry Institute, Sonoma County Orthopedic/ Podiatric Specialists, Santa Rosa, California

EDITOR

LAWRENCE M. OLOFF, DPM, FACFAS
Present Affiliations: Team Podiatrist San Francisco Giants, Podiatry Residency Director St Marys Medical Center, San Francisco, California; Teaching Staff, Silicon Valley Reconstructive Foot and Ankle Fellowship Program, Private Practice, Palo Alto Medical Foundation, Burlingame, California; Clinical Professor, College of Podiatric Medicine, Western University of Health Sciences, Pomona, California. Past Affiliations: Team Podiatrist San Francisco 49ers, Team Podiatrist Stanford University Athletics, Team Podiatrist Santa Clara University Athletics, Team Podiatrist US Decathlon, Team Podiatrist San Jose Ballet, Consultant Golden State Warriors

AUTHORS

RICHARD L. BLAKE, DPM, MS
Instructor, California School of Podiatric Medicine, Samuel Merritt University, Past President, American Academy of Podiatric Sports Medicine, Staff Podiatrist, Orthopedic and Sports Institute, Saint Francis Memorial Hospital, San Francisco, California

MAJID CHALIAN, MD
Section Chief and Assistant Professor of Radiology, Musculoskeletal Imaging and Intervention, University of Washington, Seattle, Washington

THOMAS CHANG, DPM
Podiatrist, Redwood Orthopedic Surgery Associates, Santa Rosa, California

SHIRLEY CHEN, DPM, AACFAS
Palo Alto Medical Foundation, Palo Alto Foundation Medical Group, Mountain View, California

MATTHEW D. DOYLE, DPM, FACFAS
Foot and Ankle Surgeon, Silicon Valley Reconstructive Foot and Ankle Fellowship, Palo Alto Medical Foundation, Mountain View, California

NASTARAN HOSSEINI, MD
Postdoctoral Research Fellow, Musculoskeletal Imaging and Intervention, University of Washington, Seattle, Washington

MEGAN A. ISHIBASHI, DPM, AACFAS
Fellow, Silicon Valley Reconstructive Foot and Ankle Fellowship, Palo Alto Medical Foundation, Mountain View, California

VARSHA IVANOVA, DPM
Second Year Foot and Ankle Surgery Resident, Kaiser Permanente, Santa Clara, California

MEAGAN M. JENNINGS, DPM, FACFAS
Director, Silicon Valley Foot and Ankle Reconstructive Fellowship, Palo Alto Foundation Medical Group/Sutter Health, Mountain View, California

EMILY KHUC, DPM
Podiatry Resident, Saint Mary's Medical Center San Francisco, San Francisco, California

BRANDON KIM, DPM
Kaiser Santa Clara Foot and Ankle Residency Program, Department of Orthopedics and Podiatric Surgery, Kaiser Foundation Hospitals, Santa Clara, California

CHRISTY M. KING, DPM, FACFAS, ABPM
Residency Director, Kaiser San Francisco Bay Area Foot and Ankle Residency Program, Kaiser Oakland Foundation Hospital, Attending Surgeon, Foot and Ankle Surgery, Orthopedics and Podiatry Department, Kaiser Oakland, Oakland, California

ZACHARY KRAMER, DPM, AT
Foot and Ankle Surgeon, Scripps Memorial Hospital, Encinitas, California

CRAIG E. KRCAL, JR, DPM
Resident, Kaiser San Francisco Bay Area Foot and Ankle Residency Program, Oakland, California

CHANDLER J. LIGAS, DPM
Fellow, Silicon Valley Reconstructive Foot and Ankle Fellowship, Palo Alto Medical Foundation, Mountain View, California, USA

LAWRENCE M. OLOFF, DPM, FACFAS
Present Affiliations: Team Podiatrist San Francisco Giants, Podiatry Residency Director St Marys Medical Center, San Francisco, California; Teaching Staff, Silicon Valley Reconstructive Foot and Ankle Fellowship Program, Private Practice, Palo Alto Medical Foundation, Burlingame, California; Clinical Professor, College of Podiatric Medicine, Western University of Health Sciences, Pomona, California. Past Affiliations: Team Podiatrist San Francisco 49ers, Team Podiatrist Stanford University Athletics, Team Podiatrist Santa Clara University Athletics, Team Podiatrist US Decathlon, Team Podiatrist San Jose Ballet, Consultant Golden State Warriors

CHRISTINA MA, DPM
PGY-II, Staint Mary's Foot and Ankle Surgical Residency Program, San Francisco, California

AMELIA MOSTOVOY, DPM
2nd Year Resident, St. Mary's Medical Center, San Francisco, California

ATEFE POOYAN, MD, MPH
Postdoctoral Research Fellow, Musculoskeletal Imaging and Intervention, University of Washington, Seattle, Washington

RYAN SHERRICK, DPM
Foot and Ankle Surgeon, Foot and Ankle Surgery, Innovative Medical Solutions Foot and Ankle Institute, Los Angeles, California

ERIC SHI, DPM, FACFAS
Sutter East Bay Medical Foundation, Castro Valley, Castro Valley, California

FIROOZEH SHOMAL ZADEH, MD
Postdoctoral Research Fellow, Musculoskeletal Imaging and Intervention, University of Washington, Seattle, Washington

KANWARDEEP SINGH, MD
Musculoskeletal Fellow, Department of Radiology, University of Washington, Seattle, Washington

NICHOLAS W. TODD, DPM, FACFAS
Associate Medical Director of Innovation, Palo Alto Medical Foundation, Palo Alto Foundation Medical Group, Mountain View Center, Mountain View, California

MHER VARTIVARIAN, DPM, FACFAS, ABPM
Assistant Professor, California School of Podiatric Medicine at Samuel Merritt University, Oakland, California; Associate Residency Program Director, St. Mary's Medical Center Residency Program, Attending Surgeon, University of California San Francisco, Center for Limb Preservation, Regional Chief Medical Officer-San Francisco Bay Area, Balance Health, San Francisco, California

NISHIT S. VORA, DPM
Chief Resident, Saint Mary's Medical Center, San Francisco, California

TENAYA A. WEST, DPM, FACFAS
Department of Orthopedics and Podiatric Surgery, Palo Alto Medical Foundation, Mountain View, California

ISAAC WILHELM, DPM
Resident, St. Mary's Medical Center, San Francisco, California

SAMANTHA WILLIAMS, DPM, AACFAS
Palo Alto Medical Foundation, Palo Alto Foundation Medical Group, Mountain View, California

YESSIKA WOO LEE, DPM
Foot and Ankle Surgeon, Dignity Health, San Francisco, California

JESSE YURGELON, DPM, FACFAS
Palo Alto Medical Foundation Mountain View Center, Mountain View, California

Contents

> Pediatric foot and ankle fractures are common in athletic participation. Treatment of pediatric sports trauma must take into account the unique challenges this population presents, and aim to minimize long-term complications. Given the excellent remodeling potential of pediatric bone, conservative treatment can often be used. However, a thorough understanding of physeal anatomy, fracture patterns, and biomechanics is needed to guide treatment choice and determine when surgical intervention is warranted.

> There are many factors to consider when treating an Achilles tendon rupture in the acute and chronic/neglected settings. For acute rupture, operative and nonoperative management contribute to a good prognosis with low associated risks. Patient or injury characteristics can assist in the shared decision-making about treatment. In chronic rupture, MRI may help to determine rupture location, gap distance, and tissue material available for repair. Various surgical approaches are used for chronic rupture repair. Treatment of the Achilles tendon rupture generates many interesting and complex discussions on the optimal management.

> Biomechanics is a crucial component of treating lower extremity pathology. The relaxed calcaneal stance position, the Achilles flexibility, and the first ray motion and position tests are demonstrated and should be mastered. The relaxed calcaneal stance position is crucial in children's flat feet treatment, adult acquired flat feet, and all pronatory symptoms. The Achilles flexibility measurement demonstrates normality, tightness, or overflexibility. Tightness and overflexibility denote weakness owing to the contractile properties of the tendon. The first ray motion and position examination elucidates whether the first ray is normal or part of a pronatory problem or a supinatory problem.

> Understanding the types of ankle sprains is essential in determining the most appropriate treatment and preventing substantial missed time from sports. Commonly known and recognized is an acute lateral ankle sprain, however, a differentiation should also be made to understand high (syndesmotic) ankle sprains as the mechanism of injury and recovery periods differ between these two types.

The peroneal tendons play a critical role in stabilizing the foot and ankle especially in athletes with high demands on lateral ankle strength. A complete understanding of the anatomy of the lateral ankle as well as a careful physical examination is imperative to diagnosing peroneal pathology, which is commonly misdiagnosed and can lead to chronic pain and inability to perform high level sport. Although low-demand patients do well with a conservative approach, most high-demand athletes will benefit from surgical intervention.

Movement of the first metatarsophalangeal joint is an essential function of many sports. Because of the high demand on this relatively small joint, it is prone to the development of several notable pathologic derangements that can prevent full and pain-free athletic performance. A complete understanding of the joint anatomy and a careful physical examination and history collection is crucial to identifying an accurate diagnosis. Treatment should be pathology specific and should keep in mind the career expectations of the athlete.

Orthobiologics have gained much popularity in recent years but there has not been a large amount of clinical evidence to support their use. In the limited research that has been published, they have been shown to be effective and safe. They can assist in earlier return to activity with the avoidance of surgery. They can also augment current surgical practice to aid in healing and return to sport with few complications. With new medical innovation, there is unfortunately a higher cost for these products. The use of orthobiologics will only grow and so will the need for high-level clinical evidence.

Stress fractures are a common injury that present in athletes because of the high intensity and repetitive nature of many sports. These injuries require a high index of suspicion in the treating clinician to allow for timely management. Though most low-risk fractures heal well with conservative management, high-risk stress fractures as well as any fracture in the elite athlete may warrant surgical intervention as well as an augmented treatment and rehabilitation regimen.

CLINICS IN PODIATRIC MEDICINE AND SURGERY

SERIES OF RELATED INTEREST

Orthopedic Clinics
https://www.orthopedic.theclinics.com/
Clinics in Sports Medicine
https://www.sportsmed.theclinics.com/
Foot and Ankle Clinics
https://www.foot.theclinics.com/
Physical Medicine and Rehabilitation Clinics
https://www.pmr.theclinics.com/

THE CLINICS ARE AVAILABLE ONLINE!
Access your subscription at:
www.theclinics.com

Foreword

Sports Medicine

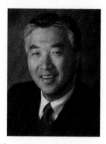

Thomas J. Chang, DPM
Consulting Editor

Many students and future Doctors of Podiatric Medicine first entered this specialty of medicine being drawn to an interest in sports-related injuries. I know that was true for me. I remember the excitement of hearing Dr George Sheehan, the world-renowned sports physician, as a student in the Sports Medicine Club during medical school. Under the guidance of Dr Howard Palamarchuk, we were also allowed to participate in the Runners Medical Tent at the Boston Marathon each year. My early exposure to the world of Sports Medicine was an exciting one.

Podiatric Physicians play a prominent role in all aspects of treating and managing foot and ankle injuries in the local, regional, and even national sports communities. Many are involved on a collegiate and professional level and have committed to being on the playing field throughout the season. I acknowledge the Sports physician careers of Drs Lowell Weil Sr and Jr, Dr. Howard Liebeskind, Dr. Robert Mohr, Dr. Patrick Deheer, and Dr. Larry Oloff, just to name a few.

Besides athletes who compete at the highest level, many of our active patients are also "athletes" in their lives. Regardless of whether your practice consists of competitive athletes, Podiatric physicians keep all levels of athletes on their feet and will always play an integral role in getting people back from injury to the playing field of life.

This issue looks at the current discussions on many topics sports related, yet is applicable to almost every patient who maintains a certain level of activity and fitness.

Clin Podiatr Med Surg 40 (2023) xiii–xiv
https://doi.org/10.1016/j.cpm.2022.10.001
0891-8422/23/© 2022 Published by Elsevier Inc.

I am grateful to Dr Oloff and his efforts in putting this tremendous group of authors together. I hope you enjoy this issue.

Thomas J. Chang, DPM
Sonoma County Orthopedic / Podiatric Specialists
3536 Mendocino Avenue, Suite 300B
Santa Rosa, CA 95403, USA

E-mail address:
thomaschang14@comcast.net

Preface

Current Concepts in Sports Medicine

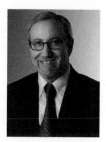

Lawrence M. Oloff, DPM, FACFAS
Editor

I have been most fortunate to have been a team podiatrist or consultant for professional and college teams in baseball, football, basketball, soccer, track and field, and dance over the last three decades. When I first entered these roles, I had thought I was well prepared to treat the variety of foot and ankle injuries that occur in sports having been in practice for some time. I soon discovered that there is no book, seminar, education, or practice background that fully prepares you for these elite athletes. When you enter this world, you will find yourself back in the role as a student. Your teachers will be the team trainers and physical therapists who practice their craft so well. I have been very lucky to work with the very best of these, and they heightened my game. I am forever grateful to them for teaching me how to treat these elite athletes and making me a better doctor.

I would also like to thank all the authors, who have graciously consented to donate time from their very busy schedules to contribute to this book. Many of them have partnered with residents so that these residents can use these articles as a teaching

Clin Podiatr Med Surg 40 (2023) xv–xvi
https://doi.org/10.1016/j.cpm.2022.09.001
0891-8422/23/© 2022 Published by Elsevier Inc.

podiatric.theclinics.com

experience. I hope that all our readers will use this *Clinics in Podiatric Medicine of North America* issue to complement their practices.

Lawrence M. Oloff, DPM, FACFAS
Present Affiliations:
Team Podiatrist San Francisco Giants
Podiatry Residency Director St Marys Medical Center
Teaching Staff Silicon Valley Reconstructive Foot and Ankle Fellowship Program
Clinical Professor, College of Podiatric Medicine, Western University of Health Sciences

Past Affiliations:
Team Podiatrist San Francisco 49ers
Team Podiatrist Stanford University Athletics
Team Podiatrist Santa Clara University Athletics
Team Podiatrist US Decathlon
Team Podiatrist San Jose Ballet
Consultant Golden State Warriors

E-mail address:
lmop11@comcast.net

Compartment Syndrome in the Foot and Leg

Samantha Williams, DPM, AACFAS[a],*, Shirley Chen, DPM, AACFAS[a],
Nicholas W. Todd, DPM, FACFAS[a]

KEYWORDS

- Exertional-related leg pain • Compartment syndrome
- Chronic exertional compartment syndrome • Sports injuries • Athletes

KEY POINTS

- Athletes with chronic exertional compartment syndrome require a comprehensive approach for proper diagnosis and treatment.
- Although chronic exertional compartment syndrome predominantly affects the lower leg, its affliction on the medial, central, and lateral compartments of the foot has also been reported.
- Intracompartmental muscle pressure readings are considered the gold standard for diagnosis, but newer noninvasive techniques are gaining popularity.
- Nonsurgical management involves anti-inflammatory medications, physical therapy modalities, and gait retraining.
- Surgical management can be achieved through an open, mini-open, or endoscopic approach to release the pathologic osteofascial compartment.

INTRODUCTION

Chronic exertional compartment syndrome (CECS) is a condition associated with strenuous exercise that can lead to debilitating pain only relieved by cessation of the causative activity.[1] The first published report of CECS was described by Mavor in 1956,[2] in which he reported bilateral anterior leg pain in a 24-year-old professional soccer player during exercise. The patient was treated successfully with a fasciotomy and fascia lata graft.[2]

The incidence of exercise-induced leg pain ranges from 14% to 27% in the literature.[3] Of these, 70% occur in the anterior leg compartment in endurance runners.[4,5] Literature regarding the relationship between CECS and gender is inconsistent. Although early reports suggested a higher male prevalence,[6,7] two more recent cohort

[a] Palo Alto Medical Foundation, Palo Alto Foundation Medical Group, 701 East El Camino Real, Mountain View, CA 94040, USA
* Corresponding author.
E-mail address: samanthawilliamsdpm@gmail.com

Clin Podiatr Med Surg 40 (2023) 1–21
https://doi.org/10.1016/j.cpm.2022.07.002

studies have proposed a female predominance.[8,9] Because those cohort studies included military and/or athlete populations, the former was most likely due to selection bias. However, a more recent heterogeneous study found an increased incidence in males.[10] As such, the current knowledge of the incidence and risk factors of CECS is largely based on small or biased cohorts, such as elite athletes or servicemen.[9,11,12]

In an effort to quantify the incidence of CECS, a large retrospective cohort study of 8.3 million service members was studied by Waterman and colleagues[9] A total of 4100 diagnosed cases of CECS were identified, which correlated to an incidence rate of 0.49 cases per 1000 person-years. Of this cohort, increased risk was seen among those with increasing age, female sex, white race, junior enlisted rank, and those within the Army branch.[9] However, de Bruijn and colleagues[10] conducted a more recent retrospective cohort study that included a more diverse patient population in terms of age and activity levels. The authors compared patients evaluated for CECS and divided their cohort into CECS diagnoses based on elevated intracompartment pressures (n = 1411) and those with normal physical examination findings (n = 153). Overall, a younger age (median age of 25 years old), male gender, bilateral symptoms, and participation in endurance running or skating were all significant predictors of CECS.[10] More studies with larger patient populations and heterogenous data are required to accurately create a predictive model for CECS.

Although the incidence of lower leg CECS is widely reported, literature on its affliction in the foot is scarce. A little scientific literature exists on incidence and predominance in relation to age, sex, and sport. Of the case reports published, the majority were male, ranging from 16 to 40 years of age, and participated in an endurance sport, such as running.[13–20] The medial compartment comprises the majority of cases, followed by the central and lateral compartments.[13–21]

ANATOMY

The leg consists of four compartments that are divided by relatively inelastic crural fascia: anterior, lateral, superficial posterior, and deep posterior. The muscles of the anterior compartment include the tibialis anterior, extensor hallucis longus, extensor digitorum longus, and peroneus tertius. The deep peroneal nerve pierces the intermuscular septum at the proximal fibula and travels within the anterior compartment of the leg. The lateral compartment includes the peroneus longus and brevis, which are accompanied by the superficial peroneal nerve and peroneal artery. The superficial peroneal nerve pierces the crural fascia on average 12.3 cm proximal to the ankle as it traverses distally, terminating in medial and intermediate dorsal cutaneous nerves 4.4 cm proximal to the ankle.[22] The posterior compartment is subdivided by the posterior intermuscular septum into superficial and deep compartments. The superficial compartment contains the gastrocnemius, soleus, and plantaris, while the deep compartment contains the popliteus, tibialis posterior, flexor hallucis longus, and flexor digitorum longus. The tibial nerve arises from the popliteal fossa and traverses distally where it gives off branches to innervate the superficial and deep compartment muscles. Some authors have postulated a "fifth" compartment of the posterior leg comprising solely the tibialis posterior muscle within its own osteofascial plane.[23] However, follow-up cadaveric studies were unable to corroborate such findings but suggest that aberrant anatomy, such as flexor digitorum longus hypertrophy can effectively compartmentalize the tibialis posterior tendon.[24] These findings corroborate the relatively high recurrence rates of CECS following posterior compartment fasciotomies. Therefore, a two-incision approach is often warranted.[23,24] Overall, approximately 60–75% of patients with CECS experience pathology in more than one compartment.[8,25,26] The anterior compartment is the most commonly affected by CECS (42.5%), followed by the lateral (35.5%), and posterior (18.9%).[8]

In total, there are nine compartments in the foot: four interossei, lateral, medial, central superficial, central deep, and calcaneal compartments. The lateral compartment consists of the abductor digiti minimi and flexor digiti minimi. The medial compartment encompasses the abductor hallucis and flexor digiti minimi brevis. In a cadaveric study focusing on the central compartment by Manoli and Weber, dyed gelatin was injected in a controlled fashion.[27] The contents of each compartment were then assessed, revealing a new compartment deep in the superficial central compartment containing only the quadratus plantae muscle. This compartment was found to communicate with the deep posterior compartment of the leg through the retinaculum posterior to the medial malleolus, thus raising the possibility of concurrent foot and leg CECS.[27,28] Infusate was monitored in a separate cadaveric study by Guyton,[29] however, challenging Manoli and Weber's[27] theory in real-time computed tomography (CT) imaging. Guyton concluded that the barrier between the flexor digitorum longus and quadratus plantae becomes incompetent at pressures less than 10 mm Hg and therefore cannot be expected to generate isolated compartment syndrome.[29] Although foot CECS is rare and limited literature is available, the majority of case reports describe pathology in the medial compartment with unilateral symptoms.[13–16,18]

PATHOPHYSIOLOGY

The etiology of CECS is much debated in the literature, but a pathologically elevated muscle compartment pressure is found as the key event in its pathogenesis. During intense exercise, muscle volume can increase by up to 20% of its resting size, which in turn causes a rise in pressure in each osteofascial compartment.[7] Contributors to this rise in pressure, however, are often multifactorial. Fascial thickening or inelasticity, microtrauma to muscle, myopathies, and vascular compromise all likely play a role in this pathologic event.[30,31]

In a case-control study published by Turnipseed in 1995, patients with CECS were found to have thicker and stiffer fascia compared with age-matched controls (0.35 mm + 0.12 mm, 109 + 65 MN/mm; vs 0.22 mm + 0.06 mm, 60.3 + 22 MN/mm).[32] Partial fascial tears can also contribute to compartment noncompliance in a similar mechanical fashion (**Fig. 1**).[32]

During intense exercise, microtrauma afflicts the muscle tissue. This, in turn, affects the biochemical and mechanical characteristics of the inelastic fascial compartment. Inflammation caused by microtrauma increases fluid flow from the capillaries to the adjacent interstitial space.[5,31] This, in turn, increases volume and pressure within the osteofascial compartment, impairing revascularization and generating pain. In multiple studies, CECS patients were shown to endure greater deoxygenation of muscles during exercise and delayed reoxygenation after activity.[31,33] This double-crush phenomenon propagates patient-reported symptoms during and immediately following activity. In a retrospective case series of 197 patients, the role of obstructed venous outflow in causing the pathology of CECS was investigated.[34] When comparing resting and stress-CT angiography, transient venous outflow obstruction was appreciated, likely caused by hypertrophied muscles in the affected compartment.[34]

With numerous conflicting studies in the literature, the distinct pathophysiology of CECS is up for debate. In a case control study by Edmundsson and colleagues,[35] biopsies from tibialis anterior muscles were obtained at the time of decompression fasciotomy and at a one-year follow-up. These authors found that patients with CECS

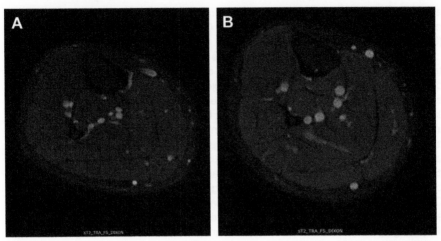

Fig. 1. Axial fat-saturated T2-weighted MRIs. (*A*) Pre-exercise imaging reveals a 1.8 cm diameter of anterior tibialis muscle belly extending 3 mm proud through an apparent fascial defect. (*B*) Post-exercise imaging has exacerbated the fascial herniation of the anterior tibialis muscle belly, which now stands 5 mm proud of fascial defect.

displayed lower capillary density (273 vs 378 capillaries/mm^2, $P = .008$), lower number of capillaries around muscle fibers (4.5 vs 5.7, $P = .004$), and a lower number of capillaries in relation to the muscle fiber area (1.1 vs 1.5, $P = .01$) compared with the control group. This study provides compelling evidence that a paucity of microcirculation is a pathogenic factor in the affected compartments of CECS.[35]

Many theories exist to explain the pain generated by the rise in intracompartmental pressures. The predominant theory is that progressive muscle hypertrophy inside a relatively inelastic osteofascial compartment comprises microcirculation, leading to ischemic pain.[36,37] Following deoxygenation of muscle tissue during exercise, there is increased cell permeability, leading to a shift of fluid in the interstitial space.[36] This results in increased intracompartmental pressures, reducing the microvascular circulation and resulting in ischemic pain. However, there are no studies to prove a causal relationship between intracompartmental pressures and ischemia. In fact, multiple studies have refuted this finding.[38,39] In a prospective blinded evaluation of 34 patients with suspected CECS, thallium-201 single-photon emission computed tomography (SPECT) was used for quantitative and qualitative assessments of perfusion between those compartments with and without CECS.[38] Overall, no compartment perfusion deficit was appreciated in those with CECS, suggesting that the pain stimulus in those patients is not related to ischemia. These nonischemic results are also concordant with the results of Amendola and colleagues[39] Utilizing MRI with methoxy isobutyl isonitrile uptake to assess perfusion to muscle in CECS patients, findings corroborated that the pathophysiology of CECS was in fact unrelated to ischemia.[39]

Other studies have proposed alternative theories for the etiology of pain in the setting of CECS.[36,40,41] The fascia itself is innervated by sensory nerves. It is proposed that in the setting of increased intracompartmental volume, sensory fibers stretch and stimulate pain.[40,41] Similar theories proposed by Humphries and colleagues[42] state that the rise in intramuscular pressure during exercise prompts a receptor-mediated cascade for pain. Finally, metabolic by-products that result from intense activity might also act as a pain mediator in CECS.[38,42]

CLINICAL EXAMINATION

Obtaining a thorough history and physical examination is critical to making an accurate diagnosis of CECS. Because it is relatively rare and underdiagnosed, there can be as much as a 22-month delay in diagnosis of this condition.[36] Typically, patients will complain of pain throughout a particular compartment of the leg at the same time or distance of a particular triggering exercise.[36,43] This nonspecific pain will persist until the cessation of the strenuous activity. Patients will generally describe this sensation as cramping, aching, or burning that begins within 15–20 minutes of the offending activity.[44]

The most common symptoms include claudication (90%), muscle group tightness (60%), and paresthesias (25%) of the affected compartment.[32] Physical examination is vital to differentiate CECS from other common causes of exercise-induced leg pain. Specifically, the patient should be examined before and after completing an activity that reproduces his/her symptoms.[36] Palpating the affected compartment may elicit pain and/or paresthesias. A general firmness can also be appreciated in the involved musculature. Gait analysis should also be conducted, as overpronation is associated with anterior compartment CECS.[45] Runners with CECS often display increased vertical ground reaction forces, longer stride length, and reduced cadence.[46]

Lower leg CECS is predominantly a bilateral syndrome.[10,11,47] In a retrospective cohort study of 1411 patients with lower leg CECS, 74% of patients had bilateral pathology. Interestingly, these findings were compartment-dependent, where 53% of lateral CECS had bilateral syndrome compared with 72% and 78% in anterior and deep-posterior CECS, respectively.[10] Patients who experienced unilateral symptoms were more likely to have a history of previous lower leg trauma (14.4% vs .9%, $P < .01$) or vascular pathology (7.2% vs 3.6%, $P < .01$) compared with patients with bilateral symptoms.[10]

Knowledge of the anatomy of each compartment is paramount to properly diagnosing CECS (**Table 1**). If the anterior compartment is primarily affected, weakness in dorsiflexion and a drop-foot gait are often observed. Weakness in eversion and plantarflexion results in lateral and posterior compartment CECS, respectively. Pedal CECS, however, is often more difficult to deduce compartment involvement. The data available in the literature suggests that CECS of the foot does not share a similar clinical picture to that of the leg. This could be because of increased compartmental musculature impacts during the causative activity.[28] According to some reports, patients with foot CECS experience pain in the affected compartment within 10–90 minutes of strenuous exercise, which subsides after 10–20 minutes of rest.[15–17,20] However, other descriptions consist of aching or cramping pain within the affected compartment within 15 minutes of activity that persists and intensifies up to 24 hours later.[13,14,18] Physical examination findings include a tense, cyanosed, protuberant compartment. Passive range of motion of digits, especially the hallux in the medial compartment of CECS, reproduces pain.

DIAGNOSIS

The diagnosis of CECS is often difficult to deduce because there are multiple etiologies with similar presentations of exercise-related foot or leg pain. This could include medial tibial stress syndrome, stress fracture, nerve entrapment, popliteal artery entrapment syndrome, claudication, or plantar fascial tear.[1] Along with a

Table 1
Lower leg compartment anatomy, signs and symptoms, and incidence of the respective compartment

Compartments	Muscles	Neurovascular	Signs/ Symptoms	Incidences (Debrujin, 2018; Velasco, 2020; Davis, 2013)
Anterior	Tibialis anterior, extensor hallucis longus, extensor digitorum longus, fibularis tertius	Deep peroneal nerve, anterior tibial artery	Dorsiflexory weakness, drop-foot	42.5–43%
Lateral	Peroneus longus, peroneus brevis	Superficial peroneal nerve, peroneal artery	Eversion weakness	19–35.5%
Superficial Posterior	Gastrocnemius, soleus, plantaris	Tibial nerve	Plantarflexion weakness	18.9–34%
Deep Posterior	Popliteus, tibialis posterior, flexor hallucis longus, flexor digitorum longus	Tibial nerve, posterior tibial artery		

comprehensive history and physical examination, there are multiple invasive and noninvasive diagnostic tools that will assist in delineating between these similar conditions.

Currently, intracompartmental pressure measurement remains the gold standard for the diagnosis of CECS. To obtain such values, a needle or catheter is inserted into the symptomatic osteofascial compartment (**Fig. 2**). Either pre- or post-exercise, the patient is placed supine on an examination table where the projected area is prepped

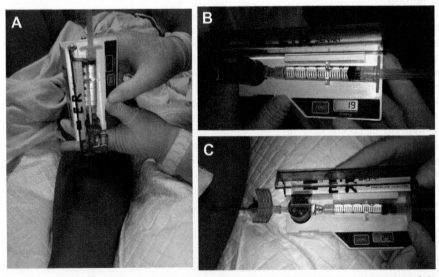

Fig. 2. (A) Indwelling slit catheter for diagnosis of CECS in the anterior compartment of the leg. (B) Pre-exercise measurement of 19 mm Hg. (C) 5 minutes post-exercise measurement of 29 mm Hg, confirming the diagnosis of CECS.

aseptically. Typically, 0.5–1 mL of lidocaine plain is raised as a skin weal along the portal site to anesthetize the skin.[26,48,49] One study concluded that the needle pain from intracompartmental pressure measurements had a median rating of 5 out of 10 with this technique, thus reducing the concern to avoid or minimize its utility in the diagnosis of CECS.[48]

The diagnostic criteria for CECS were first proposed in a retrospective study of 45 patients by Pedowitz and colleagues[7] based on intramuscular compartment pressures. When the history and physical examination are suggestive of CECS, one or more of the following objective criteria is diagnostic: (1) 15 mm Hg pre-exercise intracompartmental pressure measurement, (2) 30 mm Hg 1-minute post-exercise measurement, or (3) 20 mm Hg 5-minute post-exercise measurement.[7] It is important to note that this criterion was based solely on lower leg CECS and a majority of the patients in this cohort had anterior compartment pathology.

The validity of these criteria has been questioned by follow-up studies in the literature. In one study by Roberts and colleagues,[50] with the exception of pre-exercise pressures, many of the intracompartmental pressure measurements overlapped with healthy controls for the lateral and deep-posterior compartments. This suggests that the Pedowitz criteria may only be reasonable for diagnosing anterior compartment CECS. Another review in 2014 studied the validity of the Pedowitz criteria for the anterior compartment specifically.[51] Overall, the majority of measurements pre-, during, and post-exercise in healthy individuals were within the diagnostic range for CECS, again questioning its efficacy even within the anterior compartment.[51]

In 2020, a prospective cohort study of 864 patients ($n = 442$ with CECS; $n = 422$ healthy controls) with exertional-related leg pain was studied to better delineate a relationship between compartment-specific intramuscular pressure readings and CECS.[52] Overall, the median 1-minute post-exercise values in patients with CECS were 33 mm Hg in the deep-posterior compartment, 35 mm Hg in the superficial-posterior compartment, 40 mm Hg in the lateral compartment, and 47 mm Hg in the anterior compartment, compared with 12 mm Hg, 12 mm Hg, 14 mm Hg, and 18 mm Hg in the control group, respectively. In concordance with this study, there is robust evidence to support lower intracompartmental pressure measurements in the posterior and lateral osteofascial compartments compared with the anterior osteofascial compartment.[50–52] As such, a physician should consider lowering threshold values for the Pedowitz criteria when a patient presents with posterior and/or lateral compartment symptoms.

In contrast to acute compartment syndrome, there is no definite value that governs CECS. In a meta-analysis of 32 studies in 2012, the average pre-exercise values ranged from 7.4 mm Hg to 50.8 mm Hg in CECS patients compared with 5.7–12 mm Hg in controls.[53] During exercise, mean pressure readings ranged from 42 mm Hg to 150 mm Hg in CECS compared with 28–141 mm Hg in controls; 1-minute post-exercise values ranged from 34 mm Hg to 55.4 mm Hg and 9–19 mm Hg in CECS and control patients, respectively. Although it appears that post-exercise measurement is the most reliable value for the diagnosis of CECS, no statistically significant conclusion could be reached.[53] In 2018, Zimmerman and colleagues[48] conducted a descriptive analysis of 501 service members with exercise-related leg pain who had intracompartmental pressure measured 1 minute post-exercise. Of those diagnosed with CECS, 68% had an intracompartmental pressure measurement of >35 mm Hg. However, pain scores had a negligible correlation with compartment pressures.[48] This ultimately challenges the validity of intracompartmental pressure measurement testing and has paved the path for implementation of newer noninvasive diagnostic tools.

More recently, new techniques have emerged to assess intracompartmental pressure readings on a more dynamic scale with anthropometric data. A cohort study of 40 men ($n = 20$ with CECS; $n = 20$ healthy controls) underwent intracompartmental pressure readings continuously before, during, and after exercise.[54] Pressure readings were conducted with an indwelling transducer-tipped catheter wire inserted into the tibialis anterior muscle 3 cm distal and lateral to the tibial tuberosity. Overall, CECS patients had higher pressure measurements immediately after standing than controls (35.5 mm Hg vs 23.8 mm Hg, respectively; $P = 0.006$). During exercise, the greatest difference in pressure readings corresponded with the maximal tolerable pain in both groups (114 mm Hg in CECS vs 68.7 mm Hg in controls; $P < .001$). This corresponded to an overall greater specificity (95%) but decreased sensitivity (63%) compared with the Pedowitz criteria.[54] The authors argue that continuous pressure monitoring is better tolerated because only one stick is required for data collection. However, it is important to note that this technique requires greater physical demand to produce valid waveforms. This should be taken into consideration based on the athlete's skill level.

The new techniques emerging for the diagnosis of CECS have focused on noninvasive tools to enhance patient comfort and lower the risks that accompany catheter readings, such as bleeding and infection.[1,26] Although risks remain minimal, noninvasive measures, such as MRI, near-infrared spectroscopy (NIRS), methoxyisobutyl isonitrile (MIBI) perfusion imaging, thallous chloride scintigraphy, and triple-phase bone scan technology may prove diagnostic capability in certain patient populations. Because the pathophysiology of elevated compartment pressures is characterized by intracompartment swelling, an MRI may demonstrate diffuse high signal intensity on T2-weighted images. In one study, T2-weighted signal intensity increased by 27.5% following exercise in the anterior compartment compared with baseline.[55] This effect was not apparent in the control group and disappeared in the CECS group post-fasciotomy. MRI is also useful to rule out other differential diagnoses, including fascial defects (see **Fig. 1**), medial tibial stress syndrome, or stress fractures that may mimic exertional-related lower extremity pain. However, this may be difficult to obtain immediately following exercise in certain institutions, thus reducing its validity as a diagnostic tool.[39]

NIRS can measure tissue deoxygenation of skeletal muscles that occurs with increased intramuscular pressure in CECS. As earlier discussed, CECS pain is often associated with ischemia, and therefore NIRS has proven to be a sensitive tool for its diagnosis.[36,37,56] In one diagnostic cohort study, the sensitivity of NIRS was 85% for diagnosing CECS, which is greater in comparison to intracompartmental pressure measurement in some literature.[57] This same study, however, reported rather low sensitivity but high specificity of MRI for the diagnosis of CECS (>10%) T2-weighted signal intensity–sensitivity (40%); specificity (100%).[57]

Similar to NIRS, thallium chloride scintigraphy can demonstrate reversible ischemia in affected compartments during exercise through its SPECT scanning.[58] Takebayashi and colleagues[59] performed a quantitative analysis of post-exercise thallium chloride SPECT of the lower leg. The mean values of mean percentage uptake were 75% in the anterior compartment, 69% in the lateral compartment, 72% in the superficial-posterior compartment, and 68% in the deep-posterior compartment. However, there were discrepancies between clinical and SPECT diagnoses in 33% of these patients, thus questioning its accuracy as a diagnostic tool.[59]

MIBI perfusion involves intravenously injecting technetium-99 m to monitor its uptake in peripheral muscles. Muscle hypoxia demonstrates an inverse relationship with MIBI uptake. In some reports, a decreased concentration of MIBI is seen in the affected compartments of CECS.[60] Similarly, CECS may also become evident in dynamic bone scanning. Imaging will reveal decreased radionuclide concentration in the area of increased compartment pressure, with increased soft tissue concentration at the superior and inferior poles of the pathologic compartment. Further research is required to improve the sensitivity and specificity of noninvasive diagnostic testing of CECS.[61]

TREATMENT

There are both conservative and surgical interventions for the treatment of CECS. Conservative options include activity modification and limiting activity to a level that elicits minimal symptoms, physical therapy for stretching and strengthening of the involved muscles, massage with soft tissue release, and anti-inflammatories or orthotics for cases with excessive pronation.[62] There are also other manipulation and physical therapy techniques, such as ultrasound, myofascial release, and strain-counterstrain.[63]

Surgical intervention involving fasciotomies or fasciectomies of the affected compartment should be considered if symptoms are refractory to conservative care after a few months or if patients are experiencing extreme pressure elevation.[64,65] Only involved compartments that were measured with increased intracompartmental pressures are released. Anterior and lateral fasciotomies have a greater success rate of 80%, while deep and superficial posterior fasciotomies have lower success rates of 50%.[66,67] The decreased success of the deep posterior compartment is attributed to more complex anatomy, poor visualization, and inaccessible small muscular subdivisions.[68]

There have been multiple described incision techniques, including single, double, and triple incision fasciotomies, as well as endoscopic techniques. Regardless of the technique, all fascia hernias must be addressed with the fascial incision to adequately relieve the intracompartmental pressure. The advantages of an open fasciotomy include full visualization as well as the ability to excise a strip of the fascia during the release to decrease scarring and reoccurrence.[69] Endoscopic fasciotomies or small incision fasciotomies involve 1–3 small incisions where a subcutaneous plane overlying the fascia is made between the small incisions and the fasciotomy may be made with endoscopic guidance to confirm release of the fascia.[70,71]

TECHNIQUE
Anterior and Lateral

There is a high rate of coexistence of CECS in the anterior and lateral compartment, and both compartments may be addressed from the same incisions to gain access to both compartments.

Mark out a point approximately 11–12 cm above the tip of the fibula to mark the location of the superficial peroneal nerve. The incision is based midway between the anterior aspect of the fibula and the tibia crest (**Fig. 3**). This is an optimal position to allow both access to the lateral and anterior compartments to be released. The incision is generally between 4 cm and 6 cm. The dissection toward the anterior compartment of the leg allows visualization of the superficial peroneal nerve before incising the compartments. Full thickness skin flaps are raised bluntly and the superficial peroneal nerve is identified. The superficial peroneal nerve is then released and retracted out of the way. Variations of the nerve path must be appreciated: it may exit directly through the lateral compartment fascia posterior to the septum, through both the anterior and lateral compartments by traversing a fibrous tunnel within the intermuscular septum, or immediately anterior to the intermuscular septum from the anterior compartment alone.

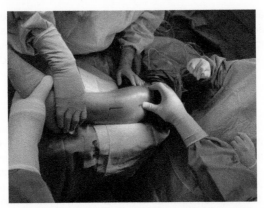

Fig. 3. Incisions for fasciotomy release of the anterior and lateral compartments are marked out. A 4–6 cm incision is made at the midline between the tibial crest and the anterior edge of the fibula 11–12 cm proximal to the distal fibula. An accessory portal is marked out at a level midway between the initial incision and Gerdy's tubercle.

The fascia is identified and a subcutaneous plane is made proximally and distally utilizing blunt instrumentation (**Fig. 4**). The fascia is then cut and released distally to the level of the extensor retinaculum with a curved scissor with the curve pointing anteriorly to avoid any damage to the superficial peroneal nerve.

An accessory incision is made proximally and dissected down to the level of the fascia. A subcutaneous plane is made distally to connect the two incisions as well as proximally to the level of the tibial tuberosity. The fascia is then incised from distal to proximal utilizing a metzenbaum scissors, hook blade, or a scalpel depending on surgeon's preference to the level of where the accessory incision is. The fascia is then further released from the accessory incision proximally to the level of Gerdy's tubercle. Through the same incisions retracted posteriorly, the lateral compartment may be released in the same fashion just 1 cm behind the anterior intermuscular septum right over the level of the peroneal tendon from the level of the distal fibula

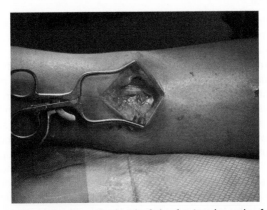

Fig. 4. Dissection is carried down to the level of the fascia where the fascia is incised and subfascial planes are created to perform the fasciotomy with care to identify and retract the superficial peroneal nerve.

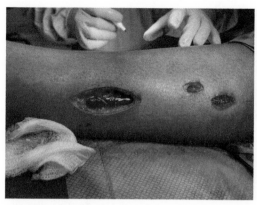

Fig. 5. Fasciotomies were completed with exposed muscle belly to confirm complete release to the anterior and lateral compartments.

to the fibular head with an additional accessory portal made more posteriorly if necessary (**Fig. 5**).

After release of the anterior and lateral compartments, the wounds are packed with moist gauze and the tourniquet should be released for visualization and control of any significant bleeding. This also allows for direct visualization to prevent damage of the saphenous vein and posterior tibial bundle when performing the superficial and deep posterior compartment releases.

Superficial Posterior

An incision is made at the middle one-third of the leg, 1 cm behind the posterior medial border of the tibia, approximately 6 cm in length (**Fig. 6**). Dissect down to the level of fascia over the gastrocnemius tendon, clearing subcutaneous tissue with blunt finger sweep dissection. The saphenous nerve and vein are visualized just medial and posterior to the medial border of the tibia overlying the deep posterior compartment of the leg and should be retracted. The fascia is then incised and released proximally to the level of the knee joint and distally to the level of the Achilles tendon, freeing up the soleus and the gastrocnemius muscles (**Fig. 7**).

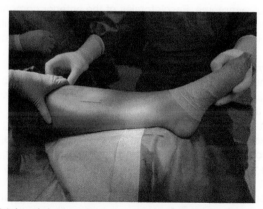

Fig. 6. The superficial and deep posterior compartments are accessed through an incision made at the middle one-third of the leg just behind the posterior medial edge of the tibia.

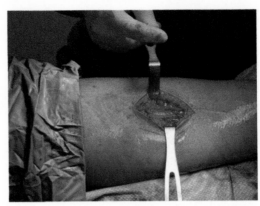

Fig. 7. Dissection is carried down to the level of the fascia overlying the gastrocnemius and soleus muscles with care to identify and retract the saphenous nerve and vein.

Deep Posterior

The deep compartment is exposed next after the superficial posterior compartment. The soleus must be released and elevated posteriorly off the posterior edge of the tibia. This exposes the deep compartment. The flexor digitorum longus can be visualized first, and the fascia can be incised and opened up. The most distal aspect can be elevated with periosteal elevators or blunt finger dissection to the level of the posterior medial malleolus. Proximally, the fascia is opened up with scissors or a periosteal elevator. When performing a deep posterior compartment release, attention must be given to adequate decompression of the tibialis posterior.[23]

Endoscopic techniques for all compartments except the deep posterior compartment are performed similarly with 2–3 stab incisions along the compartments, freeing up the subcutaneous plane utilizing blunt dissection with a periosteal elevator and releasing the fascia with a hook blade or scalpel, all with direct visualization of the fascia being released with a scope through an accessory portal.

After adequate fascial release in the affected compartments, the subcutaneous layers are closed, followed by skin closure. Simple skin incisions are closed for endoscopic procedures. A compressive dressing is applied postoperatively.

Surgical treatment of CECS has demonstrated success in returning to activity with generalized relief of symptoms. Fasciotomies of the anterior compartment of the leg have the highest success rates exceeding 85% in the literature, while deep posterior compartment fasciotomies elicit a lower success rate of approximately 70%.[72]

Postoperative course

Although an optimal post-operative rehabilitation program has not been established, there are general guidelines for returning to activity that may be monitored to cater to a patient's specific activity level. Patients may typically bear weight as tolerated and begin active and passive range of motion immediately following surgery, but crutches are often dispensed for comfort the first few days. Jazwari and colleagues[73] published a preferred protocol outlined in **Table 2**. More active walking, light jogging, and cycling are initiated when the wounds are healed at 2 weeks, and patients typically resume running training at approximately 6 weeks. Full rehabilitation and return to activities usually takes 3 months, but may be longer for patients who underwent deep posterior compartment fasciotomies.[72,74,75] Recovery and return to activity may also be assisted with physical therapy, which can be initiated 1–2 weeks after surgery.

Table 2
A postoperative rehabilitation program following compartment fasciotomies to return to sport

	Goals	Modalities	Weight-Bearing	ROM/Stretching	Exercises
Phase 1 (Day 1–14 post-operation)	Pain management, wound healing, edema control	Ice, elevation, compression	Crutches and partial weight bearing, consider CAM boot	Unrestricted non-weight bearing dorsiflexion/ plantarflexion	Unresisted ankle plantarflexion/ dorsiflexion
Phase 2 (Weeks 2–4 post-operation)	Normal ankle ROM	Ice, compression stockings	Wean crutches, progress to full weight bearing as tolerated	Begin alphabet/ankle rotation exercises, dorsiflexion towel stretches	Progression- light Theraband dorsiflexion/ plantarflexion/inversion/ eversion, pain free leg and calf press
Phase 3 (Weeks 4–6 post-operation)	Improved ankle strength, normal gait pattern maintained for 1 mile	Ice, compression stockings, scar massage	Weight bearing as tolerated	Full and unrestricted	Increase theraband resistance, mini squats to real squats, single heel raise, pain-free cardio (forward and backward treadmill), elliptical, pool running
Phase 4 (Weeks 6–12 post-operation)	45 min low impact cardio, resistance weight training at 90% normal	Ice, compression, scar massage	Unrestricted	Unrestricted	Progression of weight machines, sit ups and push ups, pain free cardio treadmill, stairmaster
Phase 5 (Weeks 12–16 post-operation)	Running normal pace, return to sports	None	Unrestricted	Unrestricted	Running progression, agility drills, plyometrics

This may be adjusted given patient's ability and activity level.

Chronic exertional compartment syndrome of the foot. Unlike CECS of the leg, whose incidence and treatment is very well documented, CECS of the foot remains underdiagnosed and is only reported in the literature on an anecdotal basis. The medial compartment is most commonly affected either bilaterally or unilaterally.[13,17] The incidence of CECS of the foot remains unclear, however, as most of the compartment syndrome of the foot that is described is an acute compartment syndrome from trauma.

The clinical signs and symptoms of CECS of the foot are more ambiguous, diverse and with a lack of consistency of its counterpart in the leg. CECS of the foot has a similar presentation consisting of pain, cramping, paresthesias, or tightness on activity that is relieved by a period of rest or cessation of activity.[14] There may also be noticeable swelling on the abductor hallucis muscle as the medial compartment of the foot is most commonly affected, or a taut compartment to the affected compartment. Foot CECS may go undiagnosed because it may look like other conditions like a Lisfranc injury, tarsal tunnel syndrome, or plantar fasciitis. Just as in the leg, the most objective investigation is a dynamic intracompartmental pressure study, which can be supplemented with clinical symptoms or advanced imaging such as MRI, demonstrating relative hypertrophy to a compartment (**Fig. 8**).

When conservative care of rest, anti-inflammatories, physical therapy or orthotics fails, surgical fasciotomy is the most effective management of CECS of the foot. Jowett and colleagues[21] published a series of five patients and seven feet with confirmed CECS of the medial compartment, surgical release of the superficial and deep fascia demonstrated significant symptom relief in all but one patient. Fasciotomies over the affected compartments can be performed either with a single incision, or endoscopically with serial stab incisions along the compartment. Endoscopic fasciotomy of the most commonly affected compartment, the medial compartment consists of three stab incisions made along the abductor hallucis muscle at equal distances (**Fig. 9**). The surgery is performed proximal to distal. The soft tissues are mobilized along the line of the abductor hallucis muscle and a fascial plane is created to connect all of the stab incisions. Next, utilizing a blunt probe to identify a layer, the cannula is inserted through the stab incision placed proximal to distal. The fascia is identified and, utilizing a small blade for the endoscopic plantar fascial release system, the fascia is perforated and cut. The muscle belly will be visualized with the scope to extrude from the fascia, clearly being under significant tension (**Fig. 10**). Once the fascia was cut all the way to the central incision, the cannula was then repositioned from

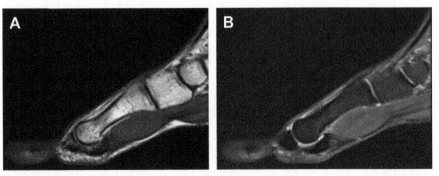

Fig. 8. Sagittal T1 (A) and T2 (B) weighted images on MRI demonstrating hypertrophy within the medial compartment to the abductor hallucis muscle belly.

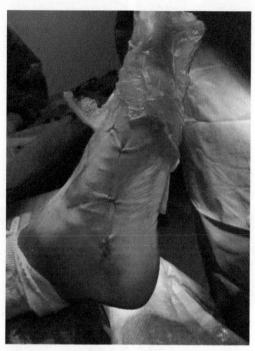

Fig. 9. Three stab incisions are made along the abductor hallucis muscle at equal distances.

the central incision to the distal incision, again being careful to be sure to be above the fascial layer and not penetrate deep. The hook blade is utilized to cut through the fascia with the muscle herniating out once the fascia is cut.

OUTCOMES/COMPLICATIONS

There have been many published studies of fasciotomies following CECS with varying results, as most studies showing the effectiveness of fasciotomy for CECS are of smaller cohort sizes. Maffuli and colleagues[76] found that in a study of 18 patients with CECS post-fasciotomy, significant improvement was seen in Short Form 36-item Health Survey and a return to preinjury or higher level of sport after minimal incision fasciotomy. Another study of 7 patients with CECS of the leg by Ballus and colleagues[77] with an ultrasound-guided fasciotomy demonstrated a decrease in pain in all patients, with all but 1 patient returning to presymptomatic exercise levels. Drexler and colleagues[78] performed a retrospective case series study of 95 legs with CECS demonstrating significant long-term improvement in postoperative activity level and quality of life after fasciotomy. Packer and colleagues[79] compared patients with CECS who were treated with conservative treatment and those who underwent operative treatment, with the operative group having higher satisfaction rates.

Common complications from fasciotomies for CECS include infection, nerve damage or entrapment, vascular injury, hemorrhage, deep vein thrombosis, chronic regional pain syndrome, or lymphocele.[80] Complication rates of fasciotomy are found to be around 11–13%.[81] In addition, a patient, particularly an active athlete, may have a recurrence of compartment syndrome after the fasciotomy, with

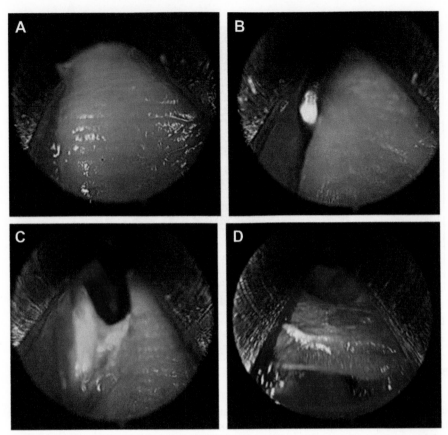

Fig. 10. (A) The cannula is inserted through the stab incisions along the fascial plane and the fascia is identified. (B) Utilizing a small hook blade from the endoscopic plantar fascial release system, the perforated. (C) The fascia is cut along the course of the medial compartment. (D) The released fascia and extruded muscle belly is identified and confirmed with the scope.

recurrence rates in the literature ranging from 6% to 11%.[82] Causes of recurrence are incomplete release of the fascia, poor rehabilitation after fasciotomy, or excessive scarring.[4,65] Although the endoscopic and smaller incision techniques have gained more favor for minimal scarring and tissue disruption as well as quicker return to activity given the smaller wound sizes, this technique has been shown to have increased complication rates, nerve damage, and symptom recurrence due to limited visualization.[64] In some instances, patients can develop an acute compartment syndrome on top of CECS.[83]

SUMMARY

CECS continues to be studied as its etiology is unclear. The evolution of alternative diagnostic options may provide more insight into the pathophysiology of the syndrome, which may provide more availability for a greater diversity of treatment options. Proper diagnosis through clinical and compartmental pressure evaluation is imperative. Conservative treatment methods may be effective early in the course of the condition, but the only definitive treatment is a surgical fasciotomy of the affected compartment. The literature demonstrates excellent success with the myriad of fasciotomy techniques that return patients and athletes back to normal, pain-free activity.

CLINICS CARE POINTS

- Chronic exertion compartment syndrome most commonly afflicts the leg, particularly the anterior compartment.
- Although chronic exertion compartment syndrome can occur with any sport, it is more common with participation in endurance running or skating.
- The most common symptoms include claudication, muscle group tightness, and paresthesias in the affected compartment.
- The gold standard for diagnosis of chronic exertion compartment syndrome is intracompartmental pressure measurement pre- and post-exercise.
- Conservative treatment for chronic exertion compartment syndrome include physical therapy, modification of activity, and NSAIDs.
- Surgical intervention involve open or endoscopic fasciotomies to release the affected compartment(s).
- Recurrence from surgical release is rare, and is most often the result of incomplete release, poor rehabilitation, and/or excessive scarring.

DISCLOSURE

The authors have nothing to disclose.

REFERENCES

1. Nwakibu U, Schwarzman G, Zimmermann WO, et al. Chronic exertional compartment syndrome of the leg management is changing: where are we and where are we going? Curr Sports Med Rep 2020;19(10):438–44.
2. Mavor GE. The anterior tibial syndrome. J Bone Joint Surg Br 1956;38-B(2): 513–7.
3. Bong MR, Polatsch DB, et al. Chronic exertional compartment syndrome: diagnosis and management. Bull NYU Hosp Jt Dis 2005. Winter-Spring.
4. Shah SN, Miller BS, Kuhn JE. Chronic exertional compartment syndrome. Am J Orthop 2004;33(7):335–41.
5. Styf J. Definitions and terminology. Etiology and pathogenesis of chronic compartment syndrome. In: Styf Jorma, editor. Compartment syndromes: diagnosis, treatment, and complications. Boca Raton (FL): CRC Press LLC; 2004.
6. Detemer DE, Sharpe K, Sufit RL, et al. Chronic compartment syndrome: diagnosis, management, and outcomes. Am J Sports Med 1985;13:162–70.
7. Pedowitz RA, Hargens AR, Mubarak SJ, et al. Modified criteria for the objective diagnosis of chronic compartment syndrome of the leg. Am J Sports Med 1990;18:35–40.
8. Davis DE, Raikin S, Garras DN, et al. Characteristics of patients with chronic exertional compartment syndrome. Foot Ankle Int 2013;34:1349–54.
9. Waterman BR, Liu J, Newcomb R, et al. Risk factors for chronic exertional compartment syndrome in a physically active military population. Am J Sports Med 2013;41:2545–9.
10. de Bruijn JA, van Zantvoort APM, van Klaveren D, et al. Factors predicting lower leg chronic exertional compartment syndrome in a large population. Int J Sports Med 2018;39(1):58–66. https://doi.org/10.1055/s-0043-119225 [Epub 2017 Nov 10. PMID: 29126337].

11. Edmundsson D, Toolanen G, Sojka P. Chronic compartment syndrome also affects nonathletic subjects: a prospective study of 63 cases with exercise-induced lower leg pain. Acta Orthop 2007;78(1):136–42.

12. Hutchinson MR, Ireland ML. Common compartment syndromes in athletes treatment and rehabilitation. Sports Med 1994;17:200–8.

13. Blacklidge DK, Kurek JB, Resto Soto AD, et al. Acute exertional compartment syndrome of the medial foot. Foot Ankle 1996;35:19–22.

14. Miozzari HM, Gerad R, Stern R, et al. Exertional medial compartment syndrome of the foot in a high level athlete. A case report. Am J Sports Med 2008;36:983–6.

15. Mollica MB. Chronic exertional compartment syndrome of the foot. J Am Podiatr Med Assoc 1998;88:21–4.

16. Muller GP, Masquelet AC. Chronic compartment syndrome of the foot. A case report. Rev Chir Orthop Reparatrice Appar Mot 1995;81:549–52.

17. Lokiec F, Siev-Ner I, Pritsch M. Chronic compartment syndrome of both feet. J Bone Joint Surg Br 1991;73:178–9.

18. Middleton DK, Johnson JE, Davies JF. Exertional compartment syndrome of bilateral feet: a case report. Foot Ankle Int 1995;16:95–6.

19. Seiler R, Guziec G. Chronic compartment syndrome of the feet. A case report. J Am Podiatr Med Assoc 1994;84:91–4.

20. Villatte G, Fadlallah E, Erivan R, et al. Bilateral simultaneous chronic exertional compartment syndrome of the lateral forefoot: a case report (compartment syndrome of the forefoot). J Orthop Surg 2019;27(2). 230949901983964.

21. Jowett A, Birks C, Blackney M. Chronic exertional compartment syndrome in the medial compartment of the foot. Foot Ankle Int 2008;29(8):838–41.

22. Blair JM, Botte MJ. Surgical anatomy of the superficial peroneal nerve in the ankle and foot. Clin Orthop Relat Res 1994;305:229–38.

23. Davey JR, Rorabeck CH, Fowler PJ. The tibialis posterior muscle compartment. Am J Sports Med 1984;12(5):391–7.

24. Ruland RT, April EW, Meinhard BP. Tibialis posterior muscle. J Orthop Trauma 1992;6(3):347–51.

25. Gill CS, Halstead ME, Matava MJ. Chronic exertional compartment syndrome of the leg in athletes: evaluation and management. Phys Sportsmed 2010;38(2): 126–32 [PubMed: 20631472].

26. Velasco TO, Leggit JC. Chronic exertional compartment syndrome: a clinical update. Curr Sports Med Rep 2020;19(9):347–52.

27. Manoli A 2nd, Weber TG. Fasciotomy of the foot: an anatomical study with special reference to release of the calcaneal compartment. Foot Ankle 1990;10(5): 267–75.

28. Padhiar N, Allen M, King JB. Chronic exertional compartment syndrome of the foot. Sports Med Arthrosc Rev 2009;17(3):198–202.

29. Guyton GP, Shearman CM, Saltzman CL. The compartments of the foot revisited. Rethinking the validity of cadaver infusion experiments. J Bone Joint Surg Br 2001;83(2):245–9.

30. Anuar K, Gurumoorthy P. Systematic review of the management of chronic compartment syndrome in the lower leg. Physiother Singapore 2006;9:2–15.

31. Schubert AG. Exertional compartment syndrome: review of the literature and proposed rehabilitation guidelines following surgical release. Int J Sports Phys Ther 2011;6(2):126–41.

32. Turnipseed WD, Hurschler C, Vanderby R. The effects of elevated compartment pressure on tibial arteriovenous flow and relationship of mechanical and

biochemical characteristics of fascia to genesis of chronic anterior compartment syndrome. J Vasc Surg 1995;21(5):810–7.

33. Fraipont MJ, Adamson GJ. Chronic exertional compartment syndrome. J Am Acad Orthop Surg 2003;11:268–76.

34. McGinley JC, Thompson TA, Ficken S, et al. Chronic Exertional compartment syndrome caused by functional venous outflow obstruction. Clin J Sport Med 2021. https://doi.org/10.1097/JSM.0000000000000929 [Epub ahead of print. PMID: 34009799].

35. Edmundsson D, Toolanen G, Thornell LE, et al. Evidence for low muscle capillary supply as a pathogenic factor in chronic compartment syndrome. Scand J Med Sci Sports 2010;20(6):805–13.

36. Tucker AK. Chronic exertional compartment syndrome of the leg. Curr Rev Musculoskelet Med 2010;3(1–4):32–7. Published 2010 Sep 2.

37. Liu B, Barrazueta G, Ruchelsman DE. Chronic exertional compartment syndrome in athletes. J Hand Surg Am 2017;42(11):917–23.

38. Trease L, van Every B, Bennell K, et al. A prospective blinded evaluation of exercise thallium-201 SPET in patients with suspected chronic exertional compartment syndrome of the leg. Eur J Nucl Med 2001;28(6):688–95.

39. Amendola A, Rorabeck CH, Vellett D, et al. The use of magnetic resonance imaging in exertional compartment syndromes. Am J Sports Med 1990;18:29–34.

40. Roraback CH, Fowler PJ. The results of fasciotomy in the management of chronic exertional compartment syndrome. Am J Sports Med 1988;16:224–7.

41. Schepsis AA, Martini D, Corbett M. Surgical management of exertional compartment syndrome of the lower leg. Long term follow-up. Am J Sports Med 1993;21: 811–7.

42. Humphries D. Exertional compartment syndromes. Medscape Gen Med 1999;3: 1–7. Available at: http://www.medscape.com/viewarticle/408500. Accessed February 3, 2022.

43. Cook S, Bruce G. Fasciotomy for chronic compartment syndrome in the lower limb. ANZ J Surg 2002;72(10):720–3.

44. Chandwani D, Varacallo M. Exertional compartment syndrome. [Updated 2021 Jul 18]. In: StatPearls [Internet]. Treasure Island (FL): StatPearls Publishing; 2022. Available at: https://www.ncbi.nlm.nih.gov/books/NBK544284/?report= classic.

45. Chatterjee R. Diagnosis of chronic exertional compartment syndrome in primary care. Br J Gen Pract 2015;65(637):e560–2.

46. Zimmermann WO, Hutchinson MR, Van den Berg R, et al. Conservative treatment of anterior chronic exertional compartment syndrome in the military with a midterm follow-up. BMJ Open Sport Exerc Med 2019;5:1–7.

47. Turnipseed WD. Diagnosis and management of chronic compartment syndrome. Surgery 2002;132(4):613–7 [discussion: 617-9].

48. Zimmermann WO, Ligthert E, Helmhout PH, et al. Intracompartmental pressure measurements in 501 service members with exercise-related leg pain. Translational J ACSM 2018;3:107–12.

49. Braver RT. Chronic exertional compartment syndrome. Clin Podiatr Med Surg 2016;33(2):219–33 [PubMed: 27013413].

50. Roberts A, Franklyn-Miller A. The validity of the diagnostic criteria used in chronic exertional compartment syndrome: a systematic review. Scand J Med Sci Sports 2012;22(5):585–95.

51. Tiidus PM. Is intramuscular pressure a valid diagnostic criterion for chronic exertional compartment syndrome? Clin J Sport Med 2014;24(1):87–8.

52. Lindorsson S, Zhang Q, Brisby H, et al. Significantly lower intramuscular pressure in the posterior and lateral compartments compared with the anterior compartment suggests alterations of the diagnostic criteria for chronic exertional compartment syndrome in the lower leg. Knee Surg Sports Traumatol Arthrosc 2021;29:1332–9.
53. Aweid O, Del Buono A, Malliaras P, et al. Systematic review and recommendations for intracompartmental pressure monitoring in diagnosing chronic exertional compartment syndrome of the leg. Clin J Sport Med 2012;22(4):356–70.
54. Roscoe D, Roberts AJ, Hulse D. Intramuscular compartment pressure measurement in chronic exertional compartment syndrome: new and improved diagnostic criteria. Am J Sports Med 2015;43(2):392–8.
55. Verleisdonk EJMM, van Gils A, van der Werken C. The diagnostic value of MRI scans for the diagnosis of chronic exertional compartment syndrome of the lower leg. Skeletal Radiol 2001;30(6):321–5.
56. Breit GA, Gross JH, Watenpaugh DE. Near-infrared spectroscopy for monitoring of tissue oxygenation of exercising skeletal muscle in a chronic compartment syndrome model. J Bone Joint Surg Am 1997;79:838–43.
57. van den Brand JG, Nelson T, Verleisdonk EJ, et al. The diagnostic value of intra-compartmental pressure measurement, magnetic resonance imaging, and near-infrared spectroscopy in chronic exertional compartment syndrome: a prospective study in 50 patients. Am J Sports Med 2005;33(5):699–704.
58. Hayes AA, Bower GD, Pitstock KL. Chronic exertional compartment syndrome of the legs diagnosed with thallous chloride scintigraphy. J Nucl Med 1995;36: 1618–24.
59. Takebayashi S, Takazawa H, Sasaki R, et al. Chronic exertional compartment syndrome in lower legs: localization and follow-up with thallium-201 SPECT imaging. J Nucl Med 1997;38(6):972–6. PMID: 9189153.
60. Owens S, Edwards P, Miles K, et al. Chronic compartment syndrome affecting the lower limb: MIBI perfusion imaging as an alternative to pressure monitoring: two case reports. Br J Sports Med 1999;33(1):49–51.
61. Matin P. Basic principles of nuclear medicine techniques for detection and evaluation of trauma and sports medicine injuries. Semin Nucl Med 1988;18(2): 90–112.
62. Wilder RP, Sethi S. Overuse injuries; tendinopathies, stress fractures, compartment syndrome and shin splints. Clin Sports Med 2004;23:55–81.
63. Brennan F, Kane S. Diagnosis, treatment options, and rehabili- tation of chronic lower leg exertional compartment syndrome. Curr Sport Med Rep 2003;2:247–50.
64. LeversedgeFJ, CaseyPJ, SeilerJG3rd, et al. Endoscopically assisted fasciotomy: description of technique and in vitro assessment of lower-leg compartment de-com- pression. Am J Sports Med 2002;30(2):272–8.
65. Tzortziou V, Maffulli N, Padhiar N. Diagnosis and management of chronic exertional compartment syndrome (CECS) in the United Kingdom. Clin J Sport Med 2006;16:209–13. DeLee JC, et al.
66. DeLee and Drez's orthopaedic sports medicine. Philadelphia: Saunders; 2003. p. 2163–70.
67. Mouhsine E, Garofalo R, Moretti B, et al. Two minimal incision fasciotomy for chronic exertional compartment syndrome of the lower leg. Knee Surg Sports Traumatol Arthrosc 2006;14:193–7.
68. Illig K, Uriel K, De Weese J, et al. Case report: a condemnation of subcutaneous fasciotomy. Mil Med 1998;163(11):794–6.

69. Matsen F, Winquist R, Krugmire R. Diagnosis and management of compartmental syndromes. J Bone Joint Surg 1980;62:286–91.
70. Hutchinson M, Bederka B, Kopplin M. Anatomic structures at risk during minimal-incision endoscopically assisted fascial compartment releases in the leg. Am J Sports Med 2003;5:764–9.
71. Kitajima I, Tachibana S, Hirota Y, et al. One-portal technique of endoscopic fasciotomy: chronic compartment syndrome of the lower leg. Arthroscopy 2001;17(8):1–3.
72. Rowden GA, Abdelkarim B, Vaca F. Compartment syndromes. Medscape 2008;(2022):1–5.
73. Dai AZ, Zacchilli M, Jejurikar N, et al. Open 4-compartment fasciotomy for chronic exertional compartment syndrome of the leg. Arthrosc Tech 2017;6(6):e2191–201.
74. Albertson K, Dammann G. The leg. In: O'Connor F, Wilder R, editors. The textbook of running medicine. New York: McGraw-Hill; 2001. p. 647–54.
75. Rorabeck CH. The diagnosis and management of chronic compartment syndromes. Instr Course Lect 1989;38:466.
76. Maffulli N, Loppini M, Spiezia F, et al. Single minimal incision fasciotomy for chronic exertional compartment syndrome of the lower leg. J Orthop Surg Res 2016;11:61.
77. Balius R, Bong DA, Ardevol J, et al. Ultrasound-guided fasciotomy for anterior chronic exertional compartment syndrome of the leg. J Ultrasound Med 2016;35:823–9.
78. Drexler M, Rutenberg TF, Rozen N, et al. Single minimal incision fasciotomy for the treatment of chronic exertional compartment syndrome: outcomes and complications. Arch Orthop Trauma Surg 2017;137:73–9.
79. Packer JD, Day MS, Nguyen JT, et al. Functional outcomes and patient satisfaction after fasciotomy for chronic exertional compartment syndrome. Am J Sports Med 2013;41:430–6.
80. Coughlin M, Mann R, Saltzman CL. Surgery of the foot and ankle. Philadelphia: Elsevier; 2007. p. 1438–44.
81. Howard J, Mohtadi N, Wiley J. Evaluation of outcomes in patients following surgical treatment of chronic exertional com- partment syndrome in the leg. Clin J Sport Med 2000;10:176–84.
82. Englund J. Chronic compartment syndrome: tips on recognizing and treating. J Fam Pract 2005;54(11):955–60.
83. Goldfarb S, Kaeding C. Bilateral acute-on-chronic exertional lateral compartment syndrome of the leg: a case report and review of the literature. Clin J Sport Med 1997;7:59–62.

Acute Syndesmosis Injuries

Matthew D. Doyle, DPM, FACFAS[a],*, Chandler J. Ligas, DPM[a],
Nishit S. Vora, DPM[b]

KEYWORDS

- Syndesmosis • Athlete • High ankle sprain

KEY POINTS

- The ankle syndesmosis is important for stability and is frequently injured during sports.
- Thorough evaluation is important for diagnosis and treatment. Advanced imaging is imperative in cases where the physical examination is inconclusive.
- Many can be treated conservatively, but instability requires surgical intervention.
- Syndesmosis injuries are a leading cause of prolonged return to sport.

INTRODUCTION/HISTORY/DEFINITIONS/BACKGROUND

Ankle syndesmosis injuries vary widely and encompass both isolated ligamentous injury as well as fractures with concomitant ligamentous injury. Syndesmotic injuries, or high ankle sprains, account for 12% of all ankle sprains.[1] In addition, it has been reported that these injuries make up 25% of ankle sprains in sports.[1-3] The incidence of syndesmotic disruption with concomitant ankle fracture has been reported to be 10%-23%, with increased prevalence in complex rotational ankle fractures.[4-6] These injuries notably cause greater dysfunction and require longer recovery and return to sport, which can make them very challenging to treat.[1] Syndesmotic injury is often misdiagnosed or not recognized at the time of presentation. Failure to recognize these injuries and treat them appropriately can lead to persistent pain, disability, and post-traumatic arthritis.[7-9] Sports injuries in elite level athletes have challenged the treatment of these injuries more recently because of operative treatment and early return to sport. Such injuries are frequent in professional football, hockey, soccer players, and basketball. In football players, these injuries occur in 0.24 per 1000 athletes and are almost 25% of all ankle sprains.[3] However, there is much debate about surgical treatment including reduction, fixation, and hardware removal.

The first case of syndesmotic injury was described by Quenu[10] in 1907 as a tibioperoneal diastasis after a ligamentous disruption and thereafter began to be studied in

a Silicon Valley Reconstructive Foot and Ankle Fellowship, Palo Alto Medical Foundation, 701 East El Camino Real, Mountain View, CA 94040, USA; b Saint Mary's Medical Center, 450 Stanyan Street, San Francisco, CA 94117, USA
* Corresponding author.
E-mail address: matthew.doyledpm@gmail.com

Clin Podiatr Med Surg 40 (2023) 23–37
https://doi.org/10.1016/j.cpm.2022.07.003
0891-8422/23/© 2022 Elsevier Inc. All rights reserved.

more depth. Historically overlooked compared with the low lateral ligamentous complex of the ankle joint, a recent study reported the incidence of syndesmotic disruption in as high as 74% of all sports injuries to the ankle.[11] This increase in trend is likely because of MRI and improvement in clinical awareness of the injury. Therefore, the practicing foot and ankle clinician should be aware of the anatomy, clinical symptoms of the injury, radiographic criteria of syndesmosis disruption, and classification/grading systems to provide a degree of severity to the syndesmosis injury in an athlete.

Anatomy

The ankle syndesmosis is an immovable joint in which bones are joined by connective tissue. The osseous structures include the concave lateral surface of the distal tibia and the convex surface of the distal medial fibula. The ligamentous structures include the interosseous (syndesmotic) ligament (IOL), the anterior inferior tibiofibular ligament (AITFL), and the posterior inferior tibiofibular ligament (PITFL), and the inferior transverse ligament (ITL) (**Fig. 1**A–C). The AITFL runs obliquely from the anterolateral surface of the distal lateral tibia (Chaput tubercle) to the anterior tubercle of the distal fibula (Wagstaffe tubercle). The PITFL runs obliquely from the posterolateral surface of the distal fibula (Volkman tubercle) to the posterior aspect of the distal fibula. The ITL is the distal-most aspect of the PITFL. The interosseous membrane connects the tibia and fibula and the distal aspect continues to become the IOL. This ligament starts about 2 cm proximal to the joint and continues distally.

The ankle joint is bicondylar. The shape of the talus with its wide anterior and the syndesmotic ligaments increase the congruence and stability of this articulation with anatomic motion. During the stance phase of gait with the ankle dorsiflexed, the fibula externally rotates and translates proximally and slightly laterally to accommodate the talus. When plantarflexed, the fibula moves distally, internally rotates, and translates anteriorly. Ogilivie-Harris et al.[7] showed that the AITFL contributes to 35% of stability, the IOL contributes to 22%, and the PITFL complex contributes to 42% of the overall stability of the syndesmosis complex.[1] Another study concluded that sequential sectioning of the syndesmotic ligaments from anterior to posterior increases instability.[12] In addition to the ligamentous strength, stability depends on the articulation of the fibula within the fibula incisura of the distal tibia. Several studies have shown that the anatomy differs and the incisura can be concave, convex, or flat.[13–15] Even very subtle changes in motion can be pathologic.[16–18] Therefore, the accurate assessment of which ligaments of the syndesmosis are involved is crucial.

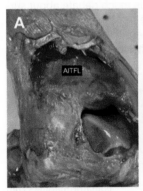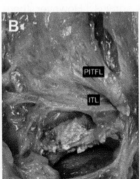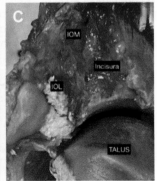

Fig. 1. ■(A-C) Ligaments comprising the ankle syndesmosis.

The vascularity of the ankle syndesmosis has been well documented.[19] The anterior branch of the peroneal artery supplies the majority of the vascularity to the anterior aspect, whereas the posterior branch supplies all of the posterior aspect. The anterior branch, due to its anatomy, is susceptible to injury, both from trauma and iatrogenically during surgery. The anterior branch perforates the interosseous membrane 3 cm above the ankle joint.

Systematic evaluation of the patient including clinical examination, radiographs, and the use of syndesmosis injury grading systems will help the clinician form an accurate assessment of which ligaments are involved and the degree of severity. The level of involvement of the ligaments can also be confirmed with the use of MRI.

Syndesmosis injuries commonly occur with external rotation and dorsiflexion of the talus with protonation, but can also occur with supination and external rotation. They are often seen in rotational ankle fractures. As the talus rotates in the mortise, it increases the force against the fibula, causing diastasis and leading to ligamentous rupture starting with the AITFL. As the talus continues to forcibly rotate externally, this leads to disruption of the IOL and then the PITFL. The fibula may also fracture at this point. Lastly, if the force continues, the deltoid ligament may rupture or there may be a fracture of the medial malleolus. In pronation-external rotation injuries, it is common to have an associated Maisonneuve fracture of the proximal fibula (**Fig. 2**A–B).

In sports, most commonly American football, athletes are at a high risk of sustaining a syndesmotic injury. In a pile or while being tackled, there is a significant force on the lower extremity with the foot in protonation and the talus externally rotated on the fibula. Running backs, wide receivers, tight ends, and linemen are common positions that sustain this injury. This can happen in several other sports such as wrestling,

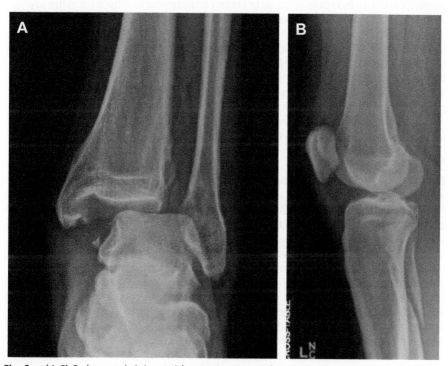

Fig. 2. ■(*A-B*) Sydnesmosis injury with a Maisonneuve fracture.

hockey, lacrosse, and rugby.[20] For athletes, this is a significant cause of missed time and can prolong return to play.[1,21,22]

Physical Examination

A thorough physical examination is of paramount importance and should include a global assessment of the ankle joint. Often patients have pain, swelling, ecchymosis, and inability or difficulty bearing weight. Patients may report having an ankle sprain or ligamentous injury. A proper history regarding the nature of the injury should be taken including the mechanism, foot/ankle position, and force of the injury. Commonly, there is pain along the anterior syndesmosis when palpating between the tibia and fibula. The proximal fibula should be assessed and palpated for pain, as well as the malleoli. Although the clinical examination can be obscured by patient guarding or pain, the physician should still isolate the syndesmosis with specialized testing and the index of suspicion should remain high. Several syndesmotic-specific tests have been described: the *External Rotation Test, Squeeze Test, Cotton Test,* and *Fibular Translation Test.* The *External Rotation Test* is performed by stabilizing the leg with the knee flexed at 90° and then externally rotating the foot, a positive test will elicit pain at the syndesmosis (when there is pain at the syndesmosis this is a positive test). This is the most reliable and has been shown to correlate with syndesmotic injury.[23,24] The *Squeeze Test* is the compression of the fibula and tibia proximal to the midpoint of the calf which causes separation at the origin and insertion sites of the AITFL, causing pain to the athlete if disrupted.[25] The *Cotton Test* applies medial and lateral forces on the talus in a neutral positioned ankle. When compared with the asymptomatic limb, the cotton test is deemed positive when this mediolateral motion is increased on the symptomatic side.[26] The *Fibular Translation Test* applies an anterior-posterior force on the fibula in hopes of finding an appreciable difference in the asymptomatic ankle compared with the symptomatic ankle. Another test that the practitioner can use is the *Double Leg Jump* Test. The inability of the patient to perform a double-leg jump over 30 cm is considered indicative of a positive functional test result. Another test is the *Stabilization Test,* which can also be done by tightly taping the patient's leg just above the ankle joint in an attempt to stabilize the syndesmosis. Toe raises, walking, and/or jumping are less painful upon taping, the test is considered positive when these symptoms of pain are resolved by taping. Although these tests can indicate a positive syndesmotic injury there is poor inter-rater reliability and these tests should be combined with the radiographic assessment of the ankle joint.

Imaging

Complete radiographic evaluation of the ankle should include anteroposterior (AP), mortise, and lateral views. Additionally, two views of tibia-fibula AP and lateral should be included to rule out a proximal fibula fracture. If the patient is able to tolerate it, weight bearing (WB) views are desired for anatomic evaluation. Radiographic examination of the ankle joint specifically addressing syndesmosis injuries should consist in evaluating the following three major criteria: the *medial clear space,* the *tibiofibular clear space* at the incisura, and the *tibiofibular overlap* between at the incisura (**Fig. 3**). The *medial clear space* should be less than or equal to 4 mm. However, it should always be stressed and compared with the contralateral limb to obtain the most exact measurements. The *tibiofibular clear space* is the most accurate of these parameters to assess diastasis at the syndesmosis.[2] Normal measurement of *tibiofibular clear space* is < 6 mm on both the AP and mortise ankle views. *Tibiofibular overlap* differs based on the ankle view: on the AP view the amount of tibiofibular overlap should be > 6 mm; the amount of tibiofibular overlap on the mortise ankle view should be > 1 mm.[23]

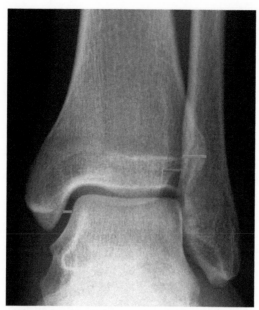

Fig. 3. ∎Radiographic evaluation of the ankle joint and syndesmosis (Blue - tibiofibular overlap; red - tibiofibular clear space; green - medial clear space).

In the office setting, stress radiography has become the mainstay of assessment when evaluating syndesmosis injuries when there is a concern and standard radiographs are equivocal.[12] Complaints of pain and guarding can make an accurate assessment of the syndesmosis difficult. Stress evaluation can be performed manually with external rotation, or by using gravity. These tests are performed under fluoroscopy while evaluating the medial clear space and tibiofibular overlap (**Fig. 4**). Both gravity and manual stress examinations have been proven to be equally accurate in determining ankle instability when there is an isolated fibula fracture.[27]

In recent reports, the specificity and sensitivity of plain film radiographs have been reported to be 44% to 58%.[28] Therefore, when faced with a subtle syndesmotic injury or subacute syndesmotic injuries, the practitioner can obtain a CT or MRI (**Fig. 5**A–B). The specific grading system for syndesmotic injuries has been graded on MRI as follows: *Grade I* is seen with edema directly adjacent to the syndesmotic ligament. *Grade II* is the thickening of the ligament with partial tearing. *Grade III* is discontinuity of the ligament and severe edema surrounding the area. These findings can be combined with classification/grading systems outlined below that will drive conservative vs. operative management of the injury in the athlete.[28] Although MRI increases sensitivity and specificity of anatomic disruption of the syndesmosis, some recent evidence suggests that the non-weightbearing (NWB) methodology of this imaging modality can lead to a degree of missed diastasis or instability of the syndesmosis in athletes.[28] Therefore, the use of WB computed tomography (CT) scans has been more recently evaluated.[29] One study that evaluated the effectiveness of WB cone beam CT scans was by del Rio and colleagues.[29] Their investigation evaluated symptomatic unstable syndesmotic injuries proven by arthroscopy and subsequently evaluated with a WBCT. The authors then compared these findings to NWB cone-beam CT scans. Thirty-nine patients were analyzed. Combined WBCT and arthroscopy were performed at a mean 22.6 days after injury. When they compared the unstable and

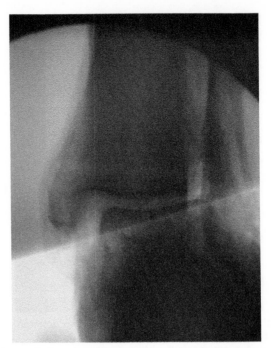

Fig. 4. ▪Stress radiograph demonstrating increase of the medial clear space.

uninjured ankles in WB for each patient, the area of the unstable ankle was a mean of 19.9% greater. When making the same comparison in NWB, the difference was less pronounced, with the unstable ankle 8.8% greater than the uninjured ankle. The difference in area observed between the unstable and uninjured ankles was thus significantly greater in WB than in NWB. Hence when a practicing physician orders a CT scan, a WBCT may increase accuracy when evaluating the syndesmosis.

Classification

Most classification systems focus on three main categories of syndesmosis injuries: congenital, acquired (atraumatic), and acquired (traumatic). The acquired traumatic syndesmosis injury which happens to athletes is broken down into an acute, subacute, and chronic time frame of syndesmosis disruption. Acute is defined as less than 3 weeks from the initial injury, subacute is defined as between 3 weeks and 3 months, and chronic being more than 3 months following initial injury. Edwards and Delee[30] identified a classification system for acute syndesmotic injuries. Type I is a sprain without diastasis, type II is a latent sprain, Type III is frank diastasis, which has been categorized into 4 specific sub-categories. Type IIIa is a frank diastasis with a lateral subluxation of the fibula with no fibula fracture. Type IIIb has a lateral subluxation of the fibula with plastic deformation of the fibula that prevents maintenance of a reduction. Type IIIc involves a posterior subluxation or dislocation of the fibula. This is a very rare form of syndesmosis injury. Type IIId is a superior subluxation, or dislocation of the talus into the ankle mortise so that it becomes wedged between the tibia and fibula without an associated fibula fracture. In the athletic population, the incidence of this degree of diastasis is less likely to be seen and the foot and ankle clinician should be more aware of the subtleties of the syndesmosis injury in the athlete.

The *West Point Ankle Grading System* provides a more accurate broad definition of the severity of ankle syndesmosis injuries.[2] Grade I ankle syndesmotic injuries occur with a sprain to the AITFL, the ankle is regarded as stable. Grade II injuries, whereby rotational forces tear the AITFL and the IOL may necessitate stabilization if the ligamentous injury is severe enough. This is the grade of injury where the *Edwards and Delee classification* is used due to the degree of diastasis present. Grade III injuries involve complete disruption of the ankle syndesmosis and present with syndesmotic instability and diastasis.

Van Dijk's classification is the most widely used system to date.[31] They classify syndesmotic injuries depending on the time elapsed since trauma as acute (less than 6 weeks), subacute (between 6 weeks and 6 months), and chronic (more than 6 months). Management of the injury will depend on the time frame. Acute injuries can be categorized into stable and unstable. Stable sprains are characterized by a lesion of the AITFL, with or without IOL, with an intact deltoid ligament. Unstable sprains also include lesions of the deltoid ligament and can be divided into latent and frank. Latent diastasis compromises AITFL lesion with or without IOL and the deltoid ligament lesion, and frank diastasis is a lesion of all syndesmotic ligaments and the deltoid ligament.

Recently there have been advances in arthroscopic assisted grading of the syndesmosis. Turky and colleagues[32] established a protocol when suspected acute and subacute syndesmotic injuries occur, the use of arthroscopy is used to grade the degree of pathology. Using standard anteromedial and anterolateral portals, they evaluated the syndesmosis with special round tip probes at varying lengths of the transverse limb. They proposed a grading system based on how far the fibula is distracted away from the tibia. Grade 0 injuries were syndesmotic ligaments that were distracted less than 2 mm. Grade I injuries were able to distract > 2 mm but less than 4 mm. Grade II injuries were distracted > 5 mm. All of these injuries were tested by stressing the anterior inferior tibiofibular and the PITFLs, but the integrity of the interosseous ligament was not tested.

Treatment

Acute traumatic, Grade I injuries or sprains are treated conservatively. In the instances of isolated syndesmosis injuries, the athlete should avoid sporting activities for a period of 4 to 8 weeks due to the weakness in the AITFL and concerns for further

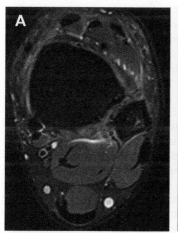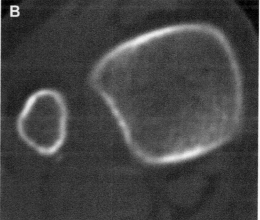

Fig. 5. ■(*A*) MRI with rupture of the AITFL. (*B*) CT scan with syndesmosis rupture.

damage if untreated. A three-staged approach to the treatment of these types of injuries.[20] Phase 1 consists of a period of limited or NWB for 1 to 2 weeks with a focus on edema control, immobilization, and gentle sagittal plane ankle range of motion exercises. Patients may be splinted or use an ankle immobilization boot with crutches during this phase. Phase II consists of functional rehabilitation for 2 weeks with progressive increases in active muscle engagement to strengthen and prevent recurrence. Generally, patients should begin with lower intensity exercises and gradually increase intensity. Once asymptomatic, they can move to Phase III. Phase III in athletes returning to sport can begin once they can hop or jog without pain. In this phase, they will focus on sport-specific strengthening and exercise. They will continue to work on endurance, balancing, agility, and can include sport-specific activities, jumping rope, aquatic therapy, and lateral movements with change of direction. The athlete can begin gravity-assisted running on specialized treadmills as well. Effective ankle bracing/taping should be provided to the athlete when returning to the sport to avoid excessive rotational forces to the syndesmosis which could cause further injury or recurrence. If the athlete has continued pain or inability to perform exercises and participate in sports, they may require surgical intervention.

Grade II injuries are treated based on the degree of diastasis present. When presented with a grade II injury without diastasis, the physician should attempt closed reduction if any fractures are present. The mechanism of injury for this grade is important to remember when reducing the deformity. Advanced imaging with a CT or MRI should be obtained to fully evaluate the amount of diastasis present. Upon successful closed reduction, the patient should spend 4 to 6 weeks of protective NWB in a CAM boot or cast. At 4 weeks, initiation of WB can begin after another WB radiograph is taken to rule out any continual instability or diastasis. The confirmed radiograph will then allow the patient to begin protected WB and initiate the rehabilitation process with the above-stated protocol.

Surgical Treatment

Acute syndesmosis diastasis that is not amenable to nonoperative management, or injuries with associated malleolar fractures, requires surgical intervention. The goal is to restore fibula to anatomic length, ankle alignment, and rotation. Fixation varies and consists of trans-syndesmotic screws, dynamic or flexible devices such as suture buttons, and/or direct repair of the AITFL ligament with suture or anchors. Screws have long been the standard type of fixation, with the size of screws typically 3.5 or 4.5 mm fully threaded screws. There has been no consensus regarding size or number of screws used. In addition, the number of cortices purchased has not been elucidated.

Percutaneous fixation can lead to malreduction of the syndesmosis, therefore fixation should be performed open. Regardless of the implant, fixation should be placed along the transmalleolar axis and parallel to the ankle joint. Syndesmosis malreduction has been reported to be as high as 52%.[33] The authors prefer direct visualization and manual palpation/reduction of the fibula and syndesmosis.[34,35] The anterolateral articular surface where the medial fibula, lateral tibia, and lateral talus meet, may provide greater accuracy in reduction. This technique involves exposing the anterior aspect of the ankle syndesmosis and direct reduction of the fibula within the incisura of the tibia. The authors do not use clamp reduction, as this can lead to malreduction. Appropriate placement of a large reduction clamp is imperative for surgeons that do use one. To decrease risk of malreduction, the medial clamp tine should be placed on the anterior one-third of the distal tibia.[36] Placing the ankle in neutral position (not dorsiflexed or plantarflexed) in the ankle

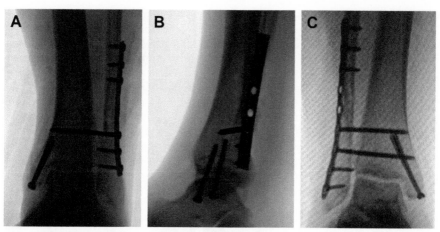

Fig. 6. ■(A-C) ORIF with use of trans-syndesmotic screws.

mortise will help prevent excessive translation of the fibula. Bumps under the ankle should be avoided to limit anterior translation of the fibula.[37] Once reduced, surgeons may place a temporary kirschner wire to maintain reduction. Fixation should be placed 2 to 3 cm proximal to the ankle joint and should not disrupt the ankle joint, a minimum of 3 cortices; however, some surgeons prefer 4 cortices and there is no overall consensus (**Fig. 6**A–C). The orientation of the screws traditionally has been thought to be 25° to 30° in the transverse plane; however, recent reports suggest syndesmotic fixation angle to be 19.7° at 2 cm and 24.8° at 3.5 cm above the tibial plafond.[38] A recent study described the center-center technique to appropriately place the syndesmotic fixation without having to obliquely orient the driver/instrumentation.[39] This technique focuses on a lateral radiograph, internally rotating the distal leg until the anterior portion of the fibula is in the center diaphysis of the tibia.

After reduction and internal fixation, the standard protocol includes a period of NWB for 4 to 6 weeks, then progressive WB with a rehabilitation program started around this time, although there are reports of early WB without loss of reduction or increased risk of complications.[40] Syndesmosis screw removal has become a widely debated topic. Retention of syndesmotic screws can lead to irritation, pain, and possible restricted motion, and in athletes, even a small amount of physiologic motion is advantageous. Screws can also break, and become prominent, causing irritation (**Fig. 7**A–B). A systematic review showed that removal of screws earlier than 3 months post-fixation can result in complications including recurrent diastasis.[41] It is recommended that if screws are removed, it should be at a minimum 3 months after open reduction internal fixation. During removal, if there is any concern for residual instability or diastasis, a flexible fixation device may be placed.

The use of dynamic, flexible fixation devices has gained popularity in recent years. These fixation options have shown biomechanical similarity to the native syndesmosis and thus the reason for increased popularity.[42] This biomechanical superiority becomes important when considering patient complaints and discomfort noted with syndesmotic screws as they begin WB. This pain is because of syndesmotic screw fixation limiting physiologic motion of the fibula in anterior to posterior translation and resistance to external rotation of the talus in the ankle mortise, thus causing stiffness and discomfort in some patients.[42] Flexible or dynamic fixation allows a more anatomic biomechanical motion of the ankle syndesmosis and can potentially decrease the need for additional surgery and avoid hardware breakage or loosening

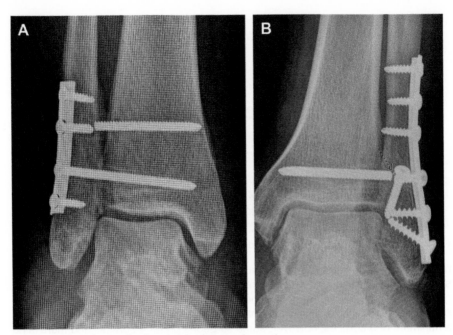

Fig. 7. ■(A-B) Radiographs showing broken syndesmotic screws.

(**Fig. 8**A–C). Additionally, it has been shown that flexible fixation devices allow improved reduction and decreased risk of malreduction, which has been well documented in prior studies.[43,44] Coetzee and colleagues[45] reported AOFAS scores comparing a cohort of 8 patients with screw fixation versus 8 patients with tightropes for the management of syndesmosis injury. They found higher AOFAS scores in the Tightrope group compared with the screw fixation group at 18.5 months

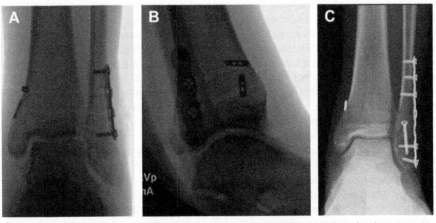

Fig. 8. ■Treatment of syndesmosis injuries with a Tightrope® XP implant (Arthrex Inc., Naples, FL). (A-B) AP and lateral radiographs post fixation of PER-type ankle fracture with syndesmosis injury. (C) AP radiograph post fixation in an SER-type ankle fracture with syndesmosis injury.

postoperatively and concluded that there was a trend toward increased ankle motion in the tightrope group. This would suggest the potential advantage of that device as it allows for more normal motion in the syndesmoses complex. Other reports have shown superiority in AOFAS scores at midterm follow-up and shorter returns to work.[46] Therefore, the demonstrated improved outcomes of the flexible fixation have led practitioners to this treatment in elite athletes. Football players are the most publicized athletes in both the media and the research world. D'Hooghe and colleagues[47] investigated 110 professional football players in their rehabilitation time following isolated syndesmotic fixation using the tightrope. Their results showed a mean time required to begin the sports-specific rehabilitation of 37 days, whereas the time to return to train with the team was 72 days. The first official match after surgical syndesmosis fixation was played on average after 103 days. Several studies have shown improved functional outcomes, patient satisfaction, decreased need for hardware removal or breakage, and maintenance of reduction.[43,47–54] Owing to these factors, it is the authors' primary method of fixation in syndesmosis injuries in athletes and young, active patients.

Direct repair of the AITFL or augmentation of the AITFL with the use of anchors and suture tape has been described recently.[55,56] AITFL repair is important in stabilizing lateral displacement and external rotation in syndesmosis injuries. Wood and colleagues[55] used a cadaveric study to show the importance of augmenting the syndesmotic repair with suture anchors by comparing normal/native ankle and injured ankle with AITFL and IOL injuries, using multiple suture buttons and suture anchor constructs. The most promising results showed greater amounts of load to failure in external rotation and fibular translation with the suture anchor construct regardless of suture button usage.

Average Return to Sport

Particular attention has been brought to the isolated syndesmotic repair and its accelerated return to sport. Although patients and athletes usually project to return to sport as early as possible, the trend is to gradually progress these athletes into full activity. Generally, athletes do return to their pre-injury level of the sport.[57] Lower grade injuries typically return to sport earlier than higher grade injuries. Although there are several instances where athletes return to professional sport within a few weeks, most require 45 to 64 days to return to pre-injury level, and this depends on the extent of injury, surgical repair, and recovery.[57] In some cases, athletes can return as early as 6 weeks after ORIF.[58] Grade IIa (Stable AITFL and IOL) injuries are treated typically nonoperatively and have an average return to the sport of 25 to 63 days based on the rehabilitation protocol described above. Grade IIb (Unstable AITFL and IOL) arthroscopically tested have a range of 27 to 104 days of return to sport if treated with tightrope fixation.[57] D'Hooghe and colleagues[47] noted a return to sport at about 4 months with treatment by dynamic flexible fixation.

SUMMARY

Syndesmosis injuries are a leading cause of prolonged return to sport for athletes. Many of these injuries can often be misdiagnosed at first presentation, unless there are concomitant fractures that require evaluation and fixation. Practitioners should have a high clinical suspicion for these injuries in athletes and should pay strict attention to the mechanism of injury and clinical testing when these patients present in the office. Prompt diagnosis and treatment will help these athletes return to sport as soon as possible, and misdiagnosis can lead to poorer outcomes and increased complications. In injuries that require surgical management, anatomic reduction is of utmost importance, and sport-specific rehabilitation and physical therapy postoperatively will help patients return to their pre-injury activity level. Controversies exist regarding type of syndesmosis fixation; however, recent literature, especially in athletes, favors flexible fixation.

CLINICS CARE POINTS

- Syndesmosis injuries are a leading cause of prolonged return to sport for athletes.
- A high clinical suspicion for these injuries in athletes is imperative during evaluation.
- Anatomic reduction improves outcomes and sport specific rehabilitation and physical therapy post operatively will help patients return to their pre-injury activity level.

DISCLOSURE

The authors have nothing to disclose.

REFERENCES

1. Waterman BR, Belmont PJ Jr, Cameron KL, et al. Risk factors for syndesmotic and medial ankle sprain: role of sex, sport, and level of competition. Am J Sports Med 2011;39(5):992–8.
2. Gerber JP, Williams GN, Scoville CR, et al. Persistent disability associated with ankle sprains: a prospective examination of an athletic population. Foot Ankle Int 1998;19(10):653–60.
3. Hunt KJ, George E, Harris AHS, et al. Epidemiology of syndesmosis injuries in intercollegiate football: incidence and risk factors from National Collegiate Athletic Association injury surveillance system data from 2004-2005 to 2008-2009. Clin J Sport Med 2013;23(4):278–82.
4. Court-Brown CM, McBirnie J, Wilson G. Adult ankle fractures: an increasing problem? Acta Orthop Scand 1998;69:43–7.
5. Beris AE, Kabbani KT, Xenakis TA, et al. Surgical treatment of malleolar fractures: a review of 144 patients. Clin Orthop Relat Res 1997;341:90–8.
6. Purvis GD. Displaced, unstable ankle fractures: classification, incidence, and management of a consecutive series. Clin Orthop Relat Res 1982;165:91–8.
7. Ogilvie-Harris DJ, Reed SC, Hedman TP. Disruption of the ankle syndesmosis: biomechanical study of the ligamentous restraints. Arthroscopy 1994;10:558–60.
8. Harper MC. Delayed reduction and stabilization of the tibiofibular syndesmosis. Foot Ankle Int 2001;22(1):15–8.
9. Brown KW, Morrison WB, Schweitzer ME, et al. MRI findings associated with distal tibiofibular syndesmosis injury. AJM Am J Roentgenol 2004;182:131–6.
10. Quenu E. Du diastasis de l'articulation tibio-peroniere inferieure. Rev Chir (Paris) 1907;36:62–90 [in French].
11. Yang Y, Zhou J, Li B. Operative exploration and reduction of syndesmosis in Weber type C ankle injury. Acta Orthop Bras 2013;21(2):103–8.
12. Xenos JS, Hopkinson WJ, Mulligan ME, et al. The tibiofibular syndesmosis: evaluation of the ligamentous structures, methods of fixation, and radiographic assessment. J Bone Joint Surg Am 1995;77:847–56.

13. Elgafy H, Semaan HB, Blessinger B, et al. Computed tomography of normal distal tibiofibular syndesmosis. Skeletal Radiol 2010;39:559.
14. Liu Q, Lin B, Guo Z, et al. Shapes of distal tibiofibular syndesmosis are associated with risk of recurrent lateral ankle sprains. Sci Rep 2017;7:6244.
15. Liu GT, Ryan E, Gustafson E, et al. Three-dimensional computed tomographic characterization of normal anatomic morphology and variations of the distal tibiofibular syndesmosis. J Foot Ankle Surg 2018;57(6):1130–6.
16. Ramsey PL, Hamilton W. Changes in tibiotalar area of contact caused by lateral talar shift. J Bone Joint Surg Am 1976;58:356–7.
17. Zindrick MR, Hopkins DE, Knight GW, et al. The effect of lateral talar shift upon the biomechanics of the ankle joint. Orthopaedic Trans 1985;9:332–3.
18. Thordarson DB, Motamed S, Hedman T, et al. The effect of fibular malreduction on contact pressures in an ankle fracture malunion model. J Bone Joint Surg Am 1997;79(12):1809–15.
19. McKeon KE, Wright RW, Johnson JE, et al. Vascular anatomy of the tibiofibular syndesmosis. J Bone Joint Surg Am 2012;94:931–8.
20. Williams GN, Jones MH, Amendola A. Syndesmotic ankle sprains in athletes. Am J Sports Med 2007;35:1197–207.
21. Waterman B, Owens B, Davey S, et al. The epidemiology of ankle sprains in the United States. J Bone Joint Surg Am 2010;92(13):2279–84.
22. Lievers WB, Adamic PF. Incidence and severity of foot and ankle injuries in men's collegiate American football. Orthop J Sports Med 2015;3(5): 2325967115581593.
23. Beumer A, Swierstra BA, Mulder PG. Clinical diagnosis of syndesmotic instability: evaluation of stress tests behind the curtains. Acta Orthop Scand 2002;73(6): 667–9.
24. Alonso A, Khoury L, Adams R. Clinical tests for ankle syndesmosis injury: reliability and prediction of return to function. J Orthop Sports Phys Ther 1998; 27(4):276–84.
25. Teitz CC, Harrington RM. A biomechanical analysis of the squeeze test for sprains of the syndesmotic ligaments of the ankle. Foot Ankle Int 1998;19:489–92.
26. Kor A. Dynamic techniques for clinical assessment of the athlete. Clin Podiatr Med Surg 2015;32(2):217–29.
27. Gill JB, Risko T, Raducan V, et al. Comparison of manual and gravity stress radiographs for the evaluation of supination-external rotation fibular fractures. J Bone Joint Surg Am 2007;89:994–9.
28. de-Las-Heras Romero J, Alvarez AML, Sanchez FM, et al. Management of syndesmotic injuries of the ankle. EFORT Open Rev 2017;2(9):403–9.
29. Del Rio A, Bewsher SM, Roshan-Zamir S, et al. Weightbearing cone-beam computed tomography of acute ankle syndesmosis injuries. J Foot Ankle Surg 2020;59(2):258–63.
30. Edwards GS Jr, DeLee JC. Ankle diastasis without fracture. Foot Ankle 1984;4: 305–12.
31. van Dijk CN, Longo UG, Loppini M, et al. Classification and diagnosis of acute isolated syndesmotic injuries: ESSKA-AFAS consensus and guidelines. Knee Surg Sports Traumatol Arthrosc 2016;24:1200–16.
32. Turky M, Menon KV, Saeed K. Arthroscopic grading of injuries of the inferior tibiofibular syndesmosis. J Foot Ankle Surg 2018;57(6):1125–9.
33. Gardner MJ, Demetrakopoulos D, Briggs SM, et al. Malreduction of the tibiofibular syndesmosis in ankle fracture. Foot Ankle Int 2006;27(10):788–92.

34. Miller AN, Carroll EA, Parker RJ, et al. Direct visualization for syndesmotic stabilization of ankle fractures. Foot Ankle Int 2009;30(5):419–26.

35. Tornetta P, Yakavonis M, Veltre D, et al. Reducing the syndesmosis under direct vision: where should I look? J Orthop Trauma 2019;33(9):450–4.

36. Cosgrove CT, Putnam SM, Cherney SM, et al. Medial clamp tine positioning affects ankle syndesmosis malreduction. J Orthop Trauma 2017;31(8):440–6.

37. Boszczyk A, Kordasiewicz B, Kicinski M, et al. Operative setup to improve sagittal syndesmotic reduction: technical tip. J Orthop Trauma 2019;33(1):e27–30.

38. Boffeli TJ, Messerly CG, Sorensen TK. Ideal angle of upper and lower syndesmotic fixation based on weightbearing computed tomographic imaging in uninjured ankles. J Foot Ankle Surg 2020;59(6):1224–8.

39. Reb CW, Brandao RA, Watson BC, et al. Medial structure injury during suture button insertion utilizing 'center-center' technique for syndesmotic stabilization. Foot Ankle Int 2018;39(8):984–9.

40. King CK, Doyle MD, Castellucci-Garza FM, et al. Early protected weightbearing after open reduction internal fixation of ankle fractures with trans-syndesmotic screws. J Foot Ankle Surg 2020;59(4):726–8.

41. Walley KC, Hofmann KJ, Velasco BT, et al. Removal of hardware after syndesmotic screw fixation: a systematic literature review. Foot Ankle Spec 2017; 10(3):252–7.

42. Clanton TO, Whitlow SR, Williams BT, et al. Biomechanical comparison of 3 current ankle syndesmosis repair techniques. Foot Ankle Int 2016;38(2):200–7.

43. Naqvi GA, Cunningham P, Lynch B, et al. Fixation of ankle syndesmotic injuries: comparison of Tightrope fixation and syndesmotic screw fixation for accuracy of syndesmotic reduction. Am J Sports Med 2012;40(12):2828–35.

44. Grassi A, Samuelsson K, D'Hooghe P, et al. Dynamic stabilization of syndesmosis injuries reduces complications and reoperations as compared with screw fixation: a meta-analysis and randomized controlled trials. Am J Sports Med 2020;48(4): 1000–13.

45. Coetzee JC, Ebeling P. Treatment of syndesmosis disruptions with Tightrope fixation. Tech Foot Ankle Surg 2008;7(3):196–202.

46. Schepers T. Acute distal tibiofibular syndesmosis injury: a systematic review of suture-button versus syndesmotic screw repair. Int Orthop 2012;36(6):1199–206.

47. D'Hooghe P, Grassi A, Alkhelaifi K, et al. Return to play after surgery for isolated unstable syndesmotic ankle injuries (West Point grade IIB and III) in 110 male professional football players: a retrospective cohort study. Br J Sports Med 2020;54(19):1168–73.

48. Cottom JM, Hyer CF, Philbin TM, et al. Treatment of syndesmotic disruptions with the : a report of 25 cases. Foot Ankle Int 2008;29(8):773–80.

49. Cottom JM, Hyer CF, Philbin TM, et al. Of the distal tibiofibular syndesmosis: comparison of an interosseous suture and endobutton to traditional screw fixation in 50 cases. J Foot Ankle Surg 2009;48(6):620–30.

50. Rigby RB, Cottom JM. Does the Arthrex Tightrope provide maintenance of the distal tibiofibular syndesmosis? A 2-year follow-up of 64 Tightropes in 37 patients. J Foot Ankle Surg 2013;52:563–7.

51. Naqvi GA, Shafqat A, Awan N. Tightrope fixation of ankle syndesmosis injuries: clinical outcome, complications, and technique modification. Injury 2012;43: 838–42.

52. Sanders D, Schneider P, Taylor M, et al. Improved reduction of the tibiofibular syndesmosis with Tightrope compared with screw fixation: results of a randomized controlled study. J Orthop Trauma 2019;33(11):531–7.

53. Laflamme M, Belzile EL, Bedard L, et al. A prospective randomized multicenter trial comparing clinical outcomes of patients treated surgically with a static or dynamic implant for acute ankle syndesmosis disruption. J Orthop Trauma 2015; 29(5):216–23.

54. DeGroot H, Al-Omari AA, Ghazaly SAE. Outcomes of suture button repair of the distal tibiofibular syndesmosis. Foot Ankle Int 2011;32(3):250–6.

55. Wood AR, Arshad SA, Kim H, et al. Kinematic analysis of combined suture-button and suture anchor augment constructs for ankle syndesmosis injuries. Foot Ankle Int 2020;41(4):463–72.

56. Kim JS, Shin HS. Suture anchor augmentation for acute unstable isolated ankle syndesmosis disruption in athletes. Foot Ankle Int 2021;42(9):1130–7.

57. Calder JD, Bamford R, Petrie A, et al. Stable versus unstable grade II high ankle sprains: a prospective study predicting the need for surgical stabilization and time to return to sports. Arthroscopy 2016;32(4):634–42.

58. Taylor DC, Tenuta JJ, Uhorchak JM, et al. Aggressive surgical treatment and early return to sports in athletes with grade III syndesmosis sprains. Am J Sports Med 2007;35(11):1833–8.

Lisfranc Injuries in the Athlete

Christina Ma, DPM^a, Meagan M. Jennings, DPM, FACFAS^{b,}*

KEYWORDS

- Lisfranc injuries athletes • Orif in lisfranc injuries • Arthrodesis in lisfranc injuries

KEY POINTS

- LisFranc injuries in the athlete can be devastating or career-ending injuries, especially if not treated appropriately.
- It is important to differentiate between a purely ligamentous LisFranc injury versus one involving fracture in order to determine appropriate treatment of the injury.
- Flexible fixation has now added another dimension to open reduction and internal fixation in subtle LisFranc injuries especially in athletes.

INTRODUCTION
Defining Lisfranc Injuries

Lisfranc injuries are injuries that affect the tarsometatarsal (TMT), intercuneiform, and naviculocuneiform joints named after a Napoleon surgeon and gynecologist who first described amputations at this level (**Table 1**). These injuries typically fall into 1 or 2 categories: (1) high-energy midfoot injuries with significant soft tissue injury and (2) low energy with ligamentous disruptions or small avulsion fractures. The low-energy injuries tend to be the pattern more frequently observed in athletes. Lisfranc injuries can become a source of persistent pain and possibly are career-ending because they can be subtle subluxations that can go undetected if not properly evaluated.[1]

Treatment of Lisfranc injuries remains controversial. Current treatment options include open reduction and internal fixation versus primary fusion. However, there continues to be debate without a clear consensus as to the optimal treatment of these injuries. Historically, treatment has progressed from closed treatment without emphasis on anatomic joint restoration to primary open reduction and stable fixation.

There is no universally accepted algorithm or criteria for the operative and nonoperative management of Lisfranc injuries. Management currently depends on the severity of the disorder. Conservative management is sufficient for nondisplaced and stable

^a Staint Mary's Foot & Ankle Surgical Residency Program, 450 Stanyan Street, San Francisco, CA 94117, USA; ^b Silicon Valley Foot & Ankle Reconstructive Fellowship, Palo Alto Foundation Medical Group / Sutter Health, 701 East EL Camino Real, Mountain View, CA 94040, USA
* Corresponding author.
E-mail address: MMJFOOTANKLE@GMAIL.COM

Clin Podiatr Med Surg 40 (2023) 39–54
https://doi.org/10.1016/j.cpm.2022.07.004
0891-8422/23/© 2022 Elsevier Inc. All rights reserved.

podiatric.theclinics.com

Table 1
Lisfranc articles comparing open reduction and internal fixation versus PA

Article	Number of Patients	Average Follow-up	Study Type	Summary
Kuo et al,[13] 2000	48	52 mo	Retrospective	• 15 purely ligamentous • 33 combined ligamentous and osseous Lisfranc • The purely ligamentous injury group had a combined midfoot arthrosis rate of 40% despite initial anatomic reduction and rigid internal fixation when compared with combined ligamentous and osseous injuries 18%, ($P = .011$)
Pelt et al,[14] 2011	5 matched fresh frozen pairs	n/a	Cadaveric model	• 10 cadaveric feet • Compare suture button tension vs rigid screw fixation • 3.5-mm fully threaded cortical screw was used to fixate vs Arthrex tightrope suture button • Both devices were effective in restraining motion to prefixation levels ($P = .487$) • No significant difference in cyclic loading making suture button a viable fixation device when compared screw fixation to restrain motion at the Lisfranc complex
Cottom et al,[15] 2019	84	3 y	Retrospective	• Purely ligamentous injuries • suture button vs 4.0 mm screw fixation • AOFAS scores improved from 30 postinjury to 90 postoperatively and visual analog scale scores improved from 8.4 to 1.3 postoperatively • They concluded ORIF using an intraosseous suture button had an adequate midterm patient satisfaction but notable for minimal diastasis in some patients in their 3-y follow-up in purely ligamentous Lisfranc dislocations

Study	n	Study Type	Follow-up	Findings
Dubois-Ferrier et al,[16] 2016	61	Retrospective	10 y	• 61 pts (Myerson A, n = 16; B, n = 27; C, n = 18) • 50 patients underwent an ORIF • 11 underwent a primary arthrodesis • Anatomic reduction achieved in 54 (88.5%) at follow-up. • Radiographic evidence of OA was noted in 44 (72.1%) of the patients, and symptomatic OA, in 54.1%, the latter having worse outcomes • Risk factors for symptomatic OA were the failure to obtain anatomic reduction, Myerson type–C compared with type–A fracture classification), and status as a former or current smoker at the time of surgery
Teng et al,[17] 2002	11	Retrospective	41.2 mo	• 11 patients who underwent ORIF • 10 patients had excellent anatomic reduction radiographically • 8 of 11 still had evidence of posttraumatic osteoarthritis and 9 of 11 had decreased relative range of motion • AOFAS midfoot score was found to be 71 • 73% demonstrated radiographic arthritis with in-shoe pressures similar to the uninjured side via Tek scan
Sheibani-rad et al,[20] 2012	193	Systematic review	1 y	• 6 reviews • Total of 193 patients • comparing clinical and radiographic outcomes • Of the 6, 4 concentrated on ORIF alone (n = 160) • More than half of the injuries were mixed osseous and ligamentous, and the remaining injuries were ligamentous • The most common complications across all studies were screw breakage and posttraumatic arthritis • At 1 y follow-up, AOFAS for ORIF was 72.5, whereas arthrodesis was 88. There was no significant effect of treatment group on the percentage of patients who had anatomic reduction ($P = .319$)

(continued on next page)

Table 1
(continued)

Article	Number of Patients	Average Follow-up	Study Type	Summary
Ly and Coetzee,[19] 2006	41	42.5 mo	Randomized, prospective	• Outcomes between primary arthrodesis and open reduction internal fixation for acute Lisfranc injuries who were randomly assigned • At the 2 y follow-up, 100% of patients in the ORIF had anatomic reductions with 11 requiring hardware removal due to standard protocol • The ORIF had a significantly higher revision rate than the arthrodesis (ORIF 79% vs PA 17% $P<.05$) • Functionally, short musculoskeletal function assessment (SMFA) scores demonstrated a trended improvement in PA as compared with the PORIF group at 2 y, however, not found to be statistically significant • At a 53-mo follow-up phone survey, there was no significant difference in patient satisfaction between PORIF (90%, 9/10) and PA (92%, 12/13)
Henning et al,[21] 2009	41	2 y	Randomized, prospective	• Military personnel during a 5-year period • 18 underwent ORIF • 14 underwent PA • Average age of 28 y • Patients presenting acutely underwent on open reduction internal fixation • Patients presenting after 6 wk underwent PA • Mean time to surgery for ORIF group was 18 d, and fixated with screws alone (10, 56%), screws and plate (1, 5%), and plate only (7, 39%). One had a midfoot collapse and underwent conversion to arthrodesis at 43 mo

- PA group, fixation constructs included screws alone in 8 (57%) and combined screws and plates in 6 (43%)
- Return to full-duty for fusion returned at an average of 4.5 mo
- Return to full-duty for ORIF returned on average at 6.7 mo
- Hardware removal in the ORIF group was 83% and PA group at 14%
- The PA group ran their fitness test an average of 9 s per mile slower than their preoperative average
- The ORIF group ran it an average of 39 s slower per mile ($P = .032$)
- At 35-mo follow-up though, there were no differences in FAAM scores
- They concluded ORIF and PA had similar rates of return to work in the young cohort; however, primary arthrodesis may decrease time required for return to work and improve ability to run in the short term despite no differences at the 35-mo benchmark

Cochran et al,[23] 2017	32	1 y	Level III, comparative cohort study

- Systematic review completed to compare ORIF and Primary fusion using PRISMA guidelines
- ORIF vs PA demonstrated that the risk of hardware removal is significantly higher than in arthrodesis patients (risk ratio 0.23 (95% CI, 0.11–0.45; $P < .001$)
- ORIF was not found to have a higher risk of revision with a risk ratio of 0.36 (95% CI, 0.08–1.59; $P = .18$)
- They concluded patients undergoing an open reduction internal fixation increases the risk of hardware removal allowing with associated morbidity

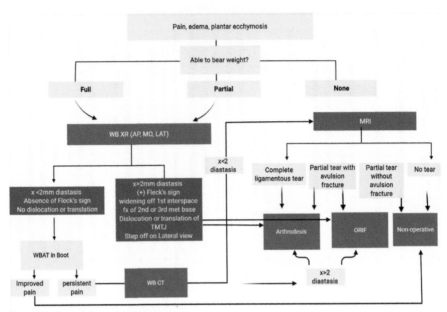

Fig. 1. Lisfranc injury algorithm.

injuries, whereas unstable and/or displaced injuries require surgical intervention with anatomic reduction.

As for Lisfranc injuries and return to sport, most studies combine bony Lisfranc and ligamentous Lisfranc injuries treated with open reduction and internal fixation. Furthermore, there is no consensus regarding return to sport after Lisfranc injury. In some studies, athletes are reported to return to sport as early as 3 to 4 months after Lisfranc injury.[2,3]

Incidence

Overall incidence of Lisfranc injuries remains unclear. Lisfranc midfoot injuries are relatively rare with incidences of 1 in 55,000 per year and make up approximately 0.2% of all fractures.[1] Midfoot sprains have been reported to affect 4% of collegiate American football players annually with 29% of injuries found in offensive lineman.[4]

Lisfranc injuries have reported to be missed approximately 20% of the time.[1] Radiographic images can often seem normal with subtle subluxations. Frequent delay can be due to underestimating the severity of the injury until the pain, swelling, and bruising persists leading to further evaluation (**Fig. 1**).

Anatomy

The Lisfranc joint complex is a unique bone structure that is responsible for the stability of the midfoot. The middle cuneiform is recessed 8-mm proximal to the medial cuneiform and 4-mm proximal to the lateral cuneiform, thus limiting translation in the coronal plane.[5] In the axial plane, the midfoot can be thought of as a transverse arch with the second metatarsal is considered the apex or keystone. The second metatarsal's recession has been noted as a form of stability. Peicha and colleagues confirmed on radiographic analysis if the mortise is shallower, the joint complex has a higher risk for injury.[6]

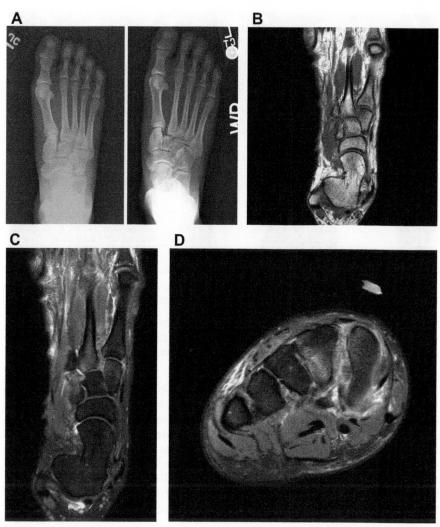

Fig. 2. A 17-year-old gymnast presents to urgent care with "foot sprain." (*A*) Nonweight-bearing images suspicious but not conclusive of Lisfranc ligamentous pathologic condition. (*B*) Weight-bearing contralateral AP films taken and reveal diastasis of left Lisfranc joint without fracture. (*C*) MR images showing bone marrow edema injury at the Lisfranc complex. (*D*) Flexible fixation due to young athlete preformed.

The Lisfranc ligament, or the oblique interosseous ligament, plays an important role in stabilizing the Lisfranc complex. It runs from the plantar base of the medial cuneiform to the plantar base of the second metatarsal and is critical to stabilizing the Lisfranc complex. The plantar ligaments have shown to be stronger than the dorsal and interosseous ligaments with the Lisfranc ligament shown to have the highest load to failure.

Mechanism of Injury

Lisfranc injuries found in athletes differ from those found in traumatic injuries. As mentioned earlier, they are lower energy in contrast to those found from motor vehicle

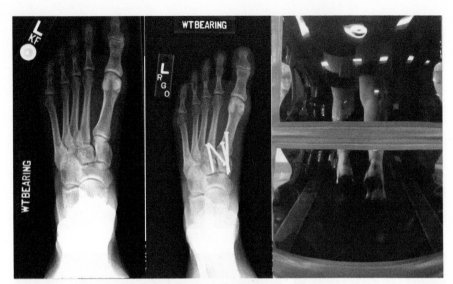

Fig. 3. 26 year old athelte with subtle Lisfranc ligamentous injury. Treated with a primary fusion and running 80% of body weight on an Alter-G treadmill at 6 weeks postop.

accidents or falls. They are often subtle diastasis from purely ligamentous injuries or with small avulsion fractures. In some cases, they can produce more severe injury patterns as seen in equestrian, soccer, or football injuries.

Direct versus indirect injuries

Direct injuries occur when force is directly applied to the foot. An example is when a heavy player steps directly on top of another player's foot. Most injuries found in athletes are indirect. The most likely position is seen from an abduction force or from a plantar flexion force. The abduction force can be seen when the foot is fixed and the body rotates over the foot, causing the foot to twist violently into an abduction and external rotation. The plantar flexion force is seen in football players or gymnasts when a force is applied to heel in line with the axis of the foot, whereas the forefoot is fixed on a playing surface. In football, this can be seen when a player falls on the heel of another player (**Figs. 2–5**).

Clinical Examination

Lisfranc injuries can vary in greatly depending on severity. Occasionally, walking is pain free while running and jumping will provoke pain, whereas for others, any sort of weight-bearing will provoke pain. Pinpoints of tenderness are often localized to the first and second metatarsal bases and can indicate subtle diastasis injuries. Ecchymosis within the plantar arch can indicate a more significant midfoot injury.

Provocation tests, which include side-to-side compression and dorsal/plantar deviation of the first metatarsal head while stabilizing the second metatarsal can help establish a diagnosis. Pronation and abduction stress of the midfoot can also elicit and reproduce the patient's symptoms.

Radiographic Evaluation

Stress and weight-bearing views

Weight-bearing images with a minimum of 3 views, including an anteroposterior (AP), a 30° oblique, and lateral view of the foot is strongly recommended if tolerated.

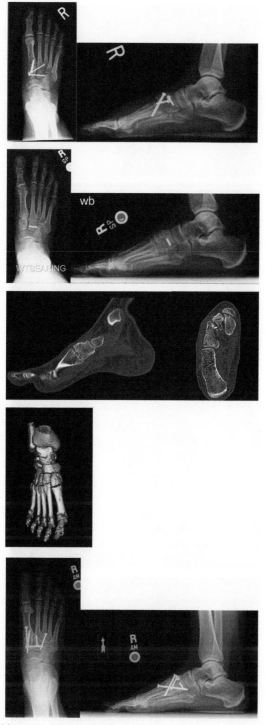

Fig. 4. A 24-year-old soccer player treated with ORIF, which was subtly malreduced. CT scan showed posttraumatic arthritis of the Post-initial. Lisfranc joint 1 to 3. Arthrodesis was then performed around 18 months postinitial ORIF.

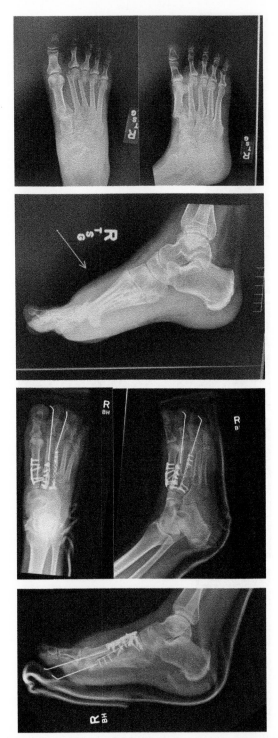

Fig. 5. A 63-year-old active woman treated with bridge-plating primary arthrodesis in a Lisfranc injury with fracture comminution and displacement of first, second, and third metatarsals after presenting 4-week status postinitial injury due to insurance issues. Significant comminution and dislocation of second and third metatarsal heads reduced with smooth k-wires.

Weight-bearing can help accentuate any deformities, especially subtle Lisfranc joint diastasis. Equal weight should be applied to both feet because guarding or preference to the uninjured side can lead to a false-negative result. Bilateral, weight-bearing AP views for comparison to the contralateral, uninjured foot are recommended whenever possible.

The AP view is most useful in assessing the first and second TMT joints. The first metatarsal aligns with the medial cuneiform both medially and laterally. A small avulsion at the lateral base of the first and medial base of the second metatarsal known as the fleck's sign can suggest a disruption of the TMT ligaments and a Lisfranc injury. Any displacement of more than 2-mm between the base of the first and second metatarsal should prompt comparison to the contralateral side. On the 30° oblique view, the medial cortex of the fourth metatarsal should line up perfectly with the medial border of the cuboid. On the lateral view, there should not be any displacement or interruption of the dorsal cortex line of the first metatarsal to the medial cuneiform. If there is any suspicion for a Lisfranc injury, a manual pronation-abduction stress view under general or local block has been more sensitive than a weight-bearing radiograph alone.[7]

Computed tomography

Computed tomography (CT) can be useful to evaluate the TMT joints in patients with ambiguous radiographic findings. Subtle subluxations as well as nondisplaced metatarsal base and cuneiform fractures not visualized on plain radiographs can be reliably detected by CT.[8] Occult fractures of the metatarsal bases and cuneiforms are often identified and increase diagnostic accuracy. Best results are obtained when the CT is taken parallel and perpendicular to the TMT joints.

MRI

MRI is an important diagnostic tool where radiographic images are inconclusive but there is a high index of suspicion for a Lisfranc injury. It is particularly useful in correlating patients with unstable fractures. The strongest predictor of instability of the Lisfranc ligament on MRI was rupture of the plantar component with a positive predictive value of 94%.[9]

Classification System

Lisfranc injuries were classified by Quénu and Küss based on radiographic findings and mechanism of injuries. The original Quénu and Küss[10] classification consists of 3 patterns of injury with modifications by Hardcastle[11] then Myerson.[12]

- Type A: total incongruity, homolateral incomplete
  - Involves all 5 TMT articulations with displacement dorsolateral as a unit.
- Type B: Partial incongruity, homolateral incomplete
  - Involves one or more but not all metatarsals. It usually involves medial displacement of the first metatarsal or dorsolateral displacement.
  - Myerson modification: distinguish between medial articulation alone (B1) or one or more lateral metatarsals (B2).
- Type C: divergent with total or partial displacements
  - Involves lateral or medial metatarsals being displaced in opposite directions or different planes.
  - Myerson modification: less than 4 lateral TMT joints involved (C1) versus all involved (C2).

Although these classification systems were descriptive and widely used, it is neither prognostic nor provides a recommended treatment algorithm.

TREATMENT OPTIONS FOR LISFRANC INJURIES
Closed Treatment

Closed treatment is rarely the treatment of choice in the athletic population. With a positive radiograph stress examination or other imaging, typically, operative treatment will be the treatment of choice unless medical comorbidities prohibit anesthesia and operative intervention.

Open Reduction and Internal Fixation

Background

The treatment of fracture dislocations of the midfoot has stressed the importance of achieving and maintaining anatomic reduction for achieving good functional outcomes. Although there have been authors who advocate closed reduction and percutaneous Kirschner-wire fixation, the current trend is toward open reduction and screw fixation.[2]

Purely ligamentous injuries have been shown to have poorer outcomes despite anatomic reduction. Kuo and colleagues in 2020 evaluated 48 patients for an overage of 52 months (13–114).[13] They found patients with anatomic reduction had a significantly better American Orthopedic Foot & Ankle Society (AOFAS; $P = .05$) and a significantly lower prevalence of secondary osteoarthritis ($P = .004$).[13] The musculoskeletal function assessment (MFA) score of 19 with 12 with arthrosis (25%) with 6 ultimately requiring arthrodesis (12.5%).[13] Ligamentous injuries were found to have higher prevalence of posttraumatic osteoarthritis compared with patients with combined ligamentous and osseous injuries (40% compared with 18%, $P = .11$).[13] Even with anatomic reduction and screw fixation, patients with purely ligamentous injury still had a higher rate of degeneration compared with combined ligamentous and osseous injuries.[13] The initial type of injury may be the determining factor of long-term outcome.[13]

Open reduction and internal fixation fixation options. Smooth Kirshner wires were initially favored for transarticular stabilization. They were easy to insert, noted to have minimal damage at the articular surface and easy to remove. The pins were often removed after 6 weeks. They are still used today, specifically during high-energy trauma with traumatized soft tissue. It allows for an unstable foot injury to be provisionally in place until the swelling resolves. After 10 to 14 days, a formal open reduction can be performed with replacement of stable screws at the first, second, and third TMT joints. Kirschner wires can continue to stabilize the fourth and fifth metatarsalcuboid joints if needed.

Cortical screw fixation (3.5 mm) has been noted to be stronger and allows a more stable construct. It is often placed from the medial cuneiform across the base of the second metatarsal and known as the "home run screw." It reduces and stabilizes the diastasis and effectively secures the keystone of the arch. Although screws provide stable fixation, it can be suboptimal in patients with suboptimal bone. It may also cause additional damage to the articular surface at the TMT joints as well as an additional surgery for removal. Bioabsorbable screws have reportedly been used to avoid a second surgery for removal; however, they are less rigid than a standard metal screw. It can successfully stabilize the joint but like the cortical screw, it can cause iatrogenic joint damage. For these reasons, they have not been widely adopted.

Dorsal bridge plates have been able to provide fixation without iatrogenic damage to the TMT joint. It provides a viable option in the setting of poor bone quality, or with comminuted metatarsal base fractures. It can allow for overall alignment and maintaining metatarsal length in high-energy traumatic injuries, as opposed to screw fixation.

However, these plates require a secondary surgery to remove them because they are not supporting arthrodesis but are serving as a form of splintage in open reduction and internal fixation (ORIF).

Suture buttons are used at the Lisfranc joints because they provide a more physiologic and less rigid fixation than the screw. Proponents suggest there is less concern for fatigue failure compared with the screw and do not require an additional surgery for removal. Recent studies by Pelt and colleagues found suture buttons are equivalent to a screw in restraining abduction.[14] Cottom and colleagues retrospectively looked at 84 patients with a 3-year minimum follow-up who underwent a suture button and 4.0-mm screw fixation at the medial and intermediate cuneiform joints.[15] They found that the AOFAS and visual analog scale scores improved from 30 and 8.4, respectfully, preoperatively to 90 and 1.3 postoperatively.[15] Moreover, although the mean preoperative step-off between the second metatarsal base and intermediate cuneiform was found to be 3.15 mm, the immediate post-reduction weight-bearing radiograph measured 0.25 mm and 0.43 mm at the final follow-up evaluation, a difference that was found to be significant without revision.[15] Although this study offers a potential improvement on ORIF, larger clinical trials will need to be performed before this is a recommended treatment option.

Failure of open reduction and internal fixation in lisfranc injuries. The failure of ORIF for Lisfranc injuries primarily has been reduced to the failure of achieving anatomic alignment on reduction. In a study by, Dubois-Ferriere and colleagues, JBJS, 2016, with follow-up at an average of 10 years, they deduced the failure of ORIF could be attributed to incomplete anatomic reduction.[16] Dubois-Ferriere also found Myerson Type C injuries also fared worse with ORIF.[16] Teng and colleagues looked at the functional outcomes following anatomic restoration of the tarso-metatarsal joint (TMTJ) fracture dislocation for nearly 3.5 years postinjury and ORIF.[17] They found an AOFAS midfoot score of 71% and 73% demonstrated radiographic arthritis with in-shoe pressures similar to the uninjured side via Tekscan.[17]

Primary fusion for LIsFranc injury. Fusion may be a valuable option in many active people. Multiple studies do demonstrate that primary arthrodesis demonstrates early return to activity compared with ORIF in short-term and medium-term data. Although we fuse the first TMT joint often times for bunion correction and medial column instability, many surgeons still have some apprehension doing a primary fusion for Lisfranc injuries even though these are considered "nonessential" joints of the foot.[18]

Certain presentation of Lisfranc injuries preclude themselves to primary arthrodesis such as comminution of joints with intra-articular involvement, when anatomic reduction is not possible otherwise, the demands of the patient are high-impact, and preexisting degenerative disease is present. Ly and Coetzee looked at the treatment of primary ligamentous Lisfranc injuries and arthrodesis versus ORIF in 2006[19] and then in 2012,[20] they did a follow-up that at 1-year follow-up, the mean AOFAS score for ORIF was 72.5 versus 88.0 for primary arthrodesis and that a slight advantage may exist in performing a primary arthrodesis for Lisfranc joint injuries in terms of clinical outcomes. Their outcomes suggested that the fusion group did better in short and medium term than ORIF.[20] Henning and colleagues in 2009 prospectively looked at ORIF versus primary arthrodesis in primarily ligamentous injury where they fused only the medial rays (1–3). Arthrodesis did significantly better than ORIF at 2 years. PA and ORIF were both satisfied with surgery; however, ORIF had a significantly higher revision rate than arthrodesis. The rate of planned and unplanned secondary surgeries including hardware removal and salvage arthrodesis between open reduction and internal fixation (ORIF) and primary arthrodesis (PA) groups was significantly different. However, at a 53-month follow-up phone survey, there was no significant difference between ORIF and PA.[21]

Other studies that evaluated ORIF versus PA demonstrated that the risk of hardware removal is significantly higher than in arthrodesis patients.[22] Cochran and colleagues looked at low-energy Lisfranc injuries in military personnel during a 5-year period.[23] Eighteen underwent ORIF and 14 underwent PA. Return to full-duty was the endpoint with the patients with fusion returned at an average of 4.5 months and those undergoing ORIF returned on average at 6.7 months. Hardware removal in the ORIF group was 83% and PA group at 14%. Although at 35-month follow-up, there were no differences in foot & ankle ability measure (FAAM) scores.[23]

In the National Football League (NFL), McHale and colleagues during a 10-year period saw 28 NFL players in which 7.1% never returned to the NFL after a Lisfranc injury and that the average return to play was 11.1 months from time of injury.[24] Attia and colleagues looked at return play after low-energy lisfranc injuries in high-demand individuals: athletes and military personnel.[25] This meta-analysis aimed to review the return-to-play and return-to-duty rates with regard to the anatomic type and the management of low-energy Lisfranc injuries in a high-demand, active population. They looked at 15 studies, which included 441 patients, and found that 86.17% were able to return to play or duty. There was no statistically significant difference in return to play or duty rates for operative versus nonoperative treatment, ORIF versus PA, or bony versus ligamentous injuries. The mean time missed from practice/duty for operative versus nonoperative treatment was 58.02 days (95% confidence interval [CI], 13.6–102.4 days; I^2 = 98.03%) and 116.4 days (95% CI, 62.4–170.4 days; I^2 = 99.45%), respectively. The mean time missed from practice/duty for bony versus ligamentous injury was 98.9 days (95% CI, 6.1–191.7 days; I^2 = 99.82%) and 76.5 days (95% CI, 37.9–115.02 days; I^2 = 99.83%), respectively, with no statistically significant differences (standardized mean difference = 3.62 days [95% CI: −5.7–13 days]; I^2 = 83.17%).[25]

POSTOPERATIVE PROTOCOLS

Postoperative protocols for both ORIF and PA typically involve and modified Jones' compression splint out of the operating room and nonweight-bearing. At 2 to 3 weeks, sutures are removed depending on skin healing. With stable fixation, most patients can go into a removable cast boot and start ankle range of motion at least 3 to 4 times per day as well as toe curls and active movement to minimize dorsal incisional adhesions. Nonweight-bearing typically follows radiographic union until between 6 and 8 weeks in which protected weight-bearing can then begin. Physical therapy can help with progressive return to activity as well as balance, strength, and ambulation and should start no later than 6 weeks from surgery or cast immobilization for closed treatment.

Athletes should be encouraged to continue core and nonweight-bearing total body exercise. With incisions healed, athletes can start water therapy with an aqua-jogging belt and water exercise safely. Stationary bicycle with low tension in a postoperative shoe is also encouraged. An Alter-G treadmill in which a patient is made a percentage of their body weight by being strapped into the treadmill itself, can typically begin after 6 weeks starting with about 20% to 30% of the athlete's body weight.

As patients return to athletic shoes first, an over-the-counter insole can help support the repair. Various slipper and sandal brands with arch support for indoor ambulation can also help support the repair and return to function. Ultimately, a custom orthotic may be helpful for patients to return to full activity.

SUMMARY

It is important to understand the pathologic condition of the injury as well as the ultimate goals of the athlete when treating these injuries. In isolated second TMTJ Lisfranc injuries, ORIF with screw or flexible fixation is a reasonable option to treat these injuries in athletes. In injuries with fractures, intra-articular comminution, or multiple levels of joint injury, primary arthrodesis may allow an earlier return to activity, work, and sport. Ultimately, the age, demands, and injury pattern should determine whether ORIF or PA is implemented as the treatment of Lisfranc injuries.

CLINICS CARE POINTS

- Thorough history of present illness (HPI) including mechanism of injury and patient demands and goals is extremely important in treating these injuries.
- Weight-bearing contralateral anteroposterior radiographs are imperative, if possible, in all suspected LisFranc injuries.
- Consider advanced imaging such as MRI and computed tomography scans to help better understand the injury and decide on appropriate treatment.

DISCLOSURE

Dr M.M. Jennings is a consultant for Depuy-Synthes and Stryker Orthopedics.

REFERENCES

1. Desmond EA, Chou LB. Current concepts review: lisfranc injuries. Foot Ankle Int 2006;27(8):653–60.
2. Curtis MJ, Myerson M, Szura B. Tarsometatarsal joint injuries in the athlete. Am J Sports Med 1993;21(4):497–501.
3. Nunley JA, Vertullo CJ. Classification, Investigation, and Management of Midfoot Sprains. Am J Sports Med 2002;30(6):871–8.
4. Meyer SA, Callaghan JJ, Albright JP, et al. Midfoot Sprains in Collegiate Football Players. Am J Sports Med 1994;22(3):392–401.
5. Sarrafian SK, editor. Anatomy of the foot and ankle: descriptive, topographic, functional. 2nd edition. Philadelphia: Lippincott; 1993. p. 204–7. Syndesmology.
6. Peicha G, Labovitz j, Seibert Fj, et al. The anatomy of the joint as a risk factor for Lisfranc dislocation and fracture dis-location. An anatomical and radiological case control study. J Bone Joint Surg Br 2002;84:981–5.
7. Kaar S. Lisfranc joint displacement following sequential ligament sectioning. J Bone Joint Surg Am 2007;89(10):2225.
8. Lu J, Ebraheim NA, Skie M, et al. Radiographic and computed tomographic evaluation of lisfranc dislocation: a cadaver study. Foot Ankle Int 1997;18(6):351–5.
9. Raikin SM, Elias I, Dheer S, et al. Prediction of midfoot instability in the subtle lisfranc injury. J Bone Joint Surg Am 2009;91(4):892–9. https://doi.org/10.2106/jbjs. h.01075.
10. Quenu E, Kuss G. Etude sur les luxations du metatarse. Rev Chir Paris 1909;39.
11. Hardcastle PH, Reschauer R, Kutscha-Lissberg E, et al. Injuries to the tarsometatarsal joint: incidence, classification and treatment. J Bone Joint Surg Br 1982; 64:349–56.

12. Myerson MS, Fisher FT, Burgess AR, et al. Fracture dislocations of the tarsome-tatarsal joints: end results correlated with pathology and treatment. Foot Ankle 1986;6:225–42.

13. Kuo RS, Tejwani NC, Digiovanni CW, et al. Outcome after open reduction and internal fixation of Lisfranc joint injuries. J Bone Joint Surg Am 2000;82(11): 1609–18.

14. Pelt CE, Bachus KN, Vance RE, et al. A Biomechanical Analysis of a Tensioned Suture Device in the Fixation of the Ligamentous Lisfranc Injury. Foot Ankle Int 2011;32(4):422–31.

15. Cottom JM, Graney CT, Sisovsky C. Treatment of lisfranc injuries using interosseous suture button: a retrospective review of 84 cases with a minimum 3-year follow-up. J Foot Ankle Surg 2020. https://doi.org/10.1053/j.jfas.2019.12.011.

16. Dubois-Ferriere V, Lu bbeke A, Chowdhary A, et al. Clinical Outcomes and Development of Symptomatic Osteoarthritis 2 to 24 Years After Surgical Treatment of Tarsometatarsal Joint Complex Injuries. J Bone Joint Surg 2016;98(9):713–20.

17. Teng AL, Pinzur MS, Lomasney L, et al. Functional outcome following anatomic restoration of tarsal-metatarsal fracture dislocation. Foot Ankle Int 2002;23(10): 922–6.

18. Hansen Jr, Sigvaard T. Functional reconstruction of the foot and ankle. Hagerstown: Lippincott Williams & Wilkins; 2000. p. 544.

19. Ly TV, Chris Coetzee J. Treatment of primarily ligamentous Lisfranc joint injuries: primary arthrodesis compared with open reduction and internal fixation: a prospective, randomized study. JBJS 2006;88(3):514–20.

20. Sheibani-Rad S, Coetzee JC, Giveans MR, et al. Arthrodesis versus ORIF for lisfranc fractures. Orthopedics 2012;35(6):868–73.

21. Henning JA, Jones CB, Sietsema DL, et al. Open reduction internal fixation vs. Primary arthrodesis for lisfranc injuries: a prospective randomized study. Foot Ankle Int 2009;30:913–22.

22. Smith N, Stone C, Furey A. Does open reduction and internal fixation versus primary arthrodesis Improve patient outcomes for lisfranc trauma? A systematic review and meta-analysis. Clin Orthop Relat Res 2016;474:1445–52.

23. Cochran G, Renninger C, Tompane T, et al. Primary arthrodesis versus open reduction and internal fixation for low-energy lisfranc injuries in a young athletic population. Foot Ankle Int 2017;38(9):957–63.

24. McHale KJ, Rozell JC, Milby AH, et al. Outcomes of lisfranc injuries in the National football League. Am J Sports Med 2016;44(7):1810–7.

25. Attia AK, Mahmoud K, Alhammoud A, et al. Return to play after low-energy lisfranc injuries in high-demand individuals: a systematic review and meta-analysis of athletes and active military personnel. Orthop J Sports Med 2021; 9(3). 2325967120988158.

Pediatric Sports Trauma

Tenaya A. West, DPM[a],*, Brandon Kim, DPM[b]

KEYWORDS

- Youth athletics • Pediatric trauma • Foot and ankle

KEY POINTS

- Epiphyseal hallux fractures are common in barefoot pediatric athletes. Although timely treatment is ideal, successful surgical outcomes can be achieved even when these fractures present in the subacute setting.
- Pediatric metatarsal fractures can often be treated successfully with conservative care even in the setting of significant displacement. In adolescent athletes, surgical fixation of Jones fractures can be considered for a more predictable return to play.
- There should be a high suspicion of a lisfranc injury in any pediatric athletic midfoot sprain. Relative radiographic norms for the lisfranc joint approach that of an adult after age six.
- Arthroscopic-assisted open reduction and internal fixation for epiphyseal pediatric ankle fractures should be considered to limit soft tissue disruption, to allow for direct visualization of periosteal debridement and anatomic articular reduction, and to optimize rehabilitation.

INTRODUCTION

Youth athletics is popular in the United States, with 60 million children aged 6 to 18 participating in organized sports and 8 million high-school students participating in interscholastic sports.[1,2] Athletic participation has numerous benefits including the promotion of healthy living habits, improvement of psychosocial health, and enhancement of academic performance.[3–5] However, the associated risk of injury is well documented in this population.[1,6,7] High-school athletes experience between 2.3 and 2.5 injuries for every 1000 exposures.[2,6] The true rate of injury is likely much higher, as up to 80% of high-school sporting injuries do not result in time loss from practice, and therefore are not captured by common inclusion criteria in the literature.[8]

Both acute and overuse injuries are common in the lower extremity. In acute youth injuries, 57% to 74% occur in the lower extremity, with up to 23% occurring in the foot or ankle.[6,9] Likewise, 73% of overuse injuries are reported in the lower extremity, with

[a] Department of Orthopedics and Podiatric Surgery, Palo Alto Medical Foundation, 701 East El Camino Real, Mountain View, CA 94040, USA; [b] Kaiser Santa Clara Foot and Ankle Residency Program, Department of Orthopedics and Podiatric Surgery, Kaiser Foundation Hospitals, 700 Lawrence Expy, Santa Clara, CA 95051, USA
* Corresponding author.
E-mail address: WestTA@sutterhealth.org

Clin Podiatr Med Surg 40 (2023) 55–73
https://doi.org/10.1016/j.cpm.2022.07.005
0891-8422/23/© 2022 Elsevier Inc. All rights reserved.

19% in the foot or ankle.[9] Multiple intrinsic and extrinsic factors contribute to the risk of injury in young athletes.[1]

Trauma in this population of athletes must be viewed separately from the adult trauma and sports medicine populations. Treatment must take into consideration the unique challenges these athletes present, including risk of early physeal arrest, parental and coach pressure, and other psychosocial factors in relation to the injury and rehabilitation. This article provides a discussion of foot and ankle fractures that may be seen with athletic participation, using the Salter–Harris (SH) classification system.[10]

DIGITAL FRACTURES

Pediatric digital fractures account for up to 18% of pediatric foot fractures and can be sustained from either direct or indirect trauma.[11] Indirect mechanisms involve hyperextension or hyperflexion combined with hyperadduction or hyperabduction, and are seen more commonly in barefoot pediatric athletes.[12] Digital physeal fractures can have complications including growth arrest, deformity, joint stiffness, pain, and loss of function.[13] In fractures of the distal phalanx the nail bed should be inspected for injury to rule out an open fracture.[11] Nondisplaced and closed reduced digital fractures can be treated with buddy splinting and a stiff-soled shoe. Operative treatment of intra-articular fractures is recommended if there is >2 mm displacement.[12]

Petnehazy and colleagues[14] compared outcomes of surgical and conservative treatment of 317 pediatric digital intra-articular fractures. Conservative treatment was used in 86% of the cohort and consisted of immobilization with a cast, buddy taping or rest alone. Operative treatment was used for 14% of the cohort and involved K-wire fixation, screw fixation, or fragment removal. In the operative group, 73% of patients had a complete resolution of symptoms compared with 65% in the conservative group; however, no statistical analysis was performed.

Special attention should be given to hallux SH III and IV fractures with lateral epiphyseal fracture fragments (**Fig. 1**). Park and colleagues[12] presented 41 children with indirect trauma to the hallux and stratified the injuries by mechanism, proposing a treatment algorithm based on injury grade. Their results suggest that lateral condyle fractures may be at higher risk of nonunion and poor functional outcomes, and surgical treatment should be considered in this subset even in those with < 2 mm displacement. Perugia and colleagues[15] followed four 13- to 15-year-old pediatric gymnasts who sustained SH type III–IV hallux fractures and were treated with open reduction and internal fixation (ORIF). All of the athletes sustained an intra-articular lateral base fracture of the hallux proximal phalanx with a hyperadduction-flexion mechanism. They underwent open reduction with K-wire fixation and had satisfactory radiological and clinical results with return to sport at 3 to 4 months and excellent AOFAS scores at the final 1-year follow-up.

Intra-articular and physeal hallux fractures may present in the subacute setting in high-level athletes who continue to train despite the pain. In these cases, excision of the fracture fragment versus ORIF must be considered. Bariteau and colleagues[16] reported excellent results in delayed ORIF of hallux intra-articular physeal fractures in two elite-level gymnasts. The gymnasts presented several months after the index injury and underwent ORIF with screw fixation. Both patients healed uneventfully and returned to full sport without limitation. At our institution we have also noted success with operative treatment of subacute displaced hallux SH III fractures in two adolescent athletes, both treated with open reduction and screw fixation. The first was a 13-year-old male track athlete who presented 5 months after his injury. The

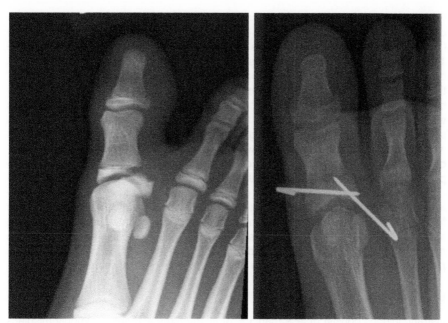

Fig. 1. Open reduction and pinning of a lateral SH III hallux fracture in a 12-year-old gymnast.

second was a 14-year-old female gymnast who had been treated conservatively at an outside facility for 4 months, with continued symptoms and inability to return to gymnastics. Both athletes had complete consolidation of the fracture postoperatively despite their delayed presentation, and returned to full sport.

Complications of digital ORIF can include physeal arrest, malunion, nonunion, infection, neurovascular embarrassment, avascular necrosis (AVN), and continued pain. Kramer and colleagues[17] presented 10 pediatric patients with a high initial complication rate of 60% however most patients were asymptomatic at final follow-up. Long-term functional and radiographic studies are needed to further compare conservative and surgical care for intra-articular and physeal digital fractures, especially in regard to lateral base fractures of the hallux.

METATARSAL FRACTURES

Metatarsal fractures are common in children, comprising 60% of all pediatric foot fractures.[18] In children greater than 5 years of age metatarsal fractures are primarily from sports-related injuries, and occur most commonly in the fifth metatarsal.[19] With increasing age, the incidence of sports-related metatarsal trauma increases. The fifth metatarsal is most commonly fractured in isolation whereas the central metatarsals 2 to 4 will typically have a concomitant fracture of the adjacent metatarsal.[19]

Metatarsal fractures can most commonly be treated conservatively with weight bearing in a cast or a stiff-soled shoe, with only a small proportion of pediatric patients requiring surgical intervention. In cases of sagittal plane displacement, or translation of greater than 75°, closed or percutaneous needle-assisted reduction or open reduction with pinning versus internal fixation should be considered.[18,20,21] Management of pediatric fifth metatarsal fractures is similar to the adult population. Herrera-Soto et al evaluated 103 pediatric patients who sustained a fifth metatarsal fracture, and patients with diaphyseal, neck, and extra-articular avulsion fractures of the base did well with conservative treatment. However, for conservatively treated metaphyseal diaphyseal (Jones) fractures, longer healing times (8–17 weeks with conservative treatment vs 5–11 weeks with screw fixation) and three refractures were noted in 15 athletic patients over 13 years of age.[22] Variation in conservative protocol was present, with eight patients receiving a short-leg walking cast and five patients receiving a non-weight-bearing cast. Mahan and colleagues[23] noted that 6 out of 32 (18.8%) pediatric patients with fractures between 20 and 40 mm from the proximal fifth metatarsal tip went on to surgery secondary to delayed healing. Conservative protocol varied in this study as well, which may limit the results. However, acute fixation of Jones fractures should be discussed as an option in pediatric athletes over the age of 13 to allow for more predictable healing and an earlier return to sport.[22,24]

Of note, the secondary ossification center of the fifth metatarsal is radiographically apparent in females 9 to 11 years of age and males 10 to 14 and can often be mistaken for a fracture.[25] The radiolucency of the apophysis will be oriented parallel to the long axis of the metatarsal, contrary to a fracture that is typically transverse. However, fifth metatarsal apophysitis can be caused by repetitive microtrauma from the pull of the peroneus brevis tendon.[26] These injuries are well managed conservatively.[27,28]

LISFRANC FRACTURES

Lisfranc injuries consist of less than 1% of all fractures and are commonly misdiagnosed in the event of subtle deformity (**Fig. 2**).[29] Sports-related injuries account for

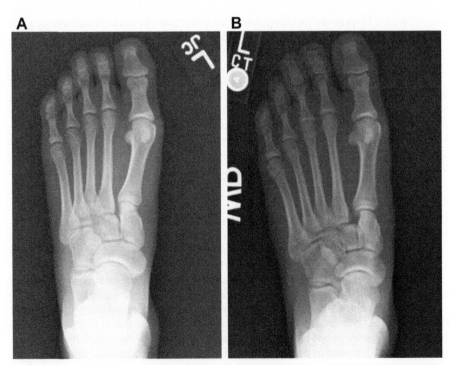

Fig. 2. Primarily ligamentous lisfranc injury in a 14-year-old gymnast initially missed by urgent care with non-weight-bearing films (A), with a clear diastasis present on weight bearing films (B).

51% of lisfranc fractures and 82% of lisfranc sprains in the pediatric population.[26] Patients with an open growth plate most commonly have an injury with tarsometatarsal joint partial incongruity and medial dislocation.[30,31] In children under the age of 6, the distance between the first and second metatarsal bases should be < 3 mm and the distance between the medial cuneiform and second metatarsal base can range between 3.1 and 7.5 mm. After the age of 6, the norms are consistent with adult values at < 2 mm for both the distance between the 1st and 2nd metatarsal bases and the distance between the medial cuneiform and second metatarsal base.[32] With diastasis and clinical correlation, a lisfranc injury should be suspected.

There is a lack of consensus on the management of lisfranc injuries in the pediatric population. In adults, displacement greater than 2 mm or lisfranc joint instability necessitates operative treatment with anatomic reduction being the most important goal.[33] In an early study by Wiley and colleagues,[34] 18 pediatric patients underwent either casting or closed reduction, with 4 out of the 7 in the closed reduction group undergoing percutaneous pinning with K-wires. Four out of 18 were noted to be mildly symptomatic after 1 year of follow-up; one was untreated due to misdiagnosis, and one had a nonanatomic reduction. The other two were not classified on initial injury severity or treatment group. On the contrary, Veijola and colleagues[35] followed seven pediatric patients who underwent Lisfranc ORIF using k-wires and screws. Six of these patients had continued postoperative discomfort to the lisfranc joint at 26-month follow-up despite the anatomic reduction. Denning and colleagues[36] compared nonoperative and operative treatment of pediatric lisfranc injuries in 41 patients who were all noted to have good to excellent long-term functional results. The nonoperative group did have higher functional scores however the authors attributed this result to selection bias. As with adult lisfranc ORIF, the most common complication with pediatric lisfranc ORIF is posttraumatic arthritis. In the adult population, 60% of patients may develop posttraumatic arthritis at 10-year follow-up even with adequate anatomic reduction.[37] Lesko and colleagues[38] followed a 10-year-old female for 5 years after undergoing a lisfranc ORIF. She had continued functional pain and required a partial fusion despite the initial adequate anatomic reduction.

Lisfranc injuries range in severity from primarily ligamentous injuries to complete displacement with comminution at the tarsometatarsal joint, and the literature has shown mixed functional outcomes in the pediatric population. With increasing severity of the injury requiring ORIF, patients may encounter continued postoperative pain which may in turn lead to eventual need for arthrodesis. Surgeon discretion should be used when deciding operative versus nonoperative care for a pediatric lisfranc injury, taking into account the injury severity and age of the child. Conservative treatment should be considered for patients under 12 years of age with uncomplicated and minimally displaced injuries.[39] The patient's family needs to be counseled at length about the severity of this injury and potential need for future surgeries.

CUBOID FRACTURES

Cuboid fractures are uncommon in the adult population with a frequency of 1.8 per 100,000 pedal fractures and are even more rare in the pediatric population.[40] These injuries are sustained through direct impact or from compression between the fourth and fifth metatarsal bases and the anterior process of the calcaneus during forced abduction in a fixed plantarflexed position ("nutcracker" fracture).[41,42] In the pediatric population this type of injury is prevalent in equestrian-related sports and can often be found in conjunction with other fractures.[42] If left untreated, patients can have detrimental long-term biomechanical outcomes because of a shortened lateral column, forefoot abduction and progressive posterior tibial tendon dysfunction and a compensatory calcaneal valgus.[43]

Cuboid fractures are commonly missed on radiographs given the bone's asymmetric shape and radiographic overlap, and are overlooked in 40%-90% of pediatric cases.[44–46] Fracture patterns are primarily linear with more than half of these injuries extending into the tarsometatarsal joint.[45] In cases where pediatric patients may have lateral column pain suspicious of an occult fracture with no obvious radiographic abnormality, advanced imaging should be considered.[42] Delayed diagnosis and treatment of cuboid injuries can double the time needed for complete healing.[47]

Conservative management should be used for minimally displaced pediatric cuboid fractures. Senaran and colleagues[47] evaluated 21 pediatric patients who were immobilized immediately following their initial presentation in either a short-leg walking cast or walking boot. All of the fractures healed completely with no complications, and the patients were asymptomatic at an average of 4.9 weeks.

Surgical intervention is indicated in the setting of severe displacement or comminution, when the lateral column is shortened or the articular surface is compromised. As with the adult population, the goals of surgical intervention are to restore articular congruency and restore the length of the lateral column thereby minimizing long-term complications. Due to increased subchondral bone strength in pediatric patients, the articular surfaces may be better preserved during injury. Therefore loss of length from trauma is often seen in the extra-articular region of the cuboid. As a result, once the bone is out to length, little to no fixation is needed in these fracture patterns.[42] In a series of horseback injuries, Ceroni followed four pediatric athletes who sustained a nutcracker cuboid fracture. The patients were treated with either an allograft bone block using no fixation or with conservative treatment.[42] Both patients who underwent surgical intervention to restore the anatomic length of the cuboid had excellent outcomes, compared with the two treated conservatively with residual lateral column shortening who were unable to return to their pre-injury level. Even in the event of intra-articular involvement, minimal fixation is needed for a successful outcome. Hsu and colleagues[48] and Holbein and colleagues[49] describe two pediatric patients with significant cuboid intra-articular impaction requiring iliac crest grafting, using k-wire fixation. At the final 2-year follow-up, both of the patients achieved an AOFAS score of 100.

Well-treated pediatric cuboid fractures can have excellent AOFAS scores ranging from 95 to 100, with lower satisfaction associated with a more severe injury pattern such as a bi-columnar fracture.[48–50] It is recommended that pediatric cuboid fractures be surgically treated if there is lateral column shortening greater than 2 to 3 mm or if there is intra-articular step off.[50]

TALUS FRACTURES

Pediatric talar fractures are uncommon given the bone's high elastic resilience. These fractures comprise 2% of all pediatric foot fractures and less than 0.08% of all pediatric fractures.[51–53] The incidence of AVN in nondisplaced talar fractures is higher in the pediatric population, as the fracture diagnosis can be more easily missed on initial presentation, leading to a delay in treatment.[54] Therefore, special attention should be given to pediatric talar injuries with the utilization of advanced imaging if there is a concern for occult injury.

Nondisplaced or minimally displaced fractures can be treated conservatively with a non-weight-bearing cast.[55] Jenson and colleagues[55] showed that with conservative treatment of nondisplaced pediatric talar fractures, approximately 91% were asymptomatic with up to 34 years of follow-up. Rammelt and colleagues[56] reported a 16% incidence of AVN in nondisplaced, conservatively treated fractures. It is important to note that the pediatric talar subchondral dome is primarily cartilaginous and a Hawkins sign will not necessarily be apparent on radiographs. If there is a concern for AVN, an MRI should be obtained.

Operative treatment is indicated in those with open fractures, residual articular displacement greater than 2 mm, or angulation. There is a correlation between age and increased displacement, with complex fracture patterns more common in children over the age of 12 as their bone morphology more similarly mirrors the adult talus.[57,58] At the age of 12, the morphology of the talus is 96% that of an adult talus in females and 88% that of an adult talus in males.[59] As a result, it is recommended that pediatric talar injuries in patients greater than the age of 10 be approached in a similar manner to the adult talus. If the talus is large enough, screws should be used; otherwise, K-wires may be used.[60] To minimize the risk of AVN, Zhang and colleagues[61] described a percutaneous technique for the treatment of pediatric neck fractures and compared outcomes with a traditional ORIF approach. They found no significant differences in rates of AVN; however, the percutaneous group had significantly higher AOFAS scores, faster union rates, and lower nonunion rates. In cases where ORIF is necessary to achieve acceptable reduction, limited and meticulous dissection should be performed to minimize the risk of AVN.

CALCANEUS FRACTURES

Pediatric calcaneal fractures are extremely rare with an incidence of 0.0001% to 0.0004% of all pediatric fractures.[62,63] These fractures are more commonly extra-articular compared with adult calcaneal fractures.[64] The posterior facet of the pediatric talus is more parallel to the ground and the lateral talar process is smaller, resulting in less impaction on the calcaneus within the subtalar joint.[60]

Nonoperative treatment of intra- and extra-articular fractures has successful clinical outcomes in the pediatric population. Mora and colleagues[65] evaluated 8 pediatric patients with calcaneal fracture displacement between 1 to 2 mm who were treated conservatively and followed for a total of 4.4 years. At final follow-up, 88% of their patients had no pain and had unrestricted foot function, with the ability to participate in competitive impact sports. Brunet and colleagues[66] had similar findings, following 19 calcaneal fractures (14 intra-articular, six with 1–2 mm of displacement, two with 3–4 mm of displacement, and six with >5 mm of displacement) treated in a brace or cast. Average AOFAS score was 96.2 with a mean final follow-up of 16.8 years. In addition, Ceccarelli and colleagues[67] followed 40 pediatric patients with calcaneal fractures with a mean follow-up of 22.8 years. They found that patients had good to excellent postoperative outcomes with no significant differences between operative and conservative care for patients under the age of 15. They also noted that patients 15 years of age and above did significantly worse with nonoperative treatment; however, the amount of initial fracture displacement was not specified. Conservative treatment of both intra- and extra-articular calcaneal fractures may be well tolerated in children under the age of 15 because of the immature talus and calcaneus having a superior capacity to remodel.[65–67]

Although conservative treatment of most calcaneal fractures in children under 15 has historically been indicated, there has been an increasing incidence of operative treatment with comparable results. Dudda and colleagues[68] evaluated 14 pediatric patients with an average age of 11.5 years old with joint depression fractures treated with ORIF with either screw or K-wire fixation, and noted an average improvement of

Bohler's angle of 14°. All patients were free of pain with normal range of motion in the subtalar joint and with no impairment of gait at 44-month follow-up. Petit and colleagues[69] and Pickle and colleagues[70] evaluated operative treatment of 14 and 7 pediatric displaced intra-articular fractures, respectively. In Pickle's cohort, all seven patients were able to return to full activities at 10 months. Five patients were noted to have decreased subtalar range of motion; however, all patients were able to compensate with no restrictions in activity, shoe gear, or notable complications at 30-month follow-up. In Petit's cohort of 14 patients, the average hindfoot AOFAS score at 67-month follow-up was 64 out of 68. Petit used lateral buttress plating that showed improved outcomes compared with screw fixation. There is no clear consensus regarding ideal fixation however with children under the age of 7, permanent hardware should be avoided given continued growth at the primary calcaneal ossification center.

Calcaneal apophyseal fractures are uncommon and can be a result of neglected calcaneal apophysitis or a primary avulsion fracture. When avulsion injuries occur, the proximal half of the apophysis will typically be involved due to the insertion of the Achilles tendon.[71] Treatment algorithms are not well defined; however, there have been multiple reported case series showing successful outcomes with surgical intervention. Wailing and colleagues and Lee and colleagues both reported case series of 4 patients who sustained an isolated calcaneal apophyseal injury as a result of neglected calcaneal apophysitis.[72,73] Their patients were treated with either fragment removal with suture repair of the Achilles tendon or definitive ORIF. All patients were able to return to sports without any restriction in activity. In addition, Imai and colleagues[74] presented a 9-year-old gymnast who was treated with two absorbable pins and bioabsorbable suture in a tension-band fashion. At a total of 2.5 years follow-up, she was asymptomatic and participating in gymnastics without restrictions or pain. Strong recommendations cannot be made regarding surgical intervention for calcaneal avulsion fractures however based on the limited case series, patients have been shown to have successful surgical outcomes.

ANKLE FRACTURES

Pediatric ankle fractures account for 5% of all pediatric fractures and 15% of all physeal injuries.[75] Normal physeal closure is typically completed around 14 years of age in girls and 16 years of age in boys. Closure occurs over a period of 18 months, starting from posterior medial, and then progressing centrally and anterolaterally, leading to characteristic fracture patterns during this period.[76] Physicians must be acutely aware of the risk of early physeal arrest, angular deformity, and joint incongruity when treating pediatric ankle fractures.

Classification

Salter–Harris I (SH I) injuries, or separation of the physeal plate, most often present with localized pain overlying the physis and are often radiographically occult. Approximately 15% of distal tibial physeal fractures are SH I injuries.[75] The prevalence and treatment of distal fibula SH I injuries is debated. Although there is often high clinical suspicion, MRI studies show that ligamentous injuries and osseous contusions are much more prevalent, and only 0% to 3% of suspected distal fibular physeal injuries actually involve the physis.[77–79]

Salter–Harris II (SH II) injuries account for approximately 40% of all distal tibial physeal injuries.[75] These fractures show a characteristic metaphyseal spike known as a Thurston Holland sign (**Fig. 3**). When these injuries occur, the periosteum tends to

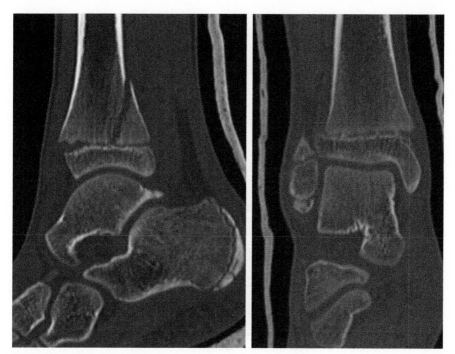

Fig. 3. Distal tibial SH II fracture in a 12-year-old soccer player.

remain attached on the metaphyseal side, but may be torn and become incarcerated on the epiphyseal side.

Salter–Harris III (SH III) fractures extend through the physis and out the epiphysis, and comprise 25% of distal tibial physeal injuries (**Fig. 4**).[75] A common subtype of SH III fractures is a juvenile Tillaux fracture, resulting from the avulsion of the anterolateral epiphysis as the anterior inferior tibiofibular ligament is stronger than the physis. These are seen during the transitional period of physeal closure generally around age 12 to 14, when the anterolateral physis is the only portion remaining open. Juvenile Tillaux fractures comprise approximately 3% to 5% of distal tibial physeal injuries.[75]

Salter–Harris IV (SH IV) fractures extend through the physis and out both the metaphysis and the epiphysis. These account for up to 25% of distal tibial physeal injuries.[75] The triplane fracture subtype occurs when the metaphyseal and epiphyseal fractures occur in different planes (**Fig. 5**). These fractures can occur medially or laterally at the physis, and can be two-part, three-part, or four-part fractures. Computed tomography (CT) imaging is often helpful to understand the more complex fracture patterns and to plan appropriate fixation. Kay and colleagues[75] wrote an excellent in-depth description of triplane subtypes. Triplane fractures comprise 5% to 7% of pediatric ankle fractures.

Salter–Harris V (SH V) injuries occur as a result of compression of the physis and are rare in the distal tibia, comprising only 1% of ankle physeal injuries.[75] These are difficult to diagnose accurately at the time of injury as they are often radiographically occult.

Management

Multiple factors must be considered in the management of pediatric ankle fractures. Initial care must focus on the reduction of gross deformity and soft tissue

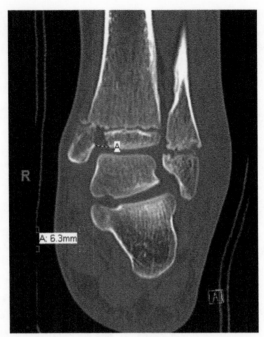

Fig. 4. SH III fracture in a 13-year-old figure skater.

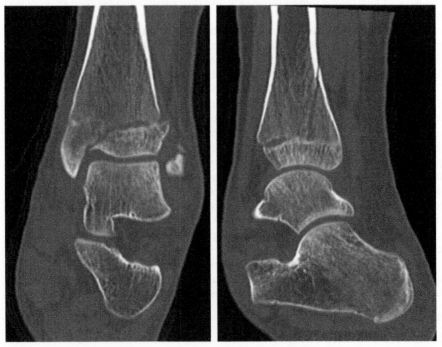

Fig. 5. Triplane ankle fracture in a 13-year-old volleyball player.

management, with immediate evaluation of neurovascular status. Attention must then be directed to more subtle displacement at the physeal plate or articular surface. Current consensus accepts 2 mm of residual displacement at the physis and 2 mm of displacement at the tibial plafond.[75] However, anatomic reduction should be considered the ultimate goal to reduce risk of premature physeal closure and joint arthrosis.[80–82]

An effort should be made to minimize radiation in the young patient. However, given the potential for long-term deleterious effects of a mistreated pediatric ankle fracture, there should be a low threshold to obtain a CT scan if there is any question regarding the amount of physeal or articular displacement, or the nature of the fracture pattern. In a blinded study, Nenopoulos and colleagues[82] found that operative treatment was recommended for 18 out of 64 pediatric ankle fractures with plain films, and 42 out of the same 64 patients with a CT scan. Similarly, in a study of 25 pediatric ankle fractures Eismann and colleagues[83] found that obtaining a CT scan resulted in radiologic and orthopedic raters to change the fracture pattern in 46% of cases, displacement from less than 2 mm to greater than 2 mm in 39% of cases, treatment from nonoperative to operative in 27% of cases, and planned fixation in 41% of cases. A CT of the foot or ankle has an effective dose of 0.07 millisieverts, which is equivalent to the exposure from 0.9 plain chest radiographs.[84] Direct communication with radiology technicians to limit the field of view and reduce the resolution to the minimum necessary can be helpful in limiting radiation in young children (**Fig. 6**).

An emphasis must be placed on the importance of quality closed reduction technique and well-molded casts, as this can often obviate the need for surgical intervention in many pediatric ankle fractures. If the first closed reduction attempt is unsuccessful, consideration for open intervention is warranted as periosteum may be blocking the reduction. Multiple closed reduction attempts should be avoided to prevent further physeal trauma. Surgical fixation is often achieved with 3.5 or

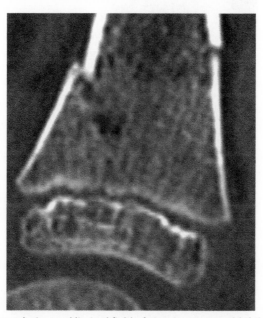

Fig. 6. CT with low resolution and limited field of view in a 6-year-old child to limit radiation

4.0 mm cortical or cannulated screws above and/or below the physis (**Fig. 7**). If fixation is needed across the physis, smooth *k*-wires should be used (**Fig. 8**).

Arthroscopic-assisted ORIF should be considered in displaced SH III and IV fractures to minimize soft tissue disruption and postoperative stiffness. This also allows for direct visualization and debridement of incarcerated periosteum, and visualization of anatomic reduction during screw placement. Advances in arthroscopy allow for 2.0 mm cameras and shavers to be used, which can be found useful in the small pediatric ankle (**Fig. 9**).

With both conservative and surgically treated fractures, immobilization is necessary for 4 to 6 weeks and must be dependent on the stability of the fracture pattern. Long-leg casting is traditionally used for SH II-IV fractures; however, the more stable fracture patterns such as standard SH II fractures may be amenable to a short-leg cast.[85] In addition, short-leg immobilization can be considered in fractures that have been stabilized surgically. Early postoperative non-weight-bearing range of motion may be considered for a compliant high-level athlete to help avoid deconditioning and cast disease. This should only be considered if there is absolute confidence in the stability of the surgical fixation and the compliance of the patient; otherwise, the benefits of early range of motion are not worth the long-term risks.

Complications

Complications from pediatric ankle fractures include early physeal arrest, limb length discrepancy, angular deformity, osteoarthritis, stiffness, and pain. Overall there is a 12% risk of osteoarthritis (mainly SH III and IV) and a 13% risk of premature physeal closure.[86,87] However, the initial severity of the injury including Salter–Harris type, amount of displacement and comminution, and quality of the reduction, influence

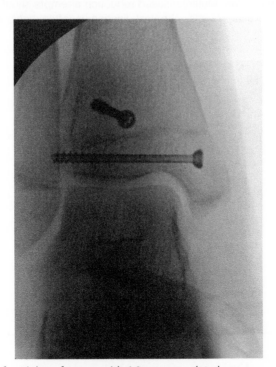

Fig. 7. Fixation of a triplane fracture with 4.0 mm cannulated screws.

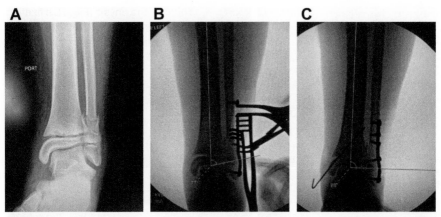

Fig. 8. Ankle fracture in an 11-year-old male involved in a high speed ATV accident (*A*). Despite bringing the fibula out to length, the ankle remained in valgus (*B*). After removal of the incarcerated periosteum on the medial aspect of the tibial physis, the ankle joint reduced to neutral (*C*). Note use of a smooth *k*-wire across the physis and spanning of the fibular physis, both later removed to allow for continued physeal growth.

outcomes significantly.[86,88] Children with physeal injuries should have serial radiographs every 6 to 12 months until there is clear evidence of symmetric growth, as evidenced by parallel Harris lines, or until physeal closure (**Fig. 10**).[88]

PSYCHOSOCIAL CONSIDERATIONS

The psychosocial aspect of pediatric sports trauma can often be overlooked when the attention is primarily directed toward treating the physical injury. It is important to remember that sports may be a large part of the child's identity and social network. Participation in sports can lead to improved self-esteem, improved social interactions, and fewer depressive symptoms.[4] An abrupt disruption in participation from an injury

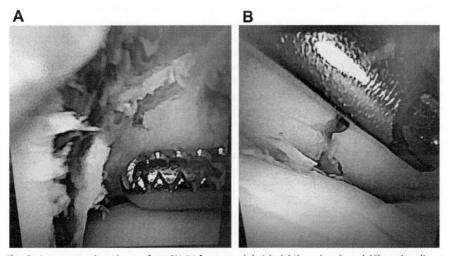

Fig. 9. Intraoperative views of an SH IV fracture debrided (*A*) and reduced (*B*) under direct visualization with use of a 2.0 mm scope and 2.0 mm shaver.

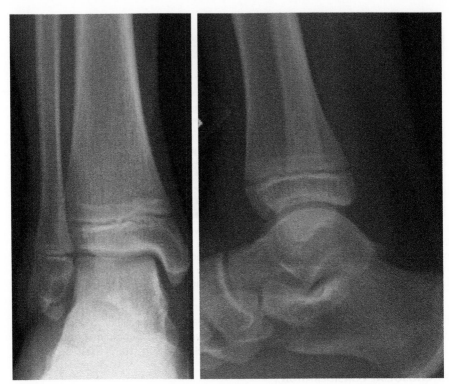

Fig. 10. Parallel Harris lines, indicating resumption of symmetric growth following an SH II fracture treated with closed reduction and short-leg casting.

can lead to a sense of identity loss, trigger or exacerbate mental health conditions, or give rise to an eating disorder.[89,90]

In youth athletes, parental pressure and emphasis by coaches on winning are related to lower confidence and may lead to maladaptive perfectionist tendencies, whereas supportive parents and mastery-oriented coach environments are related to an adaptive, healthy strive for achievement.[91] A mastery-oriented environment can be fostered in post-injury rehabilitation by providing the patient and coach with cross-training activities and exercises that are safe at each stage of rehabilitation. When possible, literature-based return-to-sport guidelines should be used, as shown in the Sweeney and colleagues[92] guide for returning to sport after gymnastics injuries. Parents should be encouraged to be supportive of their child's emotional state first, and athletic career second. There should be a low threshold to involve the child's pediatrician or a mental health professional if there is any concern regarding the patient's psychological well-being or adaptation to the injury.

DISCUSSION

Pediatric trauma must be treated meticulously with a thorough understanding of bone remodeling, physeal complications, and growth patterns. Families must be counseled at length regarding the risk of future surgery and growth disturbance when applicable, and every effort must be made to continue following the patient until normal growth has resumed.

The subset of competitive athletes must be treated with an understanding of, and protection from, external pressures in their rehabilitation. Proper patient and family education, along with clear timetables and goals, is fundamental in the treatment of the young athlete. It can be helpful to provide patients and coaches with suggestions of activities that are safe during each recovery phase. Early range of motion can be considered in amenable fracture patterns and injuries; however, long-term outcomes should always take precedent. A close relationship with a pediatric sports physical therapist is also instrumental when treating high-level athletes, and can help ensure continued compliance as the athlete graduates from the physician's care.

Further research is needed to fully evaluate the short- and long-term outcomes of conservatively and surgically treated pediatric foot and ankle fractures. The exceptional ability of the pediatric bone to remodel allows for conservative care in many fracture patterns. However, an acute understanding of biomechanical, physeal, and articular risks must be used when considering treatment choices. Above all, the safety of the child and the prevention of long-term complications should be of utmost importance when caring for pediatric fractures and sports injuries.

DISCLOSURE

The authors have nothing to disclose.

REFERENCES

1. DiFiori JP, Benjamin HJ, Brenner J, et al. Overuse injuries and Burnout in youth sports: a position Statement from the American medical Society for sports medicine. Clin J Sport Med 2014;24:3–20.
2. Comstock RD, Pierpoint LA. Summary report: National high-school sports-related injury Surveillance study, 2018-2019 school year. Cent Inj Res Policy 2019.
3. Martinsen M, Sundgot-Borgen J. Adolescent elite athletes' cigarette smoking, use of snus, and alcohol. Scand J Med Sci Sports 2012;24(2):439–46.
4. Eime R, Young J, Harvey J, et al. A systematic review of the psychological and social benefits of participation in sport for children and adolescents: informing development of a conceptual model of health through sport. Int J Behav Nutr Phys Activity 2013;10(98):1–21.
5. Jonker L, Elferink-Gemser M, Visscher C. The role of self-regulatory skills in sports and academic performances of elite youth athletes. Talent Development Excell 2011;3(2):263–75.
6. Rechel J, Yard E, Comstock R. An epidemiologic comparison of high-school sports injuries sustained in practice and competition. J Athletic Train 2008; 43(2):197–204.
7. Valasek AE, Young JA, Huang L, et al. Age and sex differences in overuse injuries presenting to pediatric sports medicine clinics. Clin Pediatr 2019;58(7):770–7.
8. Kerr Z, Lynall R, Roos K, et al. Descriptive epidemiology of non-time-loss injuries in collegiate and high-school student-athletes. J Athletic Train 2017;52(5):446–56.
9. Watkins J, Peabody P. Sports injuries in children and adolescents treated at a sports injury clinic. J Sports Med Phys Fitness 1996;36:43–8.
10. Classifications in brief: Salter-Harris classification of pediatric physeal fractures. Cepela D, Tartagilone JP, Dooley TP, Patel PN. Clin Orthop Rel Res 2016;474: 2351–537.
11. Kay RM, Tang CW. Pediatric foot fractures: evaluation and treatment. J Am Acad Orthop Surg 2001;9:308–19.

12. Park DY, Han KJ, Han SH, et al. Barefoot sports injury on hallux: a new classification by injury mechanism. J Orthop Trauma 2013;27(11):651–5.
13. Salter R, Harris WR. Injuries involving the epiphyseal plate. J Bone Joint Surg 1963;45A:587–622.
14. Petnehazy T, Schalamon J, Hartwig C, et al. Fractures of the hallux in children. Foot Ankle Int 2015;36(1):60–3.
15. Perugia D, Fabbri M, Guidi M, et al. Salter-Harris type III and IV displaced fracture of the hallux in young gymnasts: a series of four cases at 1-year follow-up. Injury 2014;45(Suppl 6):S39–42.
16. Bariteau JT, Murillo DM, Tenenbaum SA, et al. Joint salvage after neglected intra-articular physeal fracture of the hallux in high-level gymnasts. Foot Ankle Spec 2015;8(2):130–4.
17. Kramer DE, Mahan ST, Hresko MT. Displaced intra-articular fractures of the great toe in children: intervene with caution. J Pediatr Orthop 2014;34(2):144–9.
18. Rammelt S, Heineck J, Zwipp H. Metatarsal fractures. Injury 2004;35(Suppl 2): SB77–86.
19. Singer G, Cichocki M, Schalamon J, et al. A study of metatarsal fractures in children. J Bone Joint Surg Am 2008;90(4):772–6.
20. Robertson NB, Roocroft JH, Edmonds EW. Childhood metatarsal shaft fractures: treatment outcomes and relative indications for surgical intervention. J Child Orthop 2012;6(2):125–9.
21. Mahan ST, Lierhaus AM, Spencer SA, et al. Treatment dilemma in multiple metatarsal fractures: when to operate? J Pediatr Orthop B 2016;25:354–60.
22. Herrera-Soto JA, Scherb M, Duffy MF, et al. Fractures of the fifth metatarsal in children and adolescents. J Pediatr Orthop 2007;27(4):427–31.
23. Mahan ST, Hoellwarth JS, Spencer SA, et al. Likelihood of surgery in isolated pediatric fifth metatarsal fractures. J Pediatr Orthop 2015;35(3):296–302.
24. Mologne TS, Lundeen JM, Clapper MF, et al. Early screw fixation versus casting in the treatment of acute Jones fractures. Am J Sports Med 2005;33(7):970–5.
25. Dameron TB Jr. Fractures and anatomical variations of the proximal portion of the fifth metatarsal. J Bone Joint Surg [Am] 1975;57:788–92.
26. Ralph Brian G. Barrett John, Kenyhercz Christopher, DiDominico Lawrence A. Iselin's disease: a case presentation of nonunion and review of the differential diagnosis. J Foot Ankle Surg 1999;38:409–16.
27. Kishan TV, Mekala A, Bonala N, et al. Iselin's disease: Traction apophysitis of the fifth metatarsal base, a rare cause of lateral foot pain. Med J Armed Forces India 2016;72(3):299–301. https://doi.org/10.1016/j.mjafi.2015.06.015.
28. Deniz G, Kose O, Guneri B, et al. Traction apophysitis of the fifth metatarsal base in a child: Iselin's disease. BMJ Case Rep 2014;2014. https://doi.org/10.1136/bcr-2014-204687. bcr2014204687.
29. Kalia V, Fishman EK, Carrino JA, et al. Epidemiology, imaging, and treatment of Lisfranc fracture-dislocations revisited. Skeletal Radiol 2012;41:129–36.
30. Hill JF, Heyworth BE, Lierhaus A, et al. Lisfranc injuries in children and adolescents. J Pediatr Orthop B 2017;26(2):159–63.
31. Myerson MS, Fisher RT, Burgess AR, et al. Fracture dislocations of the tarsometatarsal joints: End results correlated with pathology and treatment. Foot Ankle 1986;6(5):225–42.
32. Knijnenberg LM, Dingemans SA, Terra MP, et al. Radiographic anatomy of the pediatric lisfranc joint. J Pediatr Orthop 2018;38(10):510–3.
33. Myerson MS, Cerrato R. Current management of tarsometatarsal injuries in the athlete. Instr Course Lect 2009;58:583–94.

34. Wiley JJ. Tarso-metatarsal joint injuries in children. J Pediatr Orthop 1981;1(3): 255–60.
35. Veijola K, Laine HJ, Pajulo O. Lisfranc injury in adolescents. Eur J Pediatr Surg 2013;23(4):297–303.
36. Denning JR, Butler L, Eismann EA, et al. Functional outcomes and health-related quality of life following pediatric lisfranc tarsometatarsal injury treatment. Pediatric Orthopaedic Society of North America Annual Meeting, paper 159, Atlanta, GA, 2015 - 29 Apr - 02 May, 2015, Marriott Atlanta Marquis Hotel, GA, United States (26240)
37. Dubois-Ferrière V, Lübbeke A, Chowdhary A, et al. Clinical outcomes and development of symptomatic osteoarthritis 2 to 24 years after surgical treatment of tarsometatarsal joint complex injuries. J Bone Joint Surg Am 2016;98:713–20.
38. Lesko G, Altman K, Hogue G. Midfoot Degenerative arthritis and partial fusion after pediatric lisfranc fracture-dislocation. J Am Acad Orthop Surg Glob Res Rev 2018;2(3):e004.
39. Denning JR. Complications of pediatric foot and ankle fractures. Orthop Clin North Am 2017;48:59–70.
40. Court-Brown C, Zinna S, Ekrol I. Classification and epidemiology of midfoot fractures. Foot 2006;16:138–41.
41. Hermel MB, Gershon-Cohen J. The nutcracker fracture of the cuboid by indirect violence. Radiology 1953;60:850–4.
42. Ceroni D, De Rosa V, De Coulon G, et al. Cuboid nutcracker fracture due to horseback riding in children: case series and review of the literature. J Pediatr Orthop 2007;27(5):557–61.
43. Angoules AG, Angoules NA, Georgoudis M, et al. Update on diagnosis and management of cuboid fractures. World J Orthop 2019;10(2):71–80.
44. Joo SY, Jeong C. Stress fracture of tarsal cuboid bone in early childhood. Eur J Orthop Surg Traumatol 2015;25(3):595–9. https://doi.org/10.1007/s00590-014-1543-8. Epub 2014 Sep 24. PMID: 25249481.
45. O'Dell MC, Chauvin NA, Jaramillo D, et al. MR imaging features of cuboid fractures in children. Pediatr Radiol 2018;48:680–5.
46. Simonian PT, Vahey JW, Rosenbaum DM, et al. Fracture of the cuboid in children. A source of leg symptoms. J Bone Joint Surg Br 1995;77(1):104–6.
47. Senaran H, Mason D, De Pellegrin M. Cuboid fractures in preschool children. J Pediatr Orthop 2006;26(6):741–4.
48. Hsu JC, Chang JH, Wang SJ, et al. The nutcracker fracture of the cuboid in children: a case report. Foot Ankle Int 2004;25(6):423–5.
49. Holbein O, Bauer G, Kinzl L. Fracture of the cuboid in children: case report and review of the literature. J Pediatr Orthop 1998;18(4):466–8.
50. Ruffing T, Rückauer T, Bludau F, et al. Cuboid nutcracker fracture in children: management and results. Injury 2019;50(2):607–12.
51. McCarthy JJ, Drennan JC. Drennan's the child's foot and ankle. Philadelphia: Lippincott Williams & Wilkins; 2010.
52. Linhart WE, Hollwarth ME. Fractures of the child's foot [J]. Orthopade 1986;15(3): 242–50.
53. Rammelt S, Godoy-Santos AL, Schneiders W, et al. Foot and ankle fractures during childhood: review of the literature and scientific evidence for appropriate treatment. Rev Bras Ortop 2016;51(6):630–9.
54. Rammelt S, Zwipp H, Gavlik JM. Avascular necrosis after minimally displaced talus fracture in a child. Foot Ankle Int 2000;21(12):1030–6.

55. Jensen I, JU Wester, Rasmussen F, et al. Prognosis of fracture of the talus in children. 21 (7-34)-year follow-up of 14 cases. Acta Orthop Scand 1994;65(4): 398–400.

56. Ogden J. The foot. In: Ogden J, editor. Skeletal injury in the child. New York, NY: Springer Verlag; 2000. p. 626–7.

57. Eberl R, Singer G, Schalamon J, et al. Fractures of the talus–differences between children and adolescents. J Trauma 2010;68(1):126–30.

58. Kruppa C, Snoap T, Sietsema DL, et al. Is the Midterm progress of pediatric and adolescent talus fractures stratified by age? J Foot Ankle Surg 2018;57(3):471–7.

59. Devalentine SJ. Epiphyseal injuries of the foot and ankle. Clin Podiatr Med Surg 1987;4:279–310.

60. Polyzois VD, Vasiliadis E, Zgonis T, et al. Pediatric fractures of the foot and ankle. Clin Podiatr Med Surg 2006;23(2):241–55.

61. Zhang X, Shao X, Yu Y, et al. Comparison between percutaneous and open reduction for treating paediatric talar neck fractures. Int Orthop 2017;41(12): 2581–9.

62. Wiley JJ, Profitt A. Fractures of the os calcis in children. Clin Orthop Relat Res 1984;(188):131–8.

63. Landin LA. Fracture patterns in children. Analysis of 8,682 fractures with special reference to incidence, etiology and secular changes in a Swedish urban population 1950-1979. Acta Orthop Scand Suppl 1983;202:1–109.

64. Schmidt TL, Weiner DS. Calcaneal fractures in children. An evaluation of the nature of the injury in 56 children. Clin Orthop Relat Res 1982;(171):150–5.

65. Mora S, Thordarson DB, Zionts LE, et al. Pediatric calcaneal fractures. Foot Ankle Int 2001;22(6):471–7.

66. Brunet JA. Calcaneal fractures in children. Long-term results of treatment. J Bone Joint Surg Br 2000;82(2):211–6.

67. Ceccarelli F, Faldini C, Piras F, et al. Surgical versus non-surgical treatment of calcaneal fractures in children: a long-term results comparative study. Foot Ankle Int 2000;21(10):825–32.

68. Dudda M, Kruppa C, Gebmann J, et al. Pediatric and adolescent intra-articular fractures of the calcaneus. Orthop Rev (Pavia) 2013;5(2):82–5.

69. Pickle A, Benaroch TE, Guy P, et al. Clinical outcome of pediatric calcaneal fractures treated with open reduction and internal fixation. J Pediatr Orthop 2004; 24(2):178–80.

70. Petit CJ, Lee BM, Kasser JR, et al. Operative treatment of intraarticular calcaneal fractures in the pediatric population. J Pediatr Orthop 2007;27(8):856–62.

71. Liberson A, Lieberson S, Mendes DG, et al. Remodeling of the calcaneus apophysis in the growing child. J Pediatr Orthop B 1995;4:74–9.

72. Lee KT, Young KW, Park YU, et al. Neglected Sever's disease as a cause of calcaneal apophyseal avulsion fracture: case report. Foot Ankle Int 2010;31(8):725–8.

73. Walling AK, Grogan DP, Carty CT, et al. Fractures of the calcaneal apophysis. J Orthop Trauma 1990;4(3):349–55.

74. Imai Y, Kitano T, Nakagawa K, et al. Calcaneal apophyseal avulsion fracture. Arch Orthop Trauma Surg 2007;127(5):331–3.

75. Kay RM, Matthys GA. Pediatric ankle fractures: evaluation and treatment. J Am Acad Orthop Surg 2001;9(4):268–78.

76. Dodwell ER, Kelley SP. Physeal fractures: basic science, assessment, and acute management. Orthopaedics and Trauma 2011;25(5):377–91.

77. Hofsli M, Torfing T, Al-Aubaidi Z. The proportion of distal fibula Salter-Harris type I epiphyseal fracture in the paediatric population with acute ankle injury: a prospective MRI study. J Pediatr Orthop 2016;25(2):126–32.
78. Boutis K, Plint A, Stimec J, et al. Radiograph-negative lateral ankle injuries in children: occult growth plate fracture or sprain? JAMA Pediatr 2016;170(1):e154114.
79. Boutis K, Narayanan U, Dong F, et al. Magnetic resonance imaging of clinically suspected Salter-Harris I fracture of the distal fibula 2010;41(8):852–6.
80. Leary J, Handling M, Talerico M, et al. Physeal fractures of the distal tibia. J Pediatr Orthop 2009;29:356–61.
81. Shurz M, Binder H, Platzer P, et al. Physeal injuries of the distal tibia: long-term results in 376 patients. Int Orthop 2010;34:547–52.
82. Nenopoulos A, Beslikas T, Gigis I, et al. The role of CT in diagnosis and treatment of distal tibial fracture with intra-articular involvement in children. Injury 2015; 46(11):2177–80.
83. Eismann E, Stephan Z, Mehlman C, et al. Pediatric triplane ankle fractures: impact of radiographs and computed tomography on fracture classification and treatment planning. JBJS 2015;97:995–1002.
84. Biswas D, Bible J, Bohan M, et al. Radiation exposure from musculoskeletal computerized tomographic scans. JBJS 2009;91:1882–9.
85. Dasari S, Kukushliev V, Graf A, et al. A retrospective comparison of above- vs below-the-knee cast treatment for Salter Harris-II distal tibia fractures. Foot Ankle Orthop 2022;7(1):1–8.
86. Caterini R, Farsetti P, Ippolito E. Long-term followup of physeal injury to the ankle. Foot and Ankle 1991;11(6):372–83.
87. Asad W, Younis M, Ahmed A, et al. Open versus closed treatment of distal tibia physeal fractures: a systematic review and meta-analysis. Eur J Orthop Surg Traumatol 2018;28(3):503–9.
88. Olgun Z, Maestre S. Management of pediatric ankle fractures. Curr Rev Musculoskelet Med 2018;11:475–84.
89. Sundgot-Borgen Jorunn. Risk and trigger factors for the development of eating disorders in female athletes. Med Sci Sports Exerc 1994;26(4):414–9.
90. Palisch A, Merritt L. Depressive symptoms in the young athlete after injury: recommendations for research. J Pediatr Health Care 2018;32(3):245–9.
91. Ommundsen Y, Roberts G, Lemyre P, et al. Parental and coach support or pressure on psychosocial outcomes of pediatric athletes. Clin J Sports Med 2006; 16(6):522–6.
92. Sweeney E, Howell D, James D, et al. Returning to sport after gymnastics injuries. Curr Sports Med Rep 2018;17(11):376–90.

Achilles Tendon Rupture Repair: Simple to Complex

Christy M. King, DPM, FACFAS, ABPM[a,b,]*,
Mher Vartivarian, DPM, FACFAS, ABPM[c,d,e,f]

KEYWORDS

- Acute Achilles rupture • Neglected Achilles rupture • Chronic Achilles rupture
- Ultrasound • Gap distance • Early functional rehabilitation • Allograft
- FHL tendon transfer

KEY POINTS

- Operative and nonoperative management of Achilles tendon ruptures, both using the early mobilization protocol, have a good prognosis with low associated risks.
- Primary repair of Achilles tendon rupture can be successfully achieved with small open incision or percutaneous approach.
- In an evaluation for chronic Achilles tendon rupture, an MRI can help to identify the location of the rupture and gap distance to help guide the surgical procedure selection.

INTRODUCTION

Similar to the popularity of its heroic namesake, the Achilles tendon and treatment of the unfortunate rupture is a frequently discussed and debated topic. The Achilles tendon is the strongest tendon in the body and the most commonly ruptured.[1] The incidence of Achilles tendon rupture is 5 to 37 per 100,000.[1–3] Usually, this common injury occurs in an active middle-age population with approximately 80% of the injuries occurring during physical activity.[1,2] In some cases, there can be a delayed presentation or diagnosis, improper treatment, or poor compliance with protocol that can lead to chronic or neglected Achilles tendon rupture, requiring more advanced considerations for

[a] Kaiser San Francisco Bay Area Foot & Ankle Residency Program, Kaiser Oakland Foundation Hospital, 275 MacArthur Boulevard, Clinic 17, Oakland, CA 94611, USA; [b] Foot & Ankle Surgery, Orthopedics and Podiatry Department, Kaiser Oakland, 275 MacArthur Boulevard, Clinic 17, Oakland, CA, 94611, USA; [c] California School of Podiatric Medicine at Samuel Merritt University, 3100 Telegraph Ave, Oakland, CA, 94609, USA; [d] St. Mary's Medical Center Residency Program, 450 Stanyan St. San Francisco, CA, 94117, USA; [e] University of California San Francisco, Center for Limb Preservation, 400 Parnassus- Ave, Room A-501 San Francisco, CA, 94143, USA; [f] San Francisco Bay Area, Balance Health, 2299 Post St, Suite 205, San Francisco, CA 94115, USA
* Corresponding author. 275 MacArthur Boulevard, Clinic 17, Oakland, CA 94611.
E-mail address: Christy.m.king@kp.org

Clin Podiatr Med Surg 40 (2023) 75–96
https://doi.org/10.1016/j.cpm.2022.07.006
0891-8422/23/© 2022 Elsevier Inc. All rights reserved.

podiatric.theclinics.com

treatment. The goal of any treatment of the Achilles tendon rupture repair—either acute or chronic—focuses on restoring anatomic length and physiologic tension, providing adequate strength for proper propulsion, optimizing functional return to activity, decreasing any associated pain, and decreasing potential complications.

CONSIDERATIONS: COLLAGEN TRANSFORMATION AND TENDON ELONGATION

To achieve these goals of treatment of the Achilles tendon rupture, it is important to appreciate the tendon healing process on a microscopic level. A healthy tendon is composed mainly of well-aligned type I collagen, proteoglycan, and elastin.[4] With the initiation of the inflammatory phase during injury, type III collagen is secreted by fibroblasts and other mesenchymal cells and provides the building blocks for the initial repair of acute Achilles tendon rupture.[4,5] Although type III collagen is less resistant to tensile force and more easily elongates, it can be converted to type I collagen over time (**Fig. 1**). Animal model studies reveal that the scar tissue that develops after tendon injury can convert to more normal tendon tissue with type I collagen over time.[6,7] However, the most suitable time and ideal mechanical loading in humans to allow for maximal conversion to its healthier counterpart is not fully understood (**Fig. 2**).

The degree of elongation during the healing process can contribute to the presumed success or failure of treatment and return to activity. Even in the surgical repair of an acute Achilles tendon rupture, the tendon can potentially elongate up to 1.2 cm as compared with an uninjured Achilles tendon, decreasing plantarflexion strength by 12% to 18%.[8] When directly comparing the mean volume of muscles and tendon length in Achilles tendon ruptures addressed surgically and nonsurgically for an acute Achilles tendon rupture, it was noted the tendons treated nonsurgically were 1.9 cm longer than those treated surgically.[9] MRI has shown that, after an acute Achilles tendon rupture, there is a decrease in the volume of the gastrocnemius soleus complex by 11% to 13% and the flexor hallucis longus (FHL) increases its volume to compensate for the additional plantarflexion work.[8,9]

CONTROVERSIES: ROLE OF EARLY FUNCTIONAL REHABILITATION

Ever since the early functional rehabilitation protocol was popularized by Willits et al, the ideal treatment of an acute Achilles tendon rupture with surgery versus

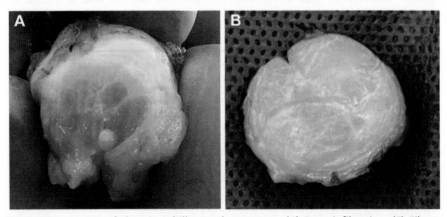

Fig. 1. Cross-section of chronic Achilles tendon rupture. (*A*) Fatty infiltration. (*B*) Fibrous deposition.

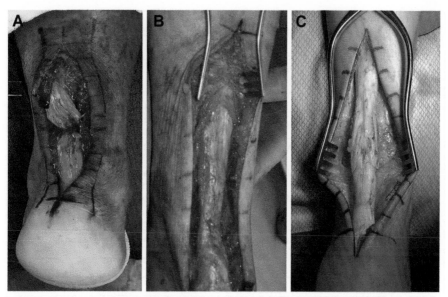

Fig. 2. (*A*) Acute Achilles tendon rupture. (*B*) Chronic Achilles tendon rupture with over-lengthening. (*C*) Chronic Achilles tendon rupture with intratendinous tear.

nonoperative immobilization, both with early functional rehabilitation, has produced many heated debates.[10,11] Classically, the risk of rerupture after surgical treatment was documented at 3%, whereas those treated with nonoperative prolonged immobilization had a rerupture rate of 12% to 13%.[10,11] Willits et al[11] revealed that, when using early functional rehabilitation, the risk of rerupture after being treated nonoperatively decreased to 4%, whereas the risk with surgical treatment was approximately 3%. Conversely, the complication rate was higher in the operative group compared with the nonoperative group, at 18% versus 8%, respectively.[11] Although the landmark study did not have a sufficient sample size to fulfill the sample size predicted by the power analysis, it stimulated an acceleration in research on the ideal treatment of Achilles tendon ruptures. In s comprehensive meta-analysis, 29 studies with 15,862 patients were evaluated, and the authors noted the rerupture rate was 2.3% in the surgical group and 3.9% in the nonoperative group, whereas the complication rate was 4.9% in operative group and 3.9% in nonoperative group.[12] However, when studies were isolated to those using the early mobilization protocol, there was no significant difference.

It has become clear that, despite the initial treatment pathway selected, early functional rehabilitation is an essential part of recovery. Building on the early functional rehabilitation protocol, we developed more specific instructions and milestones to assist in the recovery process (**Table 1**). The criteria for return to sports after anterior cruciate ligament repair were adapted for return to sport criteria in the modified protocol.[13] Although it is important for both physical and mental health to return the patient to an active lifestyle, it is necessary to set expectations, stress the importance of adherence to protocol, and encourage patients to be conscious with their activity to avoid accidents that can lead to rerupture. The patient can be more vulnerable to rerupture in the in the early recovery period between 6 and 12 weeks as

Table 1
The modified early functional rehabilitation protocol used at our facility

Phase I: Immediate Postinjury Period (0–2 to 3 Weeks)

Rehabilitation goals	Protect tendon repair
	Reduce swelling, minimize pain
	Patient education
	Keep your leg up and elevated when sitting or lying down
	Do not put weight on the injured side
	Do not pivot on your injured side
Weightbearing restrictions and precautions	Weightbearing status: Cast × 2–3 weeks, strict nonweightbearing
	Showering: Keep the cast clean and dry. You should cover it with a secure plastic wrap, so it does not get wet.
	Stairs: When climbing stairs, make sure you are leading with the noninjured side. It can be a safe alternative to go up and down the stairs on your buttocks.
Intervention	Swelling Management: Ice, compression, elevation
	Cardio: upper body ergometer
Criteria to progress	2–3 weeks

Phase II: Intermediate Postinjury Period (2 to 3–6 Weeks)

Rehabilitation goals	Continue to protect the tendon repair while allowing for early range of motion to decrease adhesions
Weightbearing restrictions	Weightbearing status: Protected weightbearing in the walking boot with 3 × 5/16 heel lifts with crutch assistance. Heel lift height may vary per person.
	Sleeping: Keep the boot on at night when sleeping
	Showering: Use shower chair
	Stairs: When climbing or going downstairs, make sure you are leading with the uninjured side
Additional interventions	Swelling control: Ice, compression, elevation
	Cardio: upper body ergometer
	Scar management (if surgically corrected)
	Massage incision site
	You can apply topical scar treatments like vitamin E oil, Mederma cream (available in pharmacies), or silicon impregnated bandages (ie, Scar away or Mepiform available online)
	Range of motion/mobility
	Active range of motion plantarflexion, inversion, eversion, dorsiflexion from maximum plantarflexion to neutral (*do not* dorsiflex past neutral)
	Strengthening
	Hip and knee strengthening
	3-way hip
	Short/long arc quads
	Prone hamstring curls
	Open chain core
Criteria to progress	6 weeks
	No wound complications
	Dorsiflexion to neutral

Phase III: Late Postinjury Period (6–8 Weeks)	
Rehabilitation goals	Start progression of weightbearing without the boot Increase dorsiflexion range of motion Safely progress strengthening Promote proper movement patterns Avoid postexercise pain and swelling Avoid activities that produce pain at injured site
Weightbearing restrictions	Weightbearing status: Protected weightbearing in the walking boot Week 6: Remove first heel lift Week 7: Remove second and third heel lifts Week 8: Start walking without the boot in supportive shoe Sleeping: You no longer need to sleep with the boot on

Additional interventions (continue with phase II interventions)	Cardio: Bike, swimming, water aerobics
	Scar management: Cross-friction massage incision site as needed
	Range of motion and mobility
	  Gentle calf stretching, nonweightbearing
	  Ankle mobilizations, as needed
	Strengthening
	  Ankle dorsiflexion, plantarflexion, inversion, eversion with resistance band
	  Progress to weightbearing hip/knee strengthening by week 8
	  Bridges, squats, step ups
	Neurological reeducation/proprioception
	  Static balance progression

Criteria to progress	Decrease in swelling and pain after exercise Dorsiflexion active range of motion to at least 5° Single leg stance for 30 seconds

Phase IV: Transitional Postinjury Period (9–12 Weeks)	
Rehabilitation goals	Achieve full dorsiflexion range of motion Safely progress calf strengthening Promote proper movement patterns Avoid postexercise pain and swelling

Additional interventions (continue with phase II–III interventions as needed)	Cardio: Bike, swimming, water aerobics, elliptical machine
	Range of motion and mobility
	  Calf stretching in weightbearing
	  Ankle mobilizations, as needed
	Strengthening
	  Initiate heel raise progression, concentric and eccentric
	  Functional movements
	    Squats → single leg squat
	    Lunges (forward, lateral, reverse)
	    Step ups, step downs
	Neurological reeducation and proprioception
	  Dynamic balance progression

Criteria to progress/return to impact training	Dorsiflexion range of motion equal to the contralateral side Ten repetitions of straight leg (SL) heel raise through 85% range of motion (contralateral side)

Phase V: Early Return to Sport Period (3–5 Months)	
Rehabilitation goals	Maintain full range of motion Initiate plyometric program Safely initiate sport specific training program Avoid postexercise pain and swelling

Additional interventions (continue with phase II–IV interventions)	Cardio: Bike, swimming, elliptical, running
	Plyometrics
	  Partial body weight with shuttle press
	  1. Bilateral hops
	  2. Alternating hops
	  3. Single leg hops
	  Frontal plane on land
	  4. Bilateral side to side
	  5. Single leg side to side
	  6. Skaters
	  Sagittal plane on land
	  7. Bilateral hops in place, forward/backward
	  8. Single leg hops in place, forward backward
	  9. Box jumps

Criteria to progress/ return to run criteria	Single leg standing heel raise test: 90% Limb Symmetry Index (10° incline1 rep:2 s rate for 60 s, no. of reps performed) Single leg hop for distance 90% Limb Symmetry Index Single leg squat 45°, 10 reps with good form

Phase VI: Unrestricted Return to Sport Period (≥6 Months)	
Rehabilitation goals	Safely return to sport

Additional interventions (continue with phase II–V interventions as needed)	Sport-specific agility and plyometric training
	  Examples:
	    Lateral shuffle, grapevine
	    Backwards running
	    Shuttle run
	    Sport cord drills
	    Ladder drills
	    T-agility
	    Box drill
	    Zig-zag run
	    Cutting and pivoting

Criteria to progress/return to unrestricted sport	Drop countermovement jump Limb Symmetry Index 90% (vertical drop from standard stair height of 20 cm) Ability to complete 1 repetition declined heel raise set at 20°

Courtesy of Christy King, DPM and Kaitlin Collins, DPT, Oakland, CA

they are given more freedom to remove the boot for exercises and start to increase movement, so it is important to encourage diligence with and adherence to the protocol.[1,11–14]

Current Evidence: Ultrasound Use

Although ultrasound examination is not necessarily needed to diagnose the presence of an Achilles tendon rupture, it can be a useful tool in evaluating the gap distance that can be used in the decision-making process. The gap distance is measured optimally with the ankle in maximum plantarflexion despite the knee extension/flexion angle.[15] Patients with a gap distance of more than 5 mm had poorer functional scores, whereas those with a gap distance of more than 10 mm had a higher risk of rerupture, greater degree of functional deficit, and poorer outcome scores(**Fig. 3**).[16–18] Amlang et al[19]

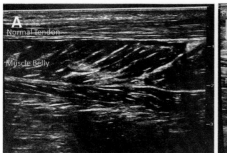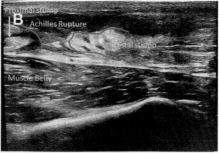

Fig. 3. Ultrasound image of the Achilles tendon. (*A*) Normal tendon with ultrasound evaluation. The nonruptured Achilles tendon shows linear fibers and the underlying muscle belly. (*B*) Achilles tendon rupture with proximal and distal stump identified. Note the less linear muscle belly; it has lost its normal tension.

proposed accounting for the location of rupture, contact of tendon rupture ends, and structure of interposition (**Fig. 4**). Ultrasound measurement of the gap distance can be used along with other patient-specific and injury factors to assist in the shared decision-making in treatment pathway.

Acute Achilles Tendon Rupture

There are various ways to approach the surgical repair of the acute Achilles tendon rupture, including open repair, small incision repair, the traditional percutaneous Achilles repair system (PARS) (Arthrex, Naples, FL), and the modified PARS with suture anchor augmentation. The most common suture techniques used are the Krakow, Kessler, and Bunnell techniques, with many variations present. The percutaneous approach to Achilles tendon repair has gained popularity over the years owing to the decreased incision size, lower potential complications, improved rates of return to baseline activity, and similar functional outcome scores.[20,21] Because the sural nerve is not visualized directly, sural nerve injury is a potential increased risk (**Fig. 5**). Because the percutaneous approach was used more frequently , modifications evolved to include additional suture anchors into the calcaneus. In a study by Cottom et al[21] evaluating the Krakow repair, traditional PARS, and modified PARS with suture anchor augmentation, it was noted that the modified PARS with suture anchor was stronger, suggesting that it may be a more reliable construct to allow for more aggressive rehabilitation and quicker return to activity. Ultimately, the goal of

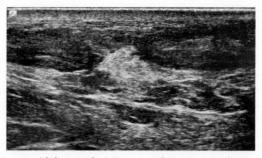

Fig. 4. Ultrasound image with hyperechoic interposed structure and an organized hematoma.

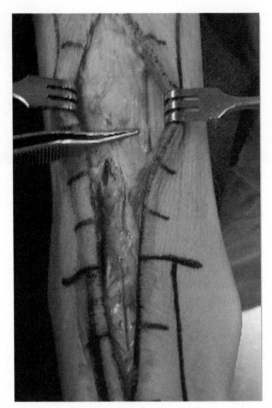

Fig. 5. It is important to be aware of the sural nerve on the lateral aspect of the incision.

open or percutaneous repair of the Achilles tendon is to restore the anatomic length, decrease adhesions, and decrease potential associated risks.

Primary repair
Pearls

- Be aware of the sural nerve; it can transverses the proximal lateral incision.
- A careful repair of the paratenon is essential because it contains a rich vascular supply. Additionally, it aids in preventing adhesions of the tendon to the skin and subcutaneous tissues.

Surgical Technique

With the patient in the prone position and appropriately padded, the injured leg is prepped in a sterile manner. The incision is made just medial to midline over the Achilles tendon (**Fig. 6**A). Care should be taken to identify the sural nerve coursing on the lateral aspect of the proximal incision (see **Fig. 5**). The paratenon is incised midline with special attention to preserve the paratenon for repair at end of the procedure (see **Fig. 6**A). The proximal and distal segments of the rupture are identified. The Krakow suture technique is most often used by the authors, which entails an interlocking suture passed separately through the proximal and distal segments of the rupture (**Fig. 6**B). Then, with the foot in maximum plantarflexion, the 2 independent suture ends are tied together (**Fig. 6**C). Complete closure of the paratenon is

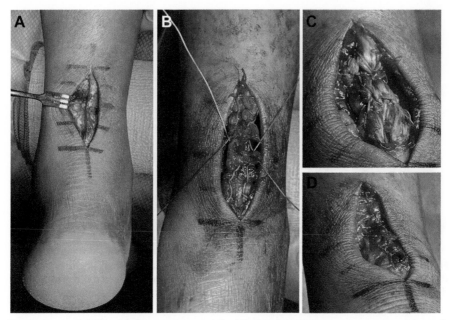

Fig. 6. Acute Achilles tendon rupture repair. (*A*) Careful dissection to protect the sural nerve. (*B*) Krakow suture pattern. (*C*) Completed repair. (*D*) Paratenon closure.

helpful to assist in decreasing adhesions and improving vascularity to the surgical site (**Fig. 6**D).

Percutaneous repair
Pearls

- Depending on the technique used, plan the incisions well to maximize access to the Achilles tendon and the minimize the surgical footprint.

Surgical Technique

Separate systems exist to assist in either traditional PARS or modified PARS with suture anchors; however, the technique described in this article can be performed without additional devices. Modifying a technique described by Carmont and Maffulli,[22] a small linear incision is made over the rupture site. Two small incisions are made proximally and distally on the medial and lateral sides of each stump (**Fig. 7**A). The Achilles tendon stumps are brought through the incision and a straight needle is used to pass a nonabsorbable suture from the rupture site through the proximal stump, exiting the proximal medial incision (**Fig. 7**B). Then, the suture is passed transversely through the proximal medial incision through the proximal lateral incision. Finally, it is passed back through the proximal stump and out the main incision (**Fig. 7**C). The same suture passing technique is passed through the distal stump. The foot is placed in maximum plantarflexion and the 2 separate ends of the sutures are tied together (**Fig. 7**D). The incisions are then sutured (**Fig. 7**E).

Postoperative Early Functional Rehabilitation Protocol

See the protocol described in **Table 1**.

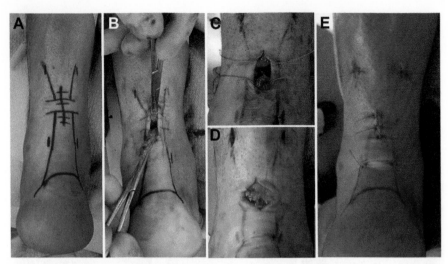

Fig. 7. Small incisional approach. (*A*) Incision planning. (*B*) Through small linear incision, the distal and proximal stumps are identified. (*C*) Placement of each suture on the proximal and distal stumps. (*D*) Tendon repair complete. (*E*) Final small incision footprint.

CHRONIC OR NEGLECTED ACHILLES TENDON RUPTURE

Swift identification and treatment contribute to a successful return to normal function; however, 25% of cases can be diagnosed late, misdiagnosed, or treated improperly, leading to chronic issues for the patient, which can include weakness in plantarflexion, decreased propulsion, dysfunctional gait, balance issues, difficulty using stairs, and, less typically, pain.[23–25] The chronic or neglected Achilles tendon rupture can be defined anywhere after 4 to 6 weeks from the initial trauma.[26] Failure to immobilize contributes to gastrocsoleal contracture, retraction of the proximal portion of the rupture, fibrous tissue, and elongation of the tendon. When the tendon heals overlengthened, there is poor energy translation from the calf to Achilles to calcaneus, leading to decreased contractile forces and strength of propulsion. Treatment of the chronic Achilles tendon rupture can be more challenging owing to adhesions, overlengthening of the tendon, and general atrophy of the gastrocsoleal complex.

Evaluation

In evaluating a chronic rupture, the traditionally used Thompson test or calf squeeze with plantarflexion of the foot is not as useful because there will be some adaptation of the remainder of the posterior compartment that will produce some plantarflexion with the Thompson test.[23–25] The Matles test with the patient prone and the knees flexed to 90° can be a useful tool in chronic Achilles tendon rupture evaluation with a sensitivity of 0.88 (**Fig. 8**).[27] Once a chronic Achilles tendon rupture is suspected, further imaging assists in surgical procedure decision-making.

Evaluation: MRI Use

Although MRI is used less commonly for the identification or treatment of acute Achilles tendon ruptures, it is valuable in evaluating the gap distance and location of the chronic Achilles tendon rupture (**Fig. 9**). Two classification systems have been

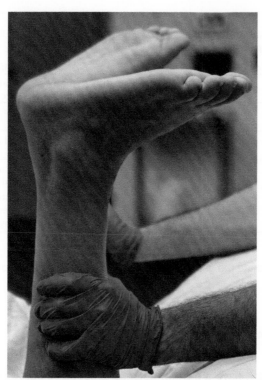

Fig. 8. Matles test with the patient prone and knees flexed to 90°. The ruptured side will sit in neutral (near) and the uninjured side is positioned in resting plantarflexion (far).

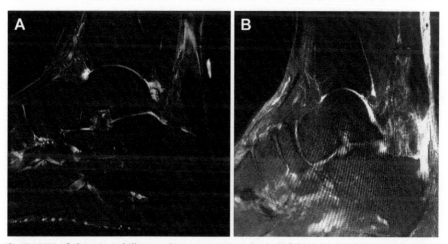

Fig. 9. MRI of chronic Achilles tendon ruptures can be helpful to measure gap distance and location of rupture. (*A*) Midsubstance Achilles tendon rupture. (*B*) Insertional Achilles tendon rupture.

Table 2
Myerson and Kuwada Classification Systems with comparison of the gap distance measured on MRI and corresponding treatment recommendations

	Myerson Classification			Kuwada Classification	
	Gap Distance	Treatment Recommendation		Gap Distance	Treatment Recommendation
Type I	1–2 cm	End to end with posterior compartment fasciotomy	Type I	Partial	Cast immobilization
Type II	2–5 cm	V-Y lengthening with or without tendon transfer	Type II	<3 cm	End to end repair
Type III	>5 cm	Tendon transfer ± V–Y advancement	Type III	3–6 cm	Autograft or Allograft
			Type IV	>6 cm	Gastrocnemius recession allograft or autograft

developed to correlate the gap distance measured on MRI and the procedure options (**Table 2**).[28,29]

General Surgical Approach

Pearls

- Before surgery, have a plan for potential procedures based on the location of rupture, the quality of the tendon tissue, and the gap distance noted on the MRI.
- The sural nerve and saphenous vein should be identified and protected.

Similar to the treatment of an acute rupture, the goal of a chronic Achilles tendon rupture repair is to restore anatomic length and physiologic tension, provide adequate strength for proper ambulation, optimize functional return, decrease pain associated with the injury or overwork of other parts of the body, and decrease associated complications. The surgical treatment options can be grouped into general categories, including resection of the scar tissue with direct end to end repair (transverse, Z-shortening), tendon advancements (V-Y advancement), tendon transfers (FHL, flexor digitorum longus, peroneus brevis), allograft reconstruction, and autograft reconstruction (**Table 3**).

For the following surgical procedures, the general surgical approach is described here with features unique to the specific technique described elsewhere in this article. The patient is placed in a prone position with appropriate padding. The surgical site is prepared in a sterile manner. The incision is made just medial to midline and care should be taken to identify and protect the sural nerve. In contrast with the approach to the paratenon in acute Achilles tendon rupture repair, a full-thickness flap is often used to assist in optimizing blood supply and tendon repair coverage. In most surgical techniques the unhealthy and/or overlengthened tendon is debrided. The ankle is placed in maximum plantarflexion and the knee can be flexed to 30° as the gap distance is measured. A posterior compartment fasciotomy can be used to provided increased vascularity to the repair. After the respective neglected Achilles tendon repair, it is important to close the full-thickness layer created in the initial phases of surgery to increase vascularity to the repair, decrease adhesions, and decrease infection risk.

Table 3
Chronic Achilles tendon repair options with associated gap distance, advantages, and disadvantages

	Gap Distance	Advantages	Disadvantages
Resection of scar tissue with end to end repair, transverse or Z shortening	1–2 cm	No additional allografts or autografts needed Quicker recovery Better for tendons that have good tissue quality but are overlengthened	Depends on tissue health
V–Y advancement	2–5 cm or with an FHL	Autograft Can accommodate larger gap distances Good blood Supply	Associated with deficiency in peak torque Longest incision for access to aponeurosis
FHL tendon transfer	2–5 cm or with a V-Y advancement >5 cm	Short harvest has easy dissection Tendon is long and durable Strongest of the tendon transfer options In phase Muscle belly contributes additional vascularity	Potential loss of hallux push off strength Decrease in ankle plantarflexion strength and torque strength Decrease in ankle range of motion
Achilles allograft	>5 cm avulsion	Relatively simple technique No donor site morbidity Good mechanical strength	Increased cost Small, yet potential risk of transmission Longer remodeling phase

General Postoperative Protocol

The general postoperative protocol may vary based on the surgical procedure selection. Typically, we follow a delayed approach to the modified early functional rehabilitation protocol. The patient is protected in a splint or short leg cast nonweightbearing for the first 2 weeks. The sutures are removed, and the patient is placed in a plantarflexed cast to decrease tension on the repair site. At 6 weeks, the patient is transitioned to the walking boot with heel lifts, and they start to follow the protocol outlined in **Table 1**.

RESECTION OF SCAR TISSUE WITH DIRECT END-TO-END REPAIR
Transverse End-to-end Repair

Pearls

- Careful evaluation of the healthy and unhealthy tendon is essential to ensure best possible tendon is used in the repair.

Background

If the gap distance or transverse section of the unhealthy tendon removed from the chronic Achilles tendon is less than 2 cm, then a resection of scar tissue and primary

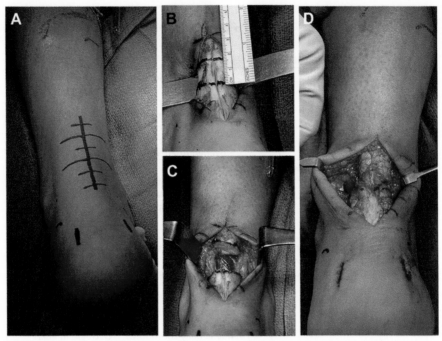

Fig. 10. Transverse resection of scar tissue. (*A*) Incision planning. (*B*) Overlengthened chronic rupture measuring less than 2 cm. (*C*) Resection of interposed scar tissue. (*D*) Krakow suture repair.

end-to-end repair of the tendon is a successful option. Yasuda et al[30] described the transverse resection of interposed scar tissue and direct repair using the Krakow technique with increase in functional scores, return to preinjury activity, and MRI results showing fusiform shape with homogenous signal supporting successful healing.

Surgical technique

After following the general surgical principles delineated in the General Surgical Approach, the zone of scar tissue and healthier tissue is palpated and visualized. This zone is measured and typically is less than 2 cm for direct repair (**Fig. 10**A). Once the unhealthy or overlengthened tendon is resected, a Krakow suture technique is placed through the distal and proximal stumps (**Fig. 10**B, C). Before completing the repair, a deep fasciotomy can be performed to increase vascularity to the repair site. The foot is placed in maximum plantarflexion, the tendon segments are well-apposed, and the suture knots are tied together (**Fig. 10**D).

Z-Shortening

Pearls

- An MRI can be useful to determine zone of healthy tendon.
- A suture and biotenodesis anchor system can be used to assist in maintaining appropriate tension.

Literature

The Z-shortening procedure can be used as an alternative to the transverse resection of a chronic Achilles tendon that is typically healed, yet overlengthened. As compared with the transverse resection of tissue, this procedure increases the overall surface area of tendon apposition for healing. The technique was described separately by Cannon et al[31] in 2003 and Maffulli et al in 2012.[32] They noted that it was a safe and effective option in the treatment of a neglected Achilles tendon rupture; however, the patient should be educated that the plantarflexion strength will likely be permanently decreased when compared with the uninjured leg.[31,32]

Surgical technique

Following the steps in the General Surgical Approach section, a linear incision is made through the zone of scar tissue into the healthy tendon both distally and proximally (**Fig. 11**B). Then, the distal medial and proximal lateral arms are created (see **Fig. 11**C). With the foot in maximum plantarflexion, equal sections are removed from each arm to complete the Z-shortening. In the experience of the authors, a nonabsorbable suture is used for repair; however, the use of an absorbable suture has also been described.[32] In some cases, a suture and anchor system can be used by attaching the proximal stump directly to the calcaneus with biotenodesis screws and integrating the distal stump into the repair to assist in maintaining the appropriate length and tension (**Fig. 11**D).

TENDON ADVANCEMENTS
V-Y Advancement

Pearls

- Prepare the V-Y to provide adequate length to close the gap, typically the arms of the V are twice the length of the rupture gap.
- Avoid disrupting the myotendinous portion from the underlying muscle.
- Complete the repair of the distal and proximal stumps of the rupture site before suturing the Y incision in the aponeurosis.

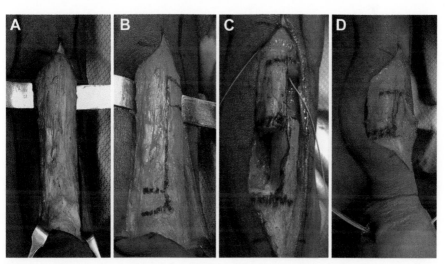

Fig. 11. Z-shortening procedure. (*A*) Achilles tendon overlengthened after previous Achilles tendon surgical repair. (*B*) Planned tendon resection. (*C*) Z-Shortening with about 1 cm removed. (*D*) Final position of the Achilles tendon with resting tension restored to the Achilles tendon.

Literature

The V-Y advancement procedure has been used for many years to address larger defects between 2 and 5 cm and can also be used in conjunction with FHL tendon transfers.[28,29] The procedure is a successful option; there is good vascularity associated with the aponeurosis and underlying muscle belly. It is important to council the patient that they can potentially see up to 30% decreased torque strength with a V-Y advancement.[33–35] The addition of an FHL transfer can potentially increase the torque strength.[35] Potential disadvantages of the procedure to consider are the generally longer length of the incision compared with other surgical options, adhesions along the incision and tendon, and deficiency in peak torque.[33–35] Advantages of the surgical option include the great blood supply associated, good healing potential, and the autograft.[33–35]

Surgical technique

Following the initial steps in the General Surgical Approach section, the incision for the V-Y is typically longer and directed more proximal than the other surgical options to gain access to the aponeurosis. Special care should be taken to identify and protect the sural nerve and saphenous vein, especially more proximally. Once the unhealthy tendon is debrided, the gap distance is measured with the foot maximally plantarflexed (**Fig. 12**A). The arms of the V are prepared to be 2 times the length of the gap distance (**Fig. 12**B). Before incision of the aponeurosis, the Krakow suture is placed in each stump of the Achilles tendon and can be gently stretched to assist in freeing adhesions and decreasing postoperative viscoelastic creep (**Fig. 12**C). Then, the incision should be made carefully through the aponeurosis and should not disturb the underlying muscle belly. As the proximal arm is gently lengthened down to the distal stump, the sutures of the Krakow pattern are tied together (**Fig. 12**D). Finally, the Y formed from the stretch of the aponeurosis is repaired.

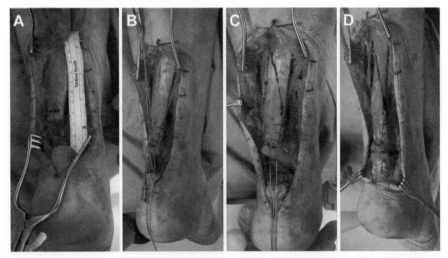

Fig. 12. V-Y tendon advancement. (*A*) Debride the scar tissue, measure the gap distance with the foot in plantarflexion. (*B*) A Krakow suture is performed. (*C*) The V is drawn on the aponeurosis with arms twice the size of the gap distance. (*D*) Complete the knot of the Krakow sutures distally and then repair the Y proximally.

TENDON TRANSFERS
Flexor Hallucis Longus

Pearls

- While performing a short harvest for the FHL tendon, take care to protect the neurovascular bundle.
- Ensure that the tendon is adequately tensioned into the calcaneus with the biotenodesis screw.

Literature

The FHL transfer is a traditional treatment for chronic Achilles tendon ruptures because it provides a relatively easy harvest, the tendon is long and durable, it is in phase, it is most similar to the axis of contraction of the Achilles tendon, and it includes a muscle to increase vascularity and optimize healing.[36,37] This procedure is typically used with any size defect. It can be used in conjunction with V-Y advancements or allograft use. A long harvest of the FHL is classically described at the knot of Henry; however, with the advent of the biotenodesis screws, the short harvest became more popular.[36] Although there are good to excellent functional scores reported, studies have shown a decrease of plantarflexion strength of 22.3% to 29.5% and a decrease in torque of 13.5% to 41.0%.[36,37] Although the FHL can engage fibers from the flexor digitorum longus at the knot of Henry, there is a potential loss of push off strength of the hallux that may not be ideal in an athletic population.[36,37]

Technique

Following the initial steps of the General Surgical Approach section, this procedure incorporates a variation as the distal incision is curved medially to gain access to the FHL as it enters the tarsal tunnel. A full-thickness incision is made down to the Achilles tendon, which is freed from underlying tissue. The deep fascia is incised and the

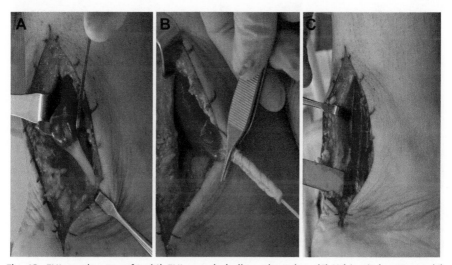

Fig. 13. FHL tendon transfer. (*A*) FHL muscle belly and tendon. (*B*) Whipstitch pattern. (*C*) Completion of the transfer into the calcaneus with a biotenodesis screw. (*Courtesy of* Dr. Lawrence Ford.)

FHL muscle belly is encountered (**Fig. 13**A). The tendon is followed into the posterior medial aspect of the ankle at the beginning of the tarsal tunnel. The ankle and hallux are plantarflexed to decrease tension and obtain the longest graft possible. Taking care to avoid the neurovascular bundle, the FHL is resected. A whipstitch with nonabsorbable suture is then placed along the FHL tendon (**Fig. 13**B). It is measured with the appropriate tendon sizer and the biotenodesis screw is selected. Then, a guidewire is drilled into the calcaneus just deep to the Achilles tendon to recreate the lever arm of the Achilles as best possible. Once placement is confirmed with intraoperative fluoroscopy, the whipstitch is carried through the calcaneus with the guidewire and secured with a biotenodesis screw with the foot is mild plantarflexion (**Fig. 13**C).

ACHILLES ALLOGRAFT RECONSTRUCTION
Pearls

- Ensure adequate apposition of the native tendon and allograft tendon.
- Suture the allograft to the native proximal tendon first, cut away the excess allograft, and finish the repair by tying this complex to the distal stump.

Literature

The Achilles cadaver allograft has gained popularity more recently because it can help to bridge larger defects, is a relatively simple technique, there is no donor site morbidity, and has similar mechanical strength.[38–41] In a study by Ofili et al[38] a nonunion of the calcaneal section attached to the allograft was noted, so it is generally recommended to remove the attached bone before use. Xenografts, synthetic grafts, and dermal matrixes have been used in allograft repair; however, Achilles cadaver allograft is the preferred material used by the authors. The potential disadvantages

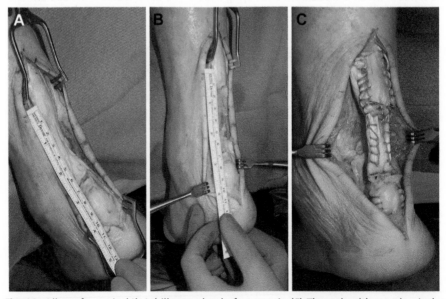

Fig. 14. Allograft repair. (*A*) Achilles tendon before repair. (*B*) The unhealthy tendon is debrided, and the gap distance is measured. (*C*) The allograft is sutured to the proximal end and then attached to distal end with the Krakow technique. (*Courtesy of* Dr. Jason Pollard.)

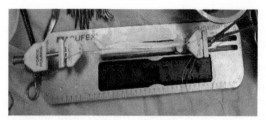

Fig. 15. The use of the graft tensioner helps to decrease viscoelastic creep that can occur in the postoperative period.

of the allograft include that it is relatively expensive, there is a small yet potential risks of disease transmission, and there is a longer remodeling phase as compared with the other surgical options. Although there is little mention of pretensioning of the allograft in foot and ankle literature, pretensioning of the anterior cruciate ligament is a

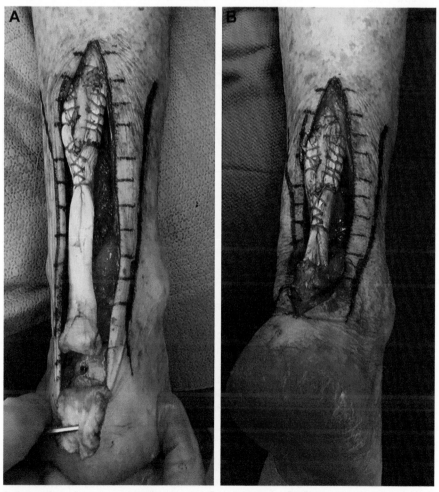

Fig. 16. Allograft use in Achilles tendon avulsion rupture. (*A*) Before using the anchors into the calcaneus. (*B*) Completed repair with maximum tension restored to the Achilles.

frequently debated topic.[42] The use of a graft tensioner may help to decrease visco-elastic creep that could lead to overlengthening in the healing process that may contribute to failure.

Surgical Technique

Following the General Surgical Approach section, the chronic Achilles tendon rupture is encountered (**Fig. 14**A). The unhealthy and or overlengthened tendon and scar tissue are debrided (**Fig. 14**B). The gap distance is measured while the Achilles allograft is prepped by thawing in saline. Following techniques adapted from the anterior cruciate ligament allograft literature, the allograft graft is stretched at 20N for 15 minutes to help settle the potential viscoelastic creep (**Fig. 15**). In our practice, the proximal native stump is wrapped with the allograft and a modified Krakow suture is used to secure the allograft to the proximal stump. Then, the foot is placed in maximum plantarflexion and the final length of the allograft is confirm and resected. A separate Krakow suture is placed in the distal stump. To finalize the repair, the Krakow suture of the proximal stump with the allograft is tied to the suture of the distal stump (**Fig. 14**C and **Fig. 16**).

CLINICS CARE POINTS

- Using patient and injury characteristics of an acute Achilles tendon rupture, like gap distance measured with ultrasound imaging, can help to guide both the practitioner and patient's ultimate decision on treatment pathway.
- Despite the technique used for chronic Achilles tendon reconstruction, the patient should be advised of general calf atrophy and potential weakness in plantarflexion as compared with the uninjured side.

DISCLOSURE

The authors have nothing to disclose.

REFERENCES

1. Park SH, Lee HS, Young KW, et al. Treatment of acute Achilles tendon rupture. Clin Orthop Surg 2020;12(1):1–8.
2. Huttunen TT, Kannus P, Rolf C, et al. Acute Achilles tendon ruptures: incidence of injury and surgery in Sweden between 2001 and 2012. Am J Sports Med 2014; 42(10):2419–23.
3. Jarvinen TA, Kannus P, Maffulli N, et al. Achilles tendon disorders: etiology and epidemiology. Foot Ankle Clin 2005;10(2):255–66.
4. Lin TW, Cardenas L, Soslowsky LJ. Biomechanics of tendon injury and repair. J Biomech 2004;37(6):865–77.
5. Nielsen MJ, Karsdal MA. in Biochemistry of Collagens. Laminins and Elastin; 2016.
6. Yasuda T, Kinoshita M, Abe M, et al. Unfavorable effect of knee immobilization on Achilles tendon healing in rabbits. Acta Orthop Scand 2000;71(1):69–73.
7. Voleti PB, Buckley MR, Soslowsky LJ. Tendon healing: repair and regeneration. Annu Rev Biomed Eng 2012;14:47–71.

8. Heikkinen J, Lantto I, Piilonen J, et al. Tendon length, calf muscle atrophy, and strength deficit after acute Achilles tendon rupture: long-term follow-up of patients in a previous study. J Bone Joint Surg Am 2017;99(18):1509–15.

9. Heikkinen J, Lantto I, Flinkkila T, et al. Soleus atrophy is common after the Nonsurgical treatment of acute Achilles tendon ruptures: a randomized Clinical trial comparing surgical and Nonsurgical functional treatments. Am J Sports Med 2017;45(6):1395–404.

10. Kocher MS, Bishop J, Marshall R, et al. Operative versus nonoperative management of acute Achilles tendon rupture: expected-value decision analysis. Am J Sports Med 2002;30(6):783–90.

11. Willits K, Amendola A, Bryant D, et al. Operative versus nonoperative treatment of acute Achilles tendon ruptures: a multicenter randomized trial using accelerated functional rehabilitation. J Bone Joint Surg Am 2010;92(17):2767–75.

12. Ochen Y, Beks RB, van Heijl M, et al. Operative treatment versus nonoperative treatment of Achilles tendon ruptures: systematic review and meta-analysis. BMJ 2019;364:k5120.

13. Reito A, Logren HL, Ahonen K, et al. Risk factors for failed nonoperative treatment and rerupture in acute Achilles tendon rupture. Foot Ankle Int 2018;39(6): 694–703.

14. Flagg KY, Karavatas SG, Thompson S Jr, et al. Current criteria for return to play after anterior cruciate ligament reconstruction: an evidence-based literature review. Ann Transl Med 2019;7(Suppl 7):S252.

15. Qureshi AA, Ibrahim T, Rennie WJ, et al. Dynamic ultrasound assessment of the effects of knee and ankle position on Achilles tendon apposition following acute rupture. J Bone Joint Surg Am 2011;93(24).

16. Kotnis R, David S, Handley R, et al. Dynamic ultrasound as a selection tool for reducing Achilles tendon reruptures. Am J Sports Med 2006;34(9):1395–400.

17. Westin O, Nilsson Helander K, Grävare Silbernagel K, et al. Acute Ultrasonography Investigation to Predict reruptures and outcomes in patients with an Achilles tendon rupture. Orthop J Sports Med 2016;4(10).

18. Yassin M, Myatt R, Thomas W, et al. Does size of tendon gap affect patient-reported outcome following Achilles tendon rupture treated with functional rehabilitation? Bone Joint J 2020;102-B(11):1535–41.

19. Amlang MH, Zwipp H, Friedrich A, et al. Ultrasonographic classification of Achilles tendon ruptures as a rationale for individual treatment selection. ISRN Orthop 2011;2011:869703.

20. Hsu AR, Jones CP, Cohen BE, et al. Clinical outcomes and complications of Percutaneous Achilles Repair System versus open technique for acute Achilles tendon ruptures. Foot Ankle Int 2015;36(11):1279–86.

21. Cottom JM, Baker JS, Richardson PE, et al. Evaluation of a New Knotless suture anchor repair in acute Achilles tendon ruptures: a biomechanical comparison of three techniques. J Foot Ankle Surg 2017;56(3):423–7.

22. Carmont MR, Maffulli N. Modified percutaneous repair of ruptured Achilles tendon. Knee Surg Sports Traumatol Arthrosc 2008;16:199–203.

23. Saini SS, Reb CW, Chapter M, et al. Achilles tendon disorders. J Am Osteopath Assoc 2015;115(11):670–6.

24. Shane AM, Reeves CL, Nguyen GB, et al. Revision surgery for the Achilles tendon. Clin Podiatr Med Surg 2020;37(3):553–68.

25. Cottom JM, Sisovsky CA. Neglected Achilles tendon ruptures. Clin Podiatr Med Surg 2021;38(2):261–77.

26. Gabel S, Manoli A 2nd. Neglected rupture of the Achilles tendon. Foot Ankle Int 1994;15(9):512–7.
27. Matles AL. Rupture of the tendo Achilles: another diagnostic sign. Bull Hosp Joint Dis 1975;36(1):48–51.
28. Kuwada GT. Classification of tendo Achilles rupture with consideration of surgical repair techniques. J Foot Surg 1990;29(4):361–5.
29. Myerson MS. Achilles tendon ruptures. Instr Course Lect 1999;48:219–30.
30. Yasuda T, Shima H, Mori K, et al. Direct repair of chronic Achilles tendon ruptures using scar tissue located between the tendon stumps. J Bone Joint Surg Am 2016;98(14):1168–75.
31. Cannon LB, Hackney RG. Operative shortening of the elongated defunctioned tendoachillies following previous rupture. J R Nav Med Serv 2003;89(3):139–41.
32. Maffulli N, Spiezia F, Longo UG, et al. Z-shortening of healed, elongated Achilles tendon rupture. Int Orthop 2012;36(10):2087–93.
33. Us AK, Bilgin SS, Aydin T, et al. Repair of neglected Achilles tendon ruptures: procedures and functional results. Arch Orthop Trauma Surg 1997;116:408–11.
34. Guclu B, Basat HC, Yildirim T, et al. Long-term results of chronic Achilles tendon ruptures repaired with V-Y tendon plasty and fascia turndown. Foot Ankle Int 2016;37:737–42.
35. Kissel CG, Blacklidge DK, Crowley DL. Repair of neglected Achilles tendon ruptures–procedure and functional results. J Foot Ankle Surg 1994;33(1):46–52.
36. Wapner KL, Hect PJ, Mills RH Jr. Reconstruction of neglected Achilles tendon injury. Orthop Clin North Am 1995;26(2):249–63.
37. Elias I, Besser M, Nazarian LN, et al. Reconstruction for missed or neglected Achilles tendon rupture with V-Y lengthening and flexor hallucis longus tendon transfer through one incision. Foot Ankle Int 2007;28(12):1238–48.
38. Ofili KP, Pollard JD, Schuberth JM. The neglected Achilles tendon rupture repaired with allograft: a review of 14 cases. J Foot Ankle Surg 2016;55(6):1245–8.
39. Nellas ZJ, Loder BG, Wertheimer SJ. Reconstruction of an Achilles tendon defect utilizing an Achilles tendon allograft. J Foot Ankle Surg 1996;35(2):144–90.
40. Lepow GM, Green JB. Reconstruction of a neglected Achilles tendon rupture with an Achilles tendon allograft: a case report. J Foot Ankle Surg 2006;45(5):351–5.
41. Park YS, Sung KS. Surgical reconstruction of chronic Achilles tendon ruptures using various methods. Orthopedics 2012;35(2):e213–8.
42. Schatzmann L, Brunner P, Staubli HU. Effect of cyclic pre-conditioning on the tensile properties of human quadriceps tendons and patellar ligaments. Knee Surg Sports Traumatol Arthrosc 1998;6(Suppl 1):S56–61.

Application of Biomechanics in Treating the Athlete

The All Important Measurements of Relaxed Calcaneal Stance Position, Achilles Flexibility, and First Ray Range of Motion

Richard L. Blake, DPM, MS

KEYWORDS

- Biomechanics • Heel • Eversion • Inversion • Achilles • Flexibility • Stability
- Examination

KEY POINTS

- Understanding biomechanics can greatly improve your treatment of patient with injuries.
- The relaxed calcaneal stance position is a key measurement of treatment of flat feet and pronation syndromes.
- The Achilles flexibility measurement is key to many lower extremity injuries.
- First ray motion and position can dictate the motion of the lower extremity for both pronatory and supinatory syndromes.

INTRODUCTION

Biomechanics is the study of the forces affecting an individual. Mitigating these forces that are causing harm to our athletes is the purpose of this article. How can you tame these forces with your knowledge of biomechanics to recognize them and treat them? I focus on 3 important measurements from the biomechanical examination we have all been taught in school. The basic biomechanical examination technique has served me well for the last 40 years. It is our foundation to the mechanical treatment of our patients. It is rounded by inflammatory and neuropathic treatments into great treatment successes. A mechanical, inflammatory, and neuropathic approach to the treatment of injuries is extremely successful. The mechanical approach, based on 3 key aspects of our biomechanical examination model, will be presented. Each of these 3 examinations can be vital in my treatment of these athletes. Each positive examination finding,

The author has nothing to disclose.
Orthopedic and Sports Institute, Saint Francis Memorial Hospital, 900 Hyde Street, San Francisco, CA 94109, USA
E-mail address: richard.blake@commonspirit.org

Clin Podiatr Med Surg 40 (2023) 97–115
https://doi.org/10.1016/j.cpm.2022.07.007
0891-8422/23/© 2022 Elsevier Inc. All rights reserved.

when reversed, can be crucial to the injury treatment and future prevention of reoccurrences. Our goal is to find the athlete's weak spots through a biomechanical examination and eliminate them to allow for longer athletic lives.

There are so many factors influencing the human body. Thus, we may feel so overwhelmed that our response is to do nothing and blame everything on a lack of time. We are partially right that time is of the essence in clinical practice. So, we must have a solid plan for the biomechanical analysis of the injured area based on our knowledge of forces. We must ask, "What increases the stress on this particular injured area?" I think if we can evaluate 3 common biomechanical components to an injury, fixing anything we find amiss, we will be way ahead of the game in helping our patients get well. This is my rule of 3. The rule of 3 means that there are typically 3 mechanical changes we can make in any injury that will both help to bring about reversal and prevent of reoccurrences. One common example of this rule of 3 is a patient presenting with running-related big toe joint pain. If we think about what would stress the first metatarsophalangeal joint intrinsically, we then look for these in our biomechanical examination. Commonly, a plantarflexed first ray would have more pressure in this area, a tight Achilles tendon would put more plantigrade force into the metatarsals, and an everted heel would put more medial force on the foot and first metatarsal in particular. This is one common example of how reversing what we find in the biomechanical examination can help our athletes for years to come. This is also the typical pattern to the examination looking for both local problems like the plantarflexed first ray, and more syndromal problems like overpronation and a tight Achilles. The more you understand the local and global forces affecting any problem, the better you will become at helping these athletes.

EVALUATIONS

The 3 evaluations that are crucial to my sports medicine practice are:

- Relaxed calcaneal stance position (RSCP)
- Achilles flexibility
- First ray range of motion

These 3 measurements are without doubt the 3 measurements I find the most useful in my day-to-day practice of sports medicine and biomechanics. Of course, I do a complete biomechanical examination at times, and, of course, most of the examinations I was taught help me to discover important clues in my diagnostic evaluation of a patient. Biomechanics actually slows you down in a very good way in the rush of modern medicine. Biomechanical findings that you can change, and educate the patient on, will help the patient for many years. The emphasis is on the measurements that I find can be easily treated and improvement can be seen. Treatment can be as simple of a varus wedge for everted heels, a valgus wedge for inverted heels, Achilles stretching for tightness, Achilles strengthening for overflexibility, Morton's extensions for metatarsus primus elevatus, or reverse Morton's (dancer's pads) for plantar flexed first rays. Measure and you will find. Do not measure and you will miss an incredible part of patient care and treatment successes.

Relaxed Calcaneal Stance Position

I start my discussion with the RCSP, heralded by Dr Ronald Valmassy as the most crucial measurement for overpronation in children's feet. In our athletes, the RCSP will document overall pronation tendencies. We will also find that asymmetrical pronation (much more everted heel for example on 1 side) makes 1 side of the body more susceptible to injury then the other side. So, let us first go over the examination.[1–3]

Always start a biomechanical examination with the patient standing in front of you both looking toward you and away from you. Observe any alignment issues, like flat feet, high arches, tibial varum or valgum, and genu varum or valgum, to name a few. In **Fig. 1**, the severe everted heels of this young patient demonstrates the RCSP at one end of the spectrum (severely pronated).

When using the RCSP on a routine basis, you can get a strong correlation between symptoms and pronation when the heel is everted past vertical, and by how much. The only severe pronators with a vertical or inverted heel in RCSP are the patients with severe tibial varum functioning maximally pronated but not everted. I have found that excessive pronation, caused by many factors, causes a myriad of symptoms that bring athletes into the office. The 27 pronation produced problems (part of the pronation syndrome) are: first metatarsophalangeal joint pain, sesamoid pain, bunions, second metatarsophalangeal joint pain, metatarsalgia, second metatarsal stress fractures, Morton's neuroma/neuritis, hammertoes, intrinsic muscle strain, plantar fasciitis, anterior tibial strain, sinus tarsi syndrome, cuboid syndrome, lateral ankle impingement, posterior tibial strain, tarsal tunnel syndrome, peroneus longus strain, Achilles strain, tibial stress fractures, medial soleus strain, lateral knee compartment pain, pes anserinus tendinitis or bursitis, patellofemoral pain, anterior cruciate ligament support when injured, medial hamstring strain, iliotibial band strain, piriformis syndrome, and some low back issues.[4] Here again, the excess pronation unearths the patient's other weak spots, and the treatment of the excess pronation helps the patient's symptoms. This is the way you learn to correlate pronation and symptoms in the real world by seeing how controlling the pronation helps their symptoms.[5]

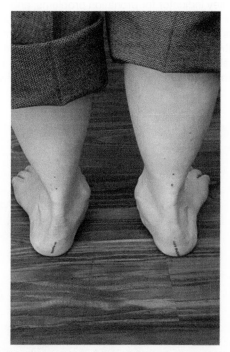

Fig. 1. Severely everted or pronated heels in a child with congenital flat feet. After age 8, according to Dr Ronald Valmassy, the heels should be vertical (within 2°) in normal development.

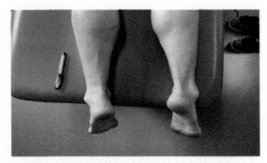

Fig. 2. We start the measurement of RCSP with the patient prone.

Excessive supination tendencies, also documented at times by the RCSP denoting inverted heels (or attached to high degrees of tibial varum), can cause 17 supination produced problems, called the supination syndrome. These supination produced problems are: hammertoes, lateral metatarsalgia, tailor's bunions, fourth or fifth metatarsal stress fractures, cuboid pain, lateral ankle instability, peroneal strain, Haglund's deformity, medial ankle impingement, fibular stress fractures, proximal tibia–fibula sprain, medial knee compartment issues, knee arthralgias, lateral knee collateral ligament sprain, lateral hamstring strain, iliotibial band syndrome, femoral stress fractures, hip arthralgias, sacroiliac joint pain, and low back pain. Again, treatment of the excessive supination, called underpronation or lateral instability or oversupination, brings these symptoms under control (**Figs. 2–6**).

Not only is RCSP a key indicator for pronation problems, and a very important part of the assessment for supination problems, but it is also important for discovering asymmetrical findings vital in treatment management. With most patients having 0° to 4° inverted neutral heel positioning (owing to a slight tibial varum), the farther away from this neutrality, the more symptoms occur owing to mechanical irritation of joints or strain in tendons attempting to center the heel. Why? It has to do with

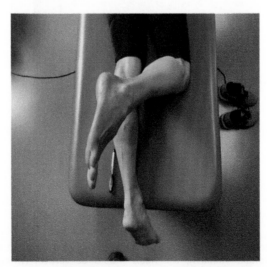

Fig. 3. Then you cross the opposite leg over to center the heel parallel with your eyes.

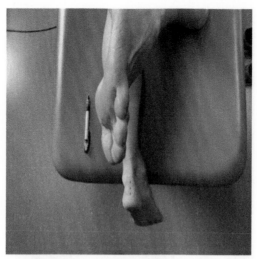

Fig. 4. Then the posterior surface of the heel is bisected at 3 points and a bisection line connects them.

both making the body stable or aligned or both. The stability that I attempt most frequently is a heel that sits vertical to 2° inverted in RCSP on my orthotic device. This heel is aligned under the leg and knee well, and the body's musculature does not have to strain to get it here. Can you see the work needed in obtaining this position in a patient who presents with posterior tibial strain and 5° everted on one side and 10° everted on the other? Can you understand which side would develop posterior tibial strain easiest?

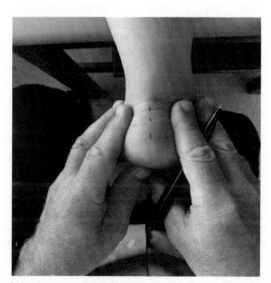

Fig. 5. A closeup of the bisection by palpating the medial and lateral borders at 3 spots. Typically heel borders diverge as they go distal.

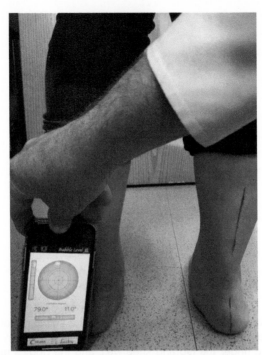

Fig. 6. I currently use an app called Bubble Level XL, after standing the patient up, to measure the RCSP. In this particular case, the left heel is reading 11° everted in extreme pronation (heel valgus).

Achilles Flexibility Evaluation

Now, we want to direct our focus on the Achilles tendon. I need not emphasize the vital function of this tendon to the well-being of our athletes. However, when the tendon gets too tight or too loose, terrible things happen to our biomechanics and to the tendon itself. The common problems with the equinus forces produced by a tight Achilles tendon are overuse of the Achilles tendon, hyperextension or excessive flexion of the knee joint, overuse of the other muscles around the ankle that help with ankle plantarflexion, excessive midfoot overload, excessive plantigrade forces on the metatarsals, excessive supination gait in propulsion, and the entire pronation syndrome. The methods of compensation will vary according to the individual patient and some can be observed in gait evaluation. The common problems seen in an Achilles tendon that is too flexible (considered extremely weak) are overuse of the Achilles tendon easily, hyperextension of the knee joint, anterior ankle impingement, and overuse of the other ankle muscles that help with plantarflexion of the ankle. Our reliable nonweightbearing Achilles tendon measurements are the gold standard to the identification and treatment of this problem.[6–8] I have summarized the examination in **Figs. 7–13**.

Understanding the effects of tight or overly flexible Achilles tendons is the key to the understanding of so many lower extremity problems. The RCSP measurement and the Achilles flexibility measurement are the 2 most important measurements you must learn, master, and develop plans to improve your abnormal findings. First of all, a tight Achilles (less than 10°–12° with the knee straight for the gastrocnemius, and less than 15°–18° with the knee bent for the soleus) has both constant and variable

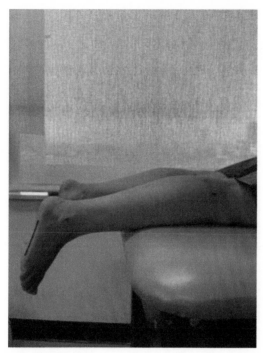

Fig. 7. We start by lying the patient in a prone position. When we measure the Achilles tendon, our reference points are the lateral side of the heel and fifth metatarsal to the bisection of the lateral malleolus to the head of the fibula.

components. The constant components of a tight Achilles are the inherent weakness of the Achilles that will strain more easily, and the increased forces on the midfoot and metatarsals causing or aggravating problems in those areas. The variable components of a tight Achilles are based on how the body choses to compensate to move weight forward. Will you excessively pronate, and thus develop pronation based symptoms? Will you have an early heel off, thus intensifying the midfoot or metatarsal symptoms? Will you have excessive out toe gait, which will torque the ankle, knee, and hip excessively? Will you develop genu recurvatum and destroy your knees?

If you measure an overly flexible Achilles tendon, you are surely seeing a very weak tendon that will strain very easily in the pursuit of sports. That weakness demands that other muscles and tendons help as the athlete attempts various activities. Therefore, weakness in the Achilles tendon, measured as overly flexible ($>13°$ with the knee straight and $>18°$ with the knee bent), can lead to strain of all of the other muscles that can help in its various functions. What does the Achilles do in gait? It plantar flexes the ankle. It helps to flex the knee with the gastrocnemius. It helps to supinate the foot (subtalar joint) in midstance and propulsion. It protects the front of the knee and ankle with its posterior balancing force. Therefore, when you measure overflexibility in the Achilles tendon, the symptoms can be to all the muscles that plantar flex the ankle—Achilles, peroneals, and posterior tibial or long flexors—and the symptoms can be to the popliteus or hamstrings that flex the knee, the symptoms can be part of the pronation syndrome foot to low back, and the symptoms can be anterior knee and ankle owing to loss of posterior joint protection. Always make your patients with an overly flexible Achilles tendon stop all their Achilles stretching, analyze all their

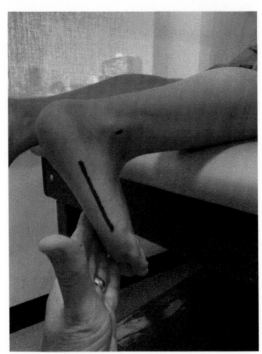

Fig. 8. It is important to slightly load the medial aspect of the foot to avoid pronating the subtalar joint while dorsiflexing the ankle after placing the subtalar joint in neutral.

activities that over dorsiflex the ankle, and develop a consistent Achilles strengthening program with double and single heel raises each evening.

First Ray Range of Motion

Let us finish our discussion by looking at our measurement of the first ray.[9,10] It is such a key measurement owing to its position at the distal end of the medial column. It needs to stabilize that medial corner of the foot (which it can not do if too elevated, called metatarsus primus elevatus) or else a cascade of pronatory issues occur all the way up the lower extremity chain[11] and/or the motion of the foot forward is blocked.[12] And, if it is too plantar flexed, it can cause a cascade of supinatory issues to occur also up the lower extremity.[13] We seek as the ideal a first metatarsal excursion of 5 to 6 mm up and 5 to 6 mm down to the stable second metatarsal head as a reference point.[14] When we are discussing first ray mechanics, why are we just focusing on the sagittal plane motion of one bone? The first ray is a complexed relationship of the navicular, first cuneiform, and first metatarsal. Yet, it is the final position of that first metatarsal in midstance that dictates normality or abnormalities in terms of the motion of the entire chain. We must reflect on the observations started by Dr Dudley Morton so many years before in discovering this significance[15] (**Figs. 14–19**).

I remember as podiatry students we all measured our thumb thickness with slight compression of the pulp. I was so happy to be approximately 10 mm, but some were 7 mm or 5 mm, and some were 11 or 12 mm. You quickly got a good idea how much excursion occurred. It served as a vital tool for surgical issues (like how would a distal metatarsal osteotomy affect the foot with its inherent metatarsal

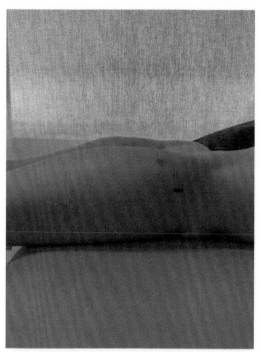

Fig. 9. It is crucial to bisect both the lateral malleolus and the head of the fibula. Also, as you dorsiflex the ankle, observe any hyperextension at the knee. This hyperextension should not occur, but may in severe equinus situations.

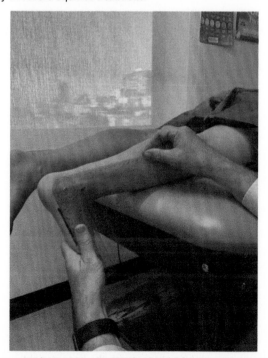

Fig. 10. It is important to have your eyes at the level of the measurement.

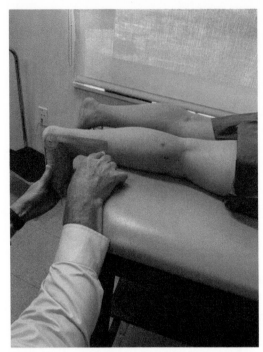

Fig. 11. My office has one-time-use paper shorts for this purpose. You must clearly be able to see the entire measurement. After dorsiflexing the ankle, ask the patient to help you while you make sure that the foot does not pronate.

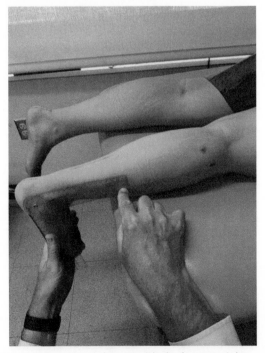

Fig. 12. Measure the gastrocnemius tightness with the knee straight.

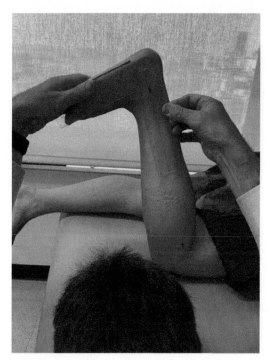

Fig. 13. Measure the soleus tightness with the knee bent.

shortening and elevating, or does the patient need a Morton's extension to help them to pronate less?).

The instabilities caused by an elevated (metatarsus primus elevatus) or plantigrade (plantarflexed first ray) are immense and so easily remedied by mechanical treatments. As I talked about the general rule of 3, it typically takes 3 issues colliding together to cause a patient to get injured in the first place, or have trouble rehabilitating. What is the biomechanical rule of 3 for sesamoid issues, or general big toe joint pain? Think about what causes stress on the tissue always. Typically, the stresses on the big toe joint are excessive pronation, a tight Achilles, and plantar flexed first rays. But, if you know mechanics, you could also say an everted RCSP, tight or weak Achilles tendons, and a plantigrade or dorsal grade first metatarsal head. "Think mechanics over angles" is the mantra that Dr Kevin Kirby taught me. Think about forces.

Therefore, when we measure the first ray motion, we are going to come up with findings summarized in the **Table 1** to discuss. Each of these findings will have a slightly different effect on the biomechanics. Normal motion and position means 5 to 6 mm dorsal excursion and 5 to 6 mm plantigrade excursion. Normal motion yet elevated means that the overall 10 to 12 mm of excursion is more dorsal than plantigrade. Limited motion but normal position means less than 10 mm overall motion, but equal up and down. Limited motion and elevated means less than 10 mm overall motion, and more dorsal than plantigrade motion. Excessive motion but normal position means more than 12 mm of overall excursion, but equal up and down.

CASE REPORT USING A TYPICAL 14-POINT BIOMECHANICAL APPROACH

History and chief complaint

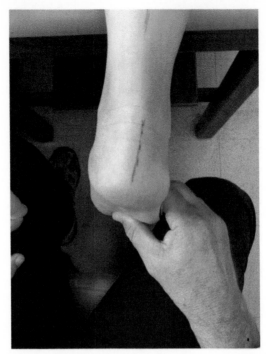

Fig. 14. The measurement of the first ray range of motion starts with placing the subtalar joint in neutral and grabbing the second metatarsal head from top to bottom. Your thumb should be parallel to the metatarsal alignment seen. The second metatarsal will not move during this measurement as it is your reference point.

- While training for his first Ironman Triathlon in Kona, Hawaii, this 40-year-old man began developing bilateral Achilles soreness with the right much worse than the left.
- He had participated in several half Ironman in his 30s and had taken a year off work to train for this event.
- The pain started while doing swimming laps with long fins, but had gradually progressed into his running.
- Only cycling was nonpainful at the time of the office visit, although he was trying to stay on the seat and not do too much hill work.
- One week before the visit, he noticed pain walking, and he has had morning soreness from day 1 arising from bed.
- There does not seem to be swelling by history.
- If he tries to run, the soreness comes on at the 2-mile mark and just gets worse.
- However, he can walk for 3 to 5 miles without any soreness.
- He reports definite bouts of Achilles issues in the past, which were always easy to pass through with icing, limited rest, and stretching.

Gait evaluation

- Limping slightly after sitting in the office, but this disappeared quickly.
- Running shoes were zero drop Altra Olympus.
- Moderate overpronation right greater than left (he was right handed) also worse running versus walking.

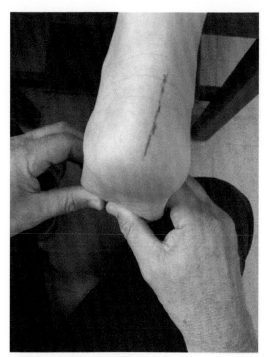

Fig. 15. The first metatarsal head is then palpated from top to bottom with the 2 plantar thumbs parallel.

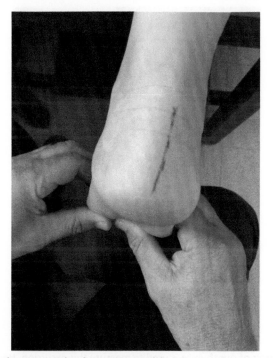

Fig. 16. Here the fingers on the first metatarsal head move the metatarsal plantigrade. without any movement of the second metatarsal.

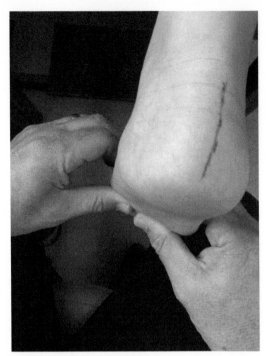

Fig. 17. Here the fingers on the first metatarsal move the metatarsal dorsally without any motion of the second metatarsal.

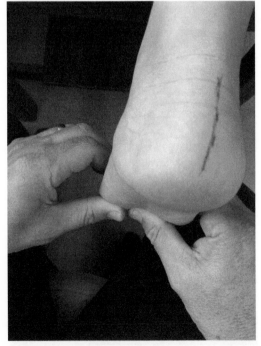

Fig. 18. The thickness of our thumbs is used to measure this excursion. Here .an 8-mm plantigrade motion is measured in the downward direction.

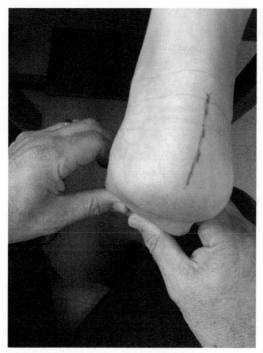

Fig. 19. There are 10 mm of dorsal motion in the upward direction.

- Slight limb dominance to right (opposite of what you expect with favoring of his much sorer right side).
- Greater internal patella rotation also right.

Physical examination

- Palpably sore in the zone of ischemia 2 to 5 cm above the Achilles attachment, right greater than left.
- Only the right side was swollen.
- No Achilles tightness noted.
- Could easily do single heel raises 2 position but only tested to 5 owing to bilateral soreness.

Cursory biomechanical examination and asymmetry noted

- Limb dominance right with ⅜-inch longer right leg.
- RCSP 8 everted right and 2 everted left.
- Ankle joint dorsiflexion right side 17° knee straight and 28° knee bent with left side 14° knee straight and 20° knee bent.
- Weak external hip rotators on both sides.
- Forefoot varus 12° right and 7° left.
- First ray range of motion 3° down 7° up right and 2° down 9° up left.

Tentative working diagnosis

- Right greater than left Achilles tendonitis with right greater than left over pronation.

Common differential diagnosis (secondary working diagnosis)

- Right Achilles tendinosis suspected.

Occam's razor and rule of 3

Table 1		
Findings commonly seen in first ray range of motion examination		
Normal motion and position	Normal motion yet elevated	Normal motion yet plantigrade
Limited motion but normal position	Limited motion and elevated	Limited motion and plantigrade
Excessive motion but normal position	Excessive motion and elevated	Excessive motion and plantigrade

- Simplest solution (Occam's razor) is to emphasize Achilles strengthening since already too flexible (normal ankle joint dorsiflexion 10°–15°).
- Rule of 3 looks deeper into the biomechanics of the stresses on the Achilles. The obvious changes are no fins during swimming owing to the torque on the Achilles, change to traditional running shoes with 14-mm heel drop and add heel lifts ($\frac{1}{4}$ inch), and begin to correct the over pronation (owing to the patient's athletic goal custom orthotic devices to be made with varus canting and Morton's extensions).

What phase of rehabilitation?

- Restrengthening (no need to immobilize and not ready to run as part of return to activity).

Should we image?

- Getting an MRI now for the swollen right Achilles makes sense owing to the patient's athletic goal.

First decision: How to reduce pain to 0 to 2

- Physical therapy could be started right now to begin to bring down the inflammation.
- Ice massage 5 minutes to each Achilles 3 times a day.
- No barefoot as stay in elevated heeled shoes as much as possible (recommended Dansko clogs for a house slipper).
- Cycling should not be increased, swimming with limited foot kicking or buoy between ankles, no running for now, and limited walking (consider a cam walker for walking if the pain over 0–2).

Second decision: Inflammation concerns

- Ice, physical therapy, and nonsteroidal anti-inflammatory drugs.

Third decision: Any nerve component?

- Not apparent.

Fourth decision: Initial mechanical changes

- Started the patient with two $\frac{1}{4}$-inch heel lifts and told him to switch shoes to Brooks Beast for higher heel and pronation control.
- An extra $\frac{1}{8}$-inch sulcus length lift given to the short left leg.
- Added Morton's extensions to shoe insert for medial support.
- Start with 2-sided toe raises to get a baseline of how many he can do before pain starts.
- Achilles taping was to be taught by the physical therapist with KinesioTape, and probably advanced in tension to Leukotape.
- Patient told to schedule for orthotic casting as varus canting to be incorporated into custom inserts.

Common mechanical changes typically used for Achilles tendon injuries

1. Cam walker.
2. Stretching for both gastrocnemius and soleus.

3. Strengthening for both gastrocnemius and soleus.
4. Heel lifts to take some pressure off the tendon.
5. Athletic shoes with heel elevation if possible.
6. Avoid negative heel positioning and stretching (where the heel is lower than the front of the foot).
7. Correction of varus or valgus heel positioning if present.
8. Taping to support the Achilles.
9. Rigid ankle–foot orthosis.

Luckily for this athlete, the MRI was negative for any acute tears, but the right Achilles was thicker than normal indicating repeated stress on the Achilles (tendinosis). The physical therapy and biomechanical changes helped to ease the stress on the Achilles. Just before the triathlon, in which he both competed and completed in 2014, he remained overly flexible in the Achilles, although improved. The progression of the treatment was:

1. Work on strength, biomechanics, and inflammation during the first 2 months (during this time both modified cycling and swimming allowed).
2. During the next 2 months, the strength gains continued and a walk–run program was initiated.
3. During the final 2 months, his running progressed to 8 to 9 miles with taping. Amazingly, at the time of the Ironman, he completed the 26.2 miles without Achilles pain, only extreme fatigue.
4. An important point during these 6 months: he was never allowed to push the pain over 0 to 2 to ensure safe progression, even when he thought he was not progressing fast enough.
5. Another very important point is that it was safe to dispense a 35° inverted right orthotic device and a 15° inverted left orthotic device because he was not running at the time, he was just restarting his running program (it would be dangerous to dispense corrective orthotic devices at a time he was increasing his running). These gave me almost complete correction of his heel valgus.

Table 2
Common injuries and corresponding biomechanics

Injury Seen	Biomechanics Discovered
Chondromalacia patellae	Everted RCSP, metatarsus primus elevatus
Shin splints (medial)	Everted RCSP, metatarsus primus elevatus, tight Achilles tendons
Achilles tendonitis	Everted RCSP, tight or over flexible Achilles tendons
Plantar fasciitis	Tight Achilles tendons
Posterior tibial tendonitis	Everted RCSP, metatarsus primus elevatus, weak Achilles tendons
Lateral ankle impingement	Everted RCSP
Metatarsal stress fractures	metatarsus primus elevatus, tight Achilles tendons
Morton's neuroma	Everted RCSP, metatarsus primus elevatus, tight Achilles tendons
Sesamoid injuries	Everted RCSP, plantar flexed first ray, tight Achilles tendons
Hallux limitus/rigidus problems	Everted RCSP, metatarsus primus elevatus, tight Achilles tendons

SUMMARY

I finish this article with a summary of the top sports medicine injuries commonly seen by podiatrists and their association with these 3 (easy to learn and master) examination findings (and a few others). The key is to master them by practice, so that you develop your skills and consistency in measurement. You measure it, change it if needed, and see how the patient responds. The key is that you know how to treat the abnormalities you find. If not, the measurements will help little in your understanding of the patient.

Table 2 demonstrates typical biomechanical findings when related to the injuries seen. It summarized the injuries caused by a biomechanical fault, which leads to more stress in the injured area, or at least aggravating the problem. Look at **Table 2** and think about the biomechanics and the injury. Try to correlate what the examination finding is implying. Remember, when a biomechanical finding can be treated or normalized, treatment of the correlating injury can occur. Treatment of biomechanics is much more than acute injury treatments. Biomechanical treatment implies speed of rehabilitation and prevention of future reoccurrences. The patient should leave your practice with a better understanding of why they got injured and how this and other injuries can be prevented in the future.

CLINICS CARE POINTS

- RCSP is the only significant measurement for documenting positive changes in children's flat feet.
- Achilles tightness can be documented to local Achilles and plantar fascial problems.
- Achilles overflexibility is not well-documented.
- First ray motion or position is not well-documented.

REFERENCES

1. Sobel E, Levitz S, Caselli M, et al. Reevaluation of the relaxed calcaneal stance position. Reliability and normal values in children and adults. J Am Podiatr Med Assoc 1999;89(5):258–64.
2. Cho Y, Park JW, Nam K. The relationship between foot posture index and resting calcaneal stance position in elementary school students. Gait Posture 2019;74: 142–7.
3. Valmassy RL. Clinical biomechanics of the lower extremities. St. Louis, Missouri: Mosby-Year Book, Inc; 1996. p. 248–9.
4. Pinto R, Souza T, Trede R, et al. Bilateral and unilateral increases in calcaneal eversion affect pelvic alignment in standing position. Man Ther 2008;13(6):513–9.
5. Cheung R, Chung R, Ng G. Efficacies of different external controls for excessive foot pronation: a meta-analysis. Br J Sports Med 2012;46(5):373.
6. Root ML, Orien WP, Weed JH. Clinical Biomech II, Normal and Abnormal Function of the Foot 1977. p. 37–40.
7. Gastwirth BW. Biomechanical examination of the foot and lower extremity. In: Valmassy, Ronald, editors. Clinical biomechanics of the lower extremities. St. Louis, Missouri: Mosby-Year Book, Inc; 1996. p. 136–7.
8. Kirby KA. Foot and lower extremity biomechanics II: precision intricast newsletters, 1997-2002, Precision Intricast, Inc, Payson (AZ): 2003; p. 81–2.

9. Root ML, Orien WP, Weed JH. Clinical Biomech II, Normal and Abnormal Function of the Foot 1977. p. 48–50.
10. Gastwirth BW. Biomechanical examination of the foot and lower extremity. In: Valmassy Ronald, editor. Clinical biomechanics of the lower extremities. St. Louis, Missouri: Mosby-Year Book, Inc.; 1996. p. 137–8.
11. Kirby KA. Foot and lower extremity biomechanics III: precision intricast newsletters, 2009-13, Precision Intricast, Inc, Payson (AZ): 2014. p. 41–42.
12. Van Gheluwe B, Dananberg H, Hagman F, et al. Effects of hallux limitus on plantar foot pressure and foot kinematics during walking. J Am Podiatr Med Assoc 2006; 96(5):428–36.
13. Root ML, Orien WP, Weed JH. Clinical Biomech II, Normal and Abnormal Function of the Foot 1977. p. 344–5.
14. Tavara-Vidalón S, Monge-Vera M, Lafuente-Sotillos G, et al. Static range of motion of the first metatarsal in the sagittal and frontal planes. J Clin Med 2018;7(11):456.
15. Glasoe W, Coughlin M. A critical analysis of Dudley Morton's concept of disordered foot function. J Foot Ankle Surg 2006;45(3):147–55.

Acute Ankle Sprains

Zachary Kramer, DPM, AT[a], Yessika Woo Lee, DPM[b],*,
Ryan Sherrick, DPM[c]

KEYWORDS

- Lateral ankle sprains • Acute sprain • High ankle sprains
- Syndesmotic ankle sprains

KEY POINTS

- This article has a clinical focus and may provide support for all health care professionals encountering patients with an acute ankle sprain.
- An acute ankle sprain is a common injury that often presents in the form of an acute lateral ankle sprain or a high ankle sprain.
- The Ottawa ankle rules provide guidance in the emergency department as to whether radiographs are necessary or can be deferred.
- We hoped to provide a useful guide to identifying and treating ankle sprains appropriately.

Abbreviations	
ALAS	Acute Lateral Ankle Sprain
ROM	Range of Motion
BMI	Body Mass Index
ATFL	Anterior Tibiofibular Ligament
CFL	Calcaneofibular Ligament
TCN	Talocalcaneonavicular
PRP	platelet-rich plasma
OCD	Osteochondral defects
AITFL	Anterior inferior tibiofibular ligament
PITFL	Posterior inferior tibiofibular ligament
TFCS	tibiofibular clear space
TFO	tibiofibular overlap

[a] Scripps Memorial Hospital, 310 Santa Fe Drive #112, Encinitas, CA 92024, USA; [b] Dignity Health, St. Mary's Medical Center, 450 Stanyan Street, San Francisco, CA 94117, USA; [c] Foot & Ankle Surgery, Innovative Medical Solutions Foot & Ankle Institute, 2080 Century Park East, STE 710, Los Angeles, CA 90067, USA
* Corresponding author.
E-mail address: yw9250@gmail.com

Clin Podiatr Med Surg 40 (2023) 117–138
https://doi.org/10.1016/j.cpm.2022.07.008
0891-8422/23/© 2022 Elsevier Inc. All rights reserved.

podiatric.theclinics.com

INTRODUCTION

Ankle sprains are among the most common injuries experienced by athletes accounting for 20% of all sports injuries in the United States.[1-4] In a period of five years an estimated 3,140,132 ankle sprains occurred for an incidence rate of 2.15 per 1000 person-years in the United States.[5] Doherty and colleagues[6] pooled data from prospective studies, reporting a cumulative incidence rate of 11.5 ankle sprains/1000 exposures and a prevalence of 11.8%. Acute ankle sprain was most common in individuals aged 10 to 19 years. Males aged 15 to 24 years sustained more ankle sprains than females in the same age range, but women older than 30 years sustained more sprains than their male counterparts.[6] Understanding the types of ankle sprain, lateral ankle sprains, medial ankle sprains, high "syndesmotic" ankle sprains, is essential in determining the most appropriate treatment and preventing substantial missed time from sports. Most commonly known and recognized is an acute lateral ankle sprain (ALAS), however, a differentiation should also be made to understand high (syndesmotic) ankle sprains as the mechanism of injury and recovery periods differ between these two types.

ALAS are the most common type of ankle sprain, frequently a result of an inversion and adduction of the foot in plantar flexion (supination). This mechanism of injury can cause damage to the lateral ankle ligaments.[7] Injury of the anterior talofibular ligament with intact medial ligaments leads to anterolateral rotary instability.[6] Additional transection of the calcaneofibular ligament adds a tilting of the talus, also known as a talar tilt.[6] In contrast, syndesmotic ankle sprains, or "high ankle" sprains, typically result from ankle dorsiflexion and foot external rotation.[8,9] In the athletic population, this is often seen in basketball, football, downhill skiing, and other field sports.[9,10] In addition, high ankle sprains have longer recovery periods, averaging 13.9 days compared with 8.1 days for lateral ankle sprains and 10.7 days for medial ankle sprains.[9]

Ankle ligament sprains are usually graded on the basis of severity. The grades assist the physician in determining the best treatment options for each patient[6] (**Table 1**). Grade I (mild) is a mild stretching of the ligaments without macroscopic rupture or joint instability. Grade II (moderate) is a partial rupture of the ligament with moderate pain and swelling. There are functional limitations and some slight to moderate instability. Typically, patients present with problems in weight bearing.[11] Grade III (severe) is a complete ligament rupture with marked pain, swelling, and hematoma. In grade III injuries, there is a significant impairment of function with instability.[11] In ALAS, classification of the ALAS in combination with a keen understanding of biological ligament healing can provide the physician with the necessary tools for successful treatment.

Biological ligament healing can be divided into three different phases: (1) the inflammatory phase (up to 10 days after trauma), (2) the proliferation phase (4th–8th week), and (3) the remodeling or maturation phase (up to 1 year after trauma).[7] The duration of the different phases may individually vary. Many treatment options have been

Table 1
Grading of ankle sprains

Ankle Sprain Grade	
Grade I	Mild stretching of the ligaments without macroscopic rupture or joint instability
Grade II	Partial rupture of the ligament with moderate pain and swelling
Grade III	Complete ligament rupture with marked pain, swelling, and hematoma

suggested: surgery, immobilization, functional treatment with bandages, tape, or different braces, balance training, or physical therapy.

Many studies have shown that ankle sprains are more serious than commonly believed since many patients develop chronic problems after injury.[12–14] The symptoms include chronic pain, recurrent swelling, and chronic instability.[12,13] Interestingly, Malliaropoulos found that low-grade ALAS result in a higher risk of reinjury than high-grade ALAS.[15] The high rate of failure after ankle sprain treatment might be explained by overlooked associated lesions, such as syndesmosis, peroneal tendon, or cartilage injuries.[6] In addition, there is strong evidence that within 1 year after injury, athletes have twice the risk of a recurrent ankle sprain.[16] Lingering symptoms, such as instability and pain, can impede or preclude a return to play. Therefore, proper initial management and detection of concomitant injuries minimizes the risk of long-term morbidity and speeds the resumption of athletic participation. The purpose of this article is to provide up-to-date treatment recommendations and current concepts for acute lateral and syndesmotic ankle sprains in the athletic population, ideally allowing the physician the ability to formulate a logical, and organized approach to treating these injuries and facilitate a patient's return to sport.

ACUTE LATERAL ANKLE SPRAINS
Predisposing Factors to Lateral Ankle Sprains in Athletes

Predisposing factors are defined as factors that increase the risk of sustaining an ALAS. Risk factors for ALAS can be classified as either intrinsic (patient-related factors, eg, proprioception) or extrinsic (eg, sports or environmental characteristics). A vital aspect that should be considered by clinicians when addressing predisposing factors is whether they can be modified or not. Modifiable risk factors may be targeted by preventive treatment.

Intrinsic risk factors

There are a number of intrinsic risk factors that substantially heighten the risk of sustaining an ALAS. These include limited dorsiflexion range of motion (ROM), reduced proprioception, and (preseason deficiencies in postural control/balance).[7] In addition, other modifiable risk factors which heighten the risk of sustaining an ALAS include body mass index (BMI) and high medial plantar pressures during running.[7] In regards to BMI, included results are conflicting as to whether a higher or lower BMI increases the risk of incurring an ALAS. A recent meta-analysis showed a greater risk of sprains in patients with a higher BMI.[7] Additional factors that may contribute to an increased risk are reduced strength, coordination, cardiorespiratory endurance, limited overall ankle joint ROM, and decreased peroneal reaction time.[17] Concerning nonmodifiable risk factors, females have a higher risk of sustaining an ALAS compared with males.[18] Additional factors correlated to an increased risk of sustaining an ALAS are physical characteristics, such as greater height, ankle joint configuration, foot posture index, and anatomical abnormalities in ankle and knee alignment.[18] As a result, several recent consensus statements and studies have advocated for treating patients with an ALAS by identifying any modifiable risk factors, such as deficiencies in proprioception and ROM, and including them in a prevention and/or rehabilitation program to reduce the risk of recurrent sprains.[18]

Another intrinsic factor that must be considered with chronic ankle sprains is the cavus foot type. Cavovarus deformity is more frequent in patients with chronic lateral ankle instability than in controls,[19] and it has been reported that up to 28% of recurrent sprains have some hindfoot varus alignment abnormalities.[20] It has been noted that a cavovarus position places lateral ankle soft-tissue structures on stretch during weight bearing and ambulation.[21] This leads to additional forces on the lateral ankle ligaments and, therefore, may perpetuate lateral ankle instability. If this cavus foot type is left undiagnosed or untreated, athletes may experience recurrent lateral ankle sprains.

Extrinsic risk factors

Despite a patient's wish to remain in a sport, the main modifiable extrinsic risk factor for ALAS appears to be the type of sport practiced. The highest incidence of ALAS was found for basketball, indoor volleyball, field sports, and climbing.[22,23]

The incidence of ALAS was dependent on the level of participation.[3] In volleyball, landing after a jump is the most important risk factor. Playing soccer on natural grass [vs artificial turf, as well as being a defender (42.3% of all sprains)] increased the incidence of ALAS.[7] Concerning shoe wear, high heels (9.5 vs 1.3 cm) heighten the risk of incurring an ALAS.[24] The only nonmodifiable factor was sex. Despite women having an increased risk of ALAS compared with men, the in-competition risk for ALAS is higher in men compared with women.[3]

Extrinsic risk factors, although outside of the patient, may provide a significant increase in the risk of sustaining an ALAS. Health care professionals involved in treating patients who sustain an ALAS should take notice especially of the type of sport practiced but also of other extrinsic risk factors, as modifications may lower the risk at future sprains and other ankle injuries.

Physical Examination

Successful treatment of an ALAS begins with a careful history and meticulous physical examination. The time since the injury, the ability to tolerate weight bearing, whether the injury is improving, and whether there have been previous sprains of the same ankle are all important components of the history. The physical examination should document the location and severity of swelling and ecchymosis. After an acute lateral ankle ligament injury, swelling, ecchymosis, and tenderness are usually noted over the anterior tibiofibular ligmaent (ATFL) and calcaneofibular ligament (CFL) in the region just anterior and distal to the tip of the fibula. However, tenderness should be checked over several different structures to look for signs that could implicate an alternative or concomitant diagnosis. Laterally, the distal syndesmosis, lateral malleolus, peroneal tendons, fifth metatarsal, anterior process of the calcaneus, and lateral process of the talus should be palpated in addition to the lateral ligament complex comprised of the anterior talofibular, calcaneofibular, and posterior talofibular ligaments. Medially, the medial malleolus, deltoid ligament, sustentaculum tali, and navicular should be examined and assessed for tenderness. Routine palpation of the Achilles tendon, tibialis anterior tendon, and midfoot articulations should also be included; injury to these structures is sometimes neglected when a diagnosis of ankle sprain is presumed. Manual muscle testing is also performed despite the effects of acute swelling and pain to verify the continuity of these structures and to aid in the detection of acute peroneal dislocation. Resistance to inversion with the ankle in a dorsiflexed everted position and circumduction of the ankle are used to improve the sensitivity of detecting peroneal dislocation. Despite the use of a careful physical examination, many findings can still be obscured by diffuse swelling and poorly localized tenderness during the first 10 to 14 days after an acute ankle inversion injury. As a result, it is important to repeat the examination 10 to 14 days later, when the findings will be more specific and revealing.[25]

Instability tests, such as the anterior drawer and talar tilt tests generally do not have a significant role in the evaluation of an acute ankle sprain. With an acute injury, the ankle is often too swollen and uncomfortable to allow an unguarded and accurate assessment of stability. The results of these tests generally do not affect the initial treatment of an acute sprain, and they should be reserved for evaluating chronic ankle instability (CAI).[25]

Evaluation for cavus foot type is also of the utmost importance when an athlete presents with a lateral ankle sprain. Initial assessment begins with a gait examination for the presence of altered gait, varus heel or obvious elevation in the medial column. In addition, a "peek-a-boo heel" has been described as another measure to assess if a varus heel exists. With this assessment, if the medial aspect of the heel cannot be seen, then it is plausible that the patient has a neutral or valgus-positioned heel. In patients who have significant heel varus, the medial heel is clearly visible.[26] The Coleman block test is also a simple test for the determination of a flexible versus rigid cavovarus foot type.[27]

Subtalar joint involvement is frequently neglected when assessing lateral ankle instability. Approximately 25% of subtalar instability is also present with an associated lateral ankle instability.[28] There is great difficulty in differentiating between acute lateral ankle instability and subtalar joint instability, though.[29] The CFL, interosseous talocalcaneal ligament, portions of the deltoid ligament, and the ligaments surrounding the talocalcaneonavicular (TCN) joint all play a role in subtalar joint instability.[28] Given this, a thorough examination of the subtalar joint and a high level of clinical suspicion are required to make an accurate diagnosis. Frequently, subtalar joint instability has similar symptoms as demonstrated in ALAS.[28,29] Unlike ALAS, though, athletes with subtalar instability may have persistent sinus tarsi symptoms and lateral hind foot pain.[30,31] These athletes frequently report a sense of instability, including a feeling of the ankle "giving way" or "rolling over."[29] The anterolateral drawer test is a specific clinical examination in the setting of subtalar instability. With this assessment, the hind foot is held by the physician in maximum dorsiflexion. This prevents inadvertent motion at the ankle level. Then a combination of inversion, internal rotation, and adduction stress is applied to the forefoot.[28,30] A positive test demonstrates an increased anterior and medial translation in addition to a varus tilt of the calcaneus under the talus. A radiographic stress examination may also be beneficial in identifying subtalar instability.[29] A lateral stress test can also be used to check for subtalar instability (Fig. 1A–C). In this case, you can radiographically demonstrate anterior translation of the calcaneus on the talus. Despite it being an underdiagnosed injury, the diagnosis of subtalar instability is critical because of its high prevalence after inversion injuries. Identifying and differentiating between lateral ankle instability and subtalar instability is of utmost importance considering both are prevalent among the athletic population.

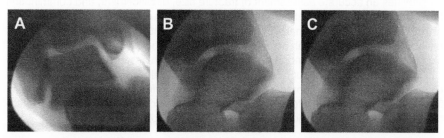

Fig. 1. A 16-year-old soccer player underwent Brostrom procedure for unstable ankle but still felt unstable post-procedure.(A) AP stress views showed no ankle instability. (B) Lateral stress showed no ankle instability. (C) 1 More force showed instability of subtalar joint. Note the anterior subluxation of calcaneus on talus.

Radiographic Evaluation

Appropriate radiographic studies are helpful for avoiding misdiagnosis and facilitating a prompt diagnosis of associated injuries. The Ottawa ankle rules provide guidance in the emergency department as to whether radiographs are necessary or can be deferred. Ankle radiographs are indicated if the presence of a fracture is suggested by tenderness along the distal 6 cm of the posterior edge of the fibula or the tip of the lateral malleolus, tenderness along the distal 6 cm of the posterior edge of the tibia or the tip of the medial malleolus, or inability to tolerate weight bearing for at least four steps. In the absence of these findings, the diagnosis is usually an acute sprain, and radiographs are unnecessary.[32] Adherence to these guidelines reduces the patient's cost, time in the emergency department, and exposure to radiation. The Ottawa ankle rules were designed for implementation and use in the emergency department. However, many patients who sustain an acute lateral ankle ligament injury are evaluated by a foot and ankle specialist in an outpatient setting several days to a few weeks after the injury.[32]

In this more specialized environment, the threshold for radiographic evaluation is lower because the definitive diagnosis and treatment plan are based on the evaluation. A foot and ankle specialist should attempt to obtain a series of weight-bearing ankle radiographs for most patients with an ALAS. Additional weight-bearing radiographs of the foot can be added when there is suspicion of a concomitant foot injury based on either the history or physical examination. Weight-bearing views provide substantially better imaging of relevant osseous structures than non-weight-bearing views and thereby minimize the possibility of missing an injury. Simulated weight-bearing views can be obtained at the initial evaluation if full weight bearing is too painful. Obtaining full weight-bearing views is delayed until symptoms improve. The anterio-posterior (AP) and mortise ankle radiographs of the ankle should be evaluated for medial clear space and syndesmotic widening, malleolar fracture, lateral process of talus fracture, and talar osteochondral fracture. The lateral views of the ankle and foot can reveal dorsal talar avulsion fractures, anterior process of the calcaneus fractures, or the presence of an os trigonum injury. The AP and oblique foot views can reveal navicular fractures, midfoot injuries, cuboid fractures, or fifth metatarsal fractures. Radiographic and physical examination findings always must be correlated to provide an accurate and complete diagnosis.[33]

Computed tomography (CT) and MRI have limited indications in the evaluation of an acute ankle sprain. On the basis of plain radiographs, CT is used to detect an associated fracture suspected; these include fracture of the lateral process of the talus and the anterior process of the calcaneus, posterior talar fracture, and osteochondral fracture. CT provides an accurate assessment of fracture size, displacement, and comminution that can ultimately guide treatment. Through visualization of the clear space in the axial plane, CT can also detect malalignment or displacement of the syndesmosis. MRI is rarely indicated to evaluate an acute ankle sprain and should be obtained only if suspicion is high for an osteochondral lesion of the talus or an associated soft-tissue injury such as an Achilles tendon rupture or peroneal tendon dislocation. MRI is useful for distinguishing a pre-existing chronic osteochondral lesion from an acute osteochondral fracture. MRI has also been found to be superior to physical examination for the detection of syndesmotic injuries in the setting of ambiguous plain radiographs.[33]

Treatment Considerations

The severity of a lateral ankle sprain affects both its treatment and prognosis. Patients with a grade I or II sprain typically do not require crutches and are able to perform activities of daily living with minimal discomfort.[34] A patient with a grade I or II sprain appears to recover best when an early rehabilitation regimen is implemented. In fact, a recent randomized controlled study demonstrated that grade I and II sprains achieve earlier recovery when an immediate functional ROM protocol is initiated compared with early immobilization.[35]

Rest, ice, compression, and elevation (RICE) is a conservative treatment method that has not been rigorously investigated, and the efficacy of this combination is questionable. The individual elements of ice and compression have been the subject of numerous scientific investigations. However, there is little scientific support for their efficacy in reducing injury-associated symptoms following an ALAS. The limited available evidence shows that the efficacy of cryotherapy for reducing an ALAS injury-associated symptoms is unclear.[34] There are no indications that the isolated use of ice can increase function as well as decrease swelling and pain at rest among individuals who have sustained an ALAS.[7]

The limited available evidence showed a low efficacy of cryotherapy for reducing acute ALAS injury-associated symptoms. However, in combination with exercise therapy, cryotherapy has a greater effect on reducing swelling compared with heat application. The combination of cryotherapy and exercise additionally results in significant improvements in ankle function in the short term, allowing patients to increase loading during weight bearing compared with standard functional treatment.[7] As a combined therapeutic modality, the use of RICE plus multimodal physiotherapy compared with RICE alone provides no additional benefits. Both treatments provide pain reduction, increase patient function, and reduce ankle swelling.[7] Overall, the evidence indicates that the individual aspects of RICE are not effective, apart from cryotherapy, if provided in combination with exercise therapy.

In addition to RICE therapy, platelet-rich plasma (PRP) injections have been gaining popularity in the sports medicine community for the treatment of ALAS. A recent randomized control trial consisted of first-time grade II ALAS treated with immobilization and PRP. This study revealed improved pain reduction and functional scores with the use of immobilization and PRP in comparison to a control group at 8 weeks. However, at the 24-week follow-up, there was no statistically significant difference between the two groups in pain and functional scores.[36] Even though there are early signs of benefits for PRP, the efficacy and clinical application of PRP have long been in question. Currently, multiple consensus statements cannot recommend PRP injections in the setting of acute ankle sprains because the scarcity of unanimous data.[37,38] Furthermore, there may be substantial financial costs associated with this therapy. PRP is frequently not covered by insurance, and the out of pocket cost to the patient may range between $500 and $2500.[39] While the cost/benefit for elite-level athletes may be valuable, the advantages for recreational athletes remain under consideration. Because of the ambiguous evidence surrounding PRP injections for ALAS, additional high-level studies are required.

Patients with a grade III injury often initially experience discomfort during ambulation and while performing activities of daily living. A period of immobilization and protected weight-bearing is often beneficial. However, the optimal length of time and the exact method of immobilization is not well established in the literature, as there have been conflicting results in various studies. A prospective randomized study compared the efficacy of four different modes of immobilization (tubular compression sleeve, walking boot, stirrup brace, and cast) for the initial treatment of an acute grade III ankle sprain.[40] Somewhat surprisingly, the results favored initial cast immobilization for a severe ankle sprain. Patients who had initial casting experienced the most rapid overall recovery, with less pain and an earlier return to activity. The use of a walking boot was found to provide no significant benefit over that of a tubular compression sleeve. In another randomized trial of acute management of lateral ankle sprains, the use of a walking boot for 3 weeks followed by progression to a functional brace was compared with immediate initiation of functional bracing treatment without any period of immobilization.[34] There was no observed difference between groups in pain or instability; however, the immediate functional bracing treatment group had better functional scores and a more rapid recovery period. In a related randomized study comparing functional bracing treatment, neuromuscular training, and a combination of these interventions for lateral ankle sprains, authors found that bracing treatment was the most cost-effective of these interventions.[41]

Although nonsurgical functional rehabilitation for a grade III ankle sprain remains the standard of care in North America, a body of evidence from Europe suggests that superior results are possible when an acute grade III sprain is surgically treated.[42,43] A meta-analysis of 27 studies revealed less giving way and overall better functional results when the initial treatment of grade III sprains was surgical rather than nonsurgical.[42] A subsequent prospective, randomized comparison of surgical treatment and functional rehabilitation in grade III ankle sprains found comparable functional results and fewer recurrent sprains in the patients treated surgically.[43] Additional high-quality studies are necessary before surgical treatment can supplant functional rehabilitation as the treatment of choice for grade III ankle sprains.

Despite the good clinical outcomes of surgery after an acute complete lateral ligament rupture, functional treatment is still the preferred method as not all patients require surgical treatment. This also helps to avoid unnecessary exposure to invasive (over) treatment and an unnecessary risk of complications.[34] However, treatment decisions have to be made on an individual basis. In professional athletes, surgical treatment may be preferred to ensure a quicker return to play and decrease recurrence.[7]

Return to Sport

The timing of the patient's return to sports activity is primarily based on the level of discomfort and the ability to perform necessary sport-specific activities. The average time to return to sport after an ALAS can range from 16 to 24 days, but a large proportion of athletes may experience reinjury or other long-term problems.[34,35,42] The emphasis of a protective brace, the initiation of peroneal strengthening and proprioceptive exercises should be aimed at preventing possible reinjury.[5]

Recurrent ankle sprains in athletes range from 12% to 47%, with junior basketball (47%), volleyball (46%), and American Football (43%) having the highest re-injury rates.[41] This CAI is characterized by recurrent ankle sprains, feelings of the ankle "giving away," and perceived instability. It is estimated that up to 40% of people develop CAI, which may also be an important mediator for post-traumatic osteoarthritis.[40]

ALAS may lead to multiple problems, such as proprioception disturbances. These disturbances seem to originate from the central nervous system above the level of the spinal reflex and may result in functional instability.[44] Additionally, delayed response time of the peroneal muscle has been detected, possibly due to traction injury of the peroneal nerve. However, motor unit insufficiencies seen after an ALAS seem to last shorter than those after other lateral ankle injuries not based on an inversion trauma mechanism.[44] Strength deficits are present following ALAS. For these reasons, early functional treatment is advised and should address proprioception, muscle response time, and muscle strength, enabling an early return to sports participation.[34]

In the recovery phase, plyometric drills should be incorporated into the rehabilitation program prior to the return to sport. Evidence supports that plyometric drills are superior to standard peroneal strengthening exercises for restoration of subjective ankle stability and resumption of athletic participation.[45] If a patient is unable to perform land-based plyometric drills due to pain or continued instability, aquatic therapy may be used to initiate the rehabilitation process.[46] The low-stress environment that aquatic therapy allows reduces axial and compressive forces on the body.[47] In return, athletes can incorporate exercises to improve or maintain ROM, strength, and cardiovascular fitness sooner. Additionally, anti-gravity treadmills have been used in athletes' recovery from injuries.[48,49] Utilizing antigravity treadmills during this rehabilitation process may preserve aerobic fitness, muscle activation patterns, and muscle mass.[50] By doing so, this may allow athletes to return to their previous level of competition sooner. High-level ongoing research is warranted to determine if aquatic therapy or antigravity treadmills impact an athlete's return to sport though.

Case series have been reported that demonstrate home-based physical therapy (PT) as an effective intervention for ALAS.[51] Recent results, though, show that supervised exercise provides better outcomes compared with nonsupervised training. According to one study, supervised exercises focusing on a variety of movements such as proprioception, strength, coordination, and function will result in a faster return to sport in patients who have had ALAS. Therefore, supervised exercise is recommended based on level 1 evidence.[34] With this in mind, physical therapists and athletic trainers play a critical role in ALAS. A study performed by Cleland and colleagues,[52] exhibited superior benefits of manual therapy with exercise compared to an at-home exercise program. Patients receiving manual therapy demonstrated greater improvements in pain and function in both the short- and long term. This only further exemplifies the importance of not only supervised rehabilitative training but interactive, hands-on intervention with a trained physical therapist or athletic trainer. While PT has been shown to be beneficial in ALAS, it is not necessary for every injury. Patients with mild symptoms may not require formal rehabilitation before their return to sport or activities of daily living. Patients must be fully evaluated and the need for physical therapy should be determined on an individual basis.

SEQUELAE OF LATERAL ANKLE SPRAINS

Acute ankle sprains have a high recurrence rate, which may ultimately develop into chronic ankle instability in athletes if not treated properly[53,54] Chronic ankle instability can be defined as insufficiency of the lateral ankle ligament complex.[55] This inadequacy can lead to chronic instability and pain and may correlate to significant loss

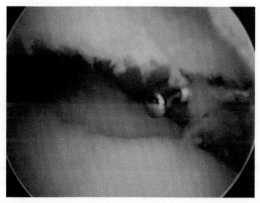

Fig. 2. Arthroscpic image showing osteochondral defect. (*Courtesy of* Lawrence Oloff, DPM, San Francisco, CA.)

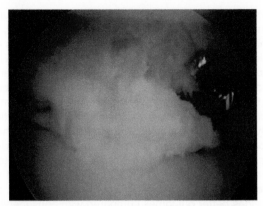

Fig. 3. Arthroscopy showing anterior ankle impingement secondary to post-ankle sprain fibrous tissue. (*Courtesy of* Lawrence Oloff, DPM, San Francisco, CA.)

of playing time for athletes. The prevalence of chronic ankle sprains has been found to be higher among individuals who participate in running, jumping, and cutting activities.[54] Considering this is a majority of the athletic population, early identification and treatment of acute ankle sprains is critical to help prevent the development of chronic instability.

Chronic lateral ankle instability has also been shown to contribute to the development of both bony and soft tissue lesions, which can be correlated to impingement syndrome.[56,57] Studies have examined patients undergoing procedures for lateral ankle instability and the prevalence of anterior impingement syndrome with arthroscopy. A retrospective case series performed in this manner found that 63% of their patients had anterior and/or anterolateral compartment intra-articular synovitis, 17% were found to have osteochondral defects (OCD) (**Fig. 2**), and 12% of their patients had anterior osseous impingement lesions (**Fig. 3**).[58] Conservative treatment in the form of ice and NSAIDs has been shown to be beneficial for impingement syndrome. In more severe cases, cast immobilization may be necessary.[59] Ultrasound-guided corticosteroid injections have also demonstrated positive outcomes and may have diagnostic uses as well.[60,61] Arthroscopic evaluation of the ankle joint and debridement has also been described as a treatment for impingement syndrome.[59,62]

Lastly, chronic lateral ankle instability may also be accompanied by OCDs affecting the talus.[58] MRI is commonly used in the assessment of OCDs. While MRI has been shown to overestimate OCD area and diameter compared with arthroscopy,[63] it still helps clinicians make decisions. MRI helps by allowing the surgeon to better

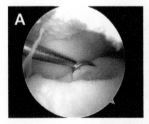
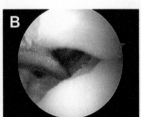
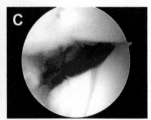

Fig. 4. (*A*) Debridement of osteochondral lesion. (*B*) Microfracture of osteochondral lesion with microfracture awl. (*C*) It is important to microfracture deep enough to promote bleeding into microfracture site to best insure production of fibrocartilage. (*Courtesy of* Lawrence Oloff, DPM, San Francisco, CA.)

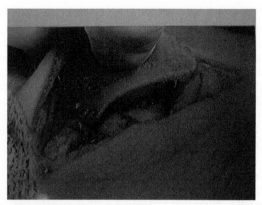

Fig. 5. Medial malleolar osteotomy to create easier access to perform OATS procedure. Two autografts are applied here due to size of lesion. (*Courtesy of* Lawrence Oloff, DPM, San Francisco, CA.)

understand the lesion characteristics and determine if any other associated injuries exist.[63] Due to the association between chronic ankle instability and OCDs of the talus, simultaneous lateral ankle reconstruction and repair of OCDs may be warranted.[64–66] Microfracture, osteochondral autograft transfer system, and other various surgical options are all available in the treatment of osteochondral defects (**Figs. 4**A–C and **5**).

HIGH "SYNDESMOTIC" ANKLE SPRAINS

Syndesmotic or high ankle sprains are more common in sports with high-speed collisions between athletes, athletes on artificial or uneven surfaces, or high torque cutting and jumping forces.[67] Unlike lateral ankle sprains, syndesmotic injuries are less common due to the mechanism of injury. Syndesmotic injuries comprise 12% of all ankle sprains but are up to 25% of ankle sprains in the athletic population.[5,67,68] As previously mentioned, the early identification and treatment of syndesmotic injuries are of utmost importance as they often require significantly longer recovery times and return to sport times.[67]

The interosseous ligament, the anterior inferior tibiofibular ligament (AITFL), the transverse tibiofibular ligament, and the posterior inferior tibiofibular ligament (PITFL) are all components of the high ankle ligaments, also known as the distal tibiofibular syndesmosis.[10,67,69] In addition, the deltoid ligaments contribute to the syndesmotic stability by preventing lateral translation of the talus.[10,67] The syndesmosis allows for coronal, sagittal and transverse plane motion and is an inherently strong articulation therefore generally only injured when the foot is forced into dorsiflexion with external rotation, resulting in abnormal stress of the syndesmotic ligaments.[9,67,69]

Mechanism of Injury

Although less frequent in the general or nonathletic population, high ankle sprains have a higher incidence in the athletic population. In a study of 25 National Collegiate Athletic Association (NCAA) sports, they found that in a period of 6 years there were 480 high ankle sprains reported, with 56.7% of them occurring during competitions compared with practices. In this same study, they found that the most common mechanism of injury was from player contact (60.4%) compared to 15.5% for noncontact and 16.9% for surface contact.[9]

External rotation has been described as the most common mechanism for high ankle sprains. However, alternative mechanisms which have been discussed in the literature include axial loading of the ankle and inversion, eversion alone or dorsiflexion forcing the widest part of the talus to separate the fibula from the tibia; all of which are mechanisms which are more common to happen in athletic competitions.[9,67,69,70] Approximately 45.5% of surface contact high ankle sprains were found in women's volleyball and 33.3% in men's lacrosse in comparison to noncontact mechanisms found mostly in men's ice hockey, which in our literature review appears to have a correlation to athletic footwear worn during some sports that would predispose athletes to high ankle sprains, such as rigid boots in ice hockey or skiing.[1,69,71,72]

Physical examination

Upon initial presentation and reviewing the mechanism of injury, there might be a suspicion of a syndesmotic injury that should be further investigated. Acutely, patients might present with diffuse swelling and global pain. However, the "tenderness length" should be established, the "squeeze test," cotton, fibular translation, external rotation, and cross-leg test should all be performed if the patient allows.[67] In a retrospective case series that studied syndesmotic injury data from three National Football League (NFL) teams, the authors found that the length of proximal tenderness was positively correlated with the grade of injury as well as time to return to practice or sport.[73] A "squeeze test" is performed by squeezing the fibula and tibia at the midcalf. A positive test would elicit pain distally over the tibial and fibular syndesmosis.[69] The cotton test involves the translation of the talus from medial to lateral in the ankle mortise, a positive result if there is an increase in motion in comparison to the opposite side or if there is pain elicited.[67] A positive external rotation test involves eliciting pain in the region of the distal ankle or interosseous membrane while having the patient dangle their affected limb over the table with the knee flexed at approximately 90 degrees, and an external rotation motion is applied while stabilizing the leg at the midshaft.[73]

In regards to the cross-leg test, the patient must sit with the injured leg crossed over the non-injured side. Next pressure is applied to the medial aspect of the proximal tibia and fibula just distal to the knee in an attempt to provide shear strain to the distal syndesmosis. The cross-leg test is considered positive if there is pain at the distal syndesmosis.[67,69] Fibular translation requires the stabilization of the tibiotalar joint with one hand and translating the fibula anterior and posterior with the other hand. A positive test would elicit an increase in movement compared with the uninjured leg or if there is pain.[67,73] Despite the usefulness of these exams, no individual test is diagnostic for a syndesmotic injury. However, a combination of each test could lead to an accurate diagnosis resulting in further workup.[67,69,73]

A Maisonneuve fracture should also be excluded in the setting of a high ankle sprain. This proximal fibular fracture is associated with rupture of the tibiofibular syndesmosis and the anterior fibers of the deltoid ligament.[74] Although rare, accounting for about 5% of the ankle fractures treated,[75] practitioners should have a high clinical suspicion for this type of injury. Clinically, athletes may experience pain at the proximal fibula, medial ankle tenderness, and a ballotable fibula.[76] Due to the close proximity of the peroneal nerve to the Maisonneuve fracture, a sensory test should also be conducted.[77]

Radiographic imaging

In addition to the aforementioned description of symptoms, mechanism of injury, and diagnostic testing, an invaluable tool to use to assess high ankle sprains is radiographic imaging modalities in the form of plain radiographs and MRI. Imaging results have been a topic of research given their importance in determining injury severity, appropriate treatment and rehab, as well as predicting return to sport times.[69] In 2012, Miller and colleagues[78] looked at collegiate football players with high ankle sprains in an attempt to determine whether musculoskeletal ultrasound compared to physical examination was more predictive of return to sport. There is a clear correlation between injury severity and physical examinations and recovery times.[10,67,69,73] The data provided by Miller and colleagues[78] suggests that physical examination has a higher predictive value than musculoskeletal ultrasound when assessing injury severity and return to unrestricted athletic activity.

Plain radiographs have proven to be a convenient and cost-effective initial radiographic modality. Most commonly, weight bearing anteroposterior views, mortise views and lateral views are obtained in order to assess the tibiofibular clear space (TFCS), tibiofibular overlap (TFO), and medial clear space. TFCS is the clear space measured between the medial border of the fibula and the floor of the incisura fibularis 1 cm above the tibial plafond[79] and considered abnormal when it is > 5 mm.[80] On an AP view the TFO is generally measured from the lateral border of the anterior tubercle of the tibia to the medial border of the fibula[79] and an overlap of <10 mm is considered abnormal.[80] The medial clear space is measured between the lateral aspect of the medial malleolus to the medial border of the talus, any measurements >4 mm is considered abnormal.[80] The identification of any one of the TFO, TFCS, or medial clear space as abnormal is considered to represent a syndesmotic injury, however, plain radiographs have been known to miss more subtle syndesmotic injuries.

Stress radiographs have also been reported to be helpful in identifying syndesmotic injuries, but they can prove to be difficult to obtain in the acute setting.[73] Additional plain radiographs that should be considered are high tibia and fibula films. As reported by Taweel, there are cases that prove the usefulness of high tibial and fibular films to help identify Maisonneuve fractures that are sometimes found with high ankle sprains.[81] A Maisonneuve fracture is a spiral fracture of the proximal third of the fibula as a result of a high energy twisting of the lower extremity and is found with high ankle sprains.[81]

A better imaging modality that can be used in the setting of an acute ankle sprain to help confirm the diagnosis is an MRI, which can help elicit not just a syndesmotic injury but also help in identifying the severity as well as help identify any additional soft tissue injuries or osteochondral injuries. In Sikka's retrospective study looking at data from three NFL teams they found that MRI was useful in defining the diagnosis along with any associated injuries that can help determine treatment, rehab, and prognosis.[73] However, further studies are needed to investigate if there is a role for MRI in predicting the return to sports time. In another professional athletic association study, Mollon and colleagues[82] reviewed the National Hockey League (NHL) injury database to better understand the diagnostic value of MRI scans and their predictive value on return to play. After reviewing 105 NHL athletes with high ankle sprains over five seasons, the authors concluded that high ankle sprains have a variation in time of recover, with an average of 45 days to recovery in comparison with an average of 28 days in the NFL and average of 1.4 days in a lateral ankle sprain.[82] Both Mollon and Sikka were able to determine that MRI scans were helpful in the definitive diagnosis of high ankle sprains and evaluating for associated injuries such as osteochondral defects or concomitant soft tissue injuries. However, this did not prove helpful in predicting return to play time for these high-level athletes.[73,82]

Treatment considerations

Clinicians should attempt conservative care for stable syndesmotic injuries without significant diastasis. Limiting external rotation should be a primary objective during the initial stages of rehabilitation. A CAM boot is useful in providing stability to the syndesmosis and is typically prescribed to reduce rotatory forces upon the ankle.[40,83] Early ROM after lateral ankle sprains is common and facilitates a quicker return to sport. With syndesmotic injuries, though, early motion may place additional stress on the syndesmosis, and by doing so, this may prolong recovery time.[84] The period of immobilization typically ranges from 1–2 weeks and is oftentimes associated with modifications in weight bearing status depending on the severity of the sprain[69,85] (Williams, Osbahr).

Adjunct treatment in the form of PRP has been gaining popularity in high ankle sprains. Laver and colleagues[86] performed ultrasound guided PRP injections to the anterior tibiofibular ligament (AITFL), which demonstrated a shorter return to play in elite level athletes when compared to a control group. Currently, though, this is the only high-quality literature that could be found that supports the use of PRP for syndesmotic injuries. Given this, PRP should be used sparingly until more research is completed and further confirms its efficacy in the use of high ankle sprains.

Syndesmotic injuries in conjunction with tibiofibular diastasis or disruption of the deltoid ligament may benefit from surgical stabilization.[87] High-grade syndesmotic injuries associated with malleolar fracture typically require surgical intervention at the fractured site. The surgical approach and fixation of the ankle syndesmosis may consist of screws, suture buttons, or a combination of the two. However, the type of repair to the syndesmosis injury remains controversial.[87]

Huber and colleagues[88] found that screw fixation resulted in potential nonphysiologic stabilization of the fibula and syndesmosis. Given the natural motion at the ankle syndesmosis, screws may loosen or break when left in place. In the athletic population, syndesmotic screws may be removed. Screw removal may be performed at a minimum of 8 weeks, but ideally should remain until 12 weeks.[89] However, screw removal is not absolute, and there is evidence to support routine screw removal in the general population.[90]

A newer construct for syndesmosis correction involves suture buttons and provides an alternative to screw fixation. A recent study by McKenzie and colleagues[91] demonstrated that the suture button resulted in a lower tendency toward malreduction and lowered reoperation rates. When compared to screw fixation, though, biomechanical studies are inconclusive regarding suture button strength. The suture button does allow the restoration of the physiologic motion between the distal tibia and fibula.[92,93] This natural syndesmotic motion may be critical in allowing athletes to return to their previous level of play.

Return to sport
A large amount of force is generally required to produce syndesmotic injuries.[94] Due to this, it typically results in missed practices and games as well as significantly longer recovery times when compared with their lateral ankle sprain counterparts. This correlates with longer treatment times for athletes to successfully return to their preinjury levels.[85,94,95] A recent study observed that NCAA athletes with high ankle sprains returned to sport on average after 13.9 days compared with 8.1 days for lateral ankle sprains.[9] Meanwhile, literature done within the National Football League (NFL) demonstrated the average return to sport time was 80.5 ± 132.9 days.[96] Lastly, a recent systematic review found that the average time to return to sport was 41.7 days for non-operative treatment and 55.2 days for operative treatment.[97] The differences in return to sport between these studies show how devastating high ankle sprains are and how difficult it can be to determine an athlete's return to sport. The athlete's sport, position within that sport, and level of competition should all be considered within this process.

Rehabilitation concepts surrounding high ankle sprains are similar to those of lateral ankle sprain regimens. The unique anatomy and biomechanics associated with these syndesmosis injuries must be kept in mind throughout therapy and play a critical role in the return to sport process. Throughout the rehabilitation period, and as mentioned previously in regards to ALAS rehabilitation, incorporating supervised and hands-on physical therapy is beneficial in allowing athletes to return to sport. The addition of manual therapy, neuromuscular, and proprioceptive training programs throughout the rehab process should be integrated. When performed correctly, they provide benefits in terms of pain reduction and functional recovery.[98–100]

Other treatments used more selectively include transcutaneous electric nerve stimulation and therapeutic ultrasound. While these modalities have been a foundational piece in the recovery of ankle sprains, the current literature does not fully support their use. These interventions have not shown a significant reduction in pain, edema, or accelerated functional recovery after an acute ankle sprain.[101,102] Considering this, these therapies cannot be recommended based on present-day research.

With the incorporation of bracing and therapy, the patient should gradually advance throughout the rehabilitation process to more challenging movements and sport-specific drills.[103] A reliable sign of healing is the athlete's ability to repeatedly perform a single leg hop 10 times without pain.[67] Once completed, the patient may transition to running, jumping, and agility drills. Abrupt lateral movements should also be included in a progressive fashion. This will not only ensure appropriate healing of the injury but also allow time for the athlete to gain confidence in using and moving the affected limb. Once these exercises are completed, pain-free sport-specific drills such as dribbling a basketball, running route patterns, etc. may be built into rehab and the athlete can slowly return to their individual sport under supervision.[69]

DISCUSSION

An acute ankle sprain is a common injury that often presents in the form of an ALAS or a high ankle sprain. Throughout these authors' literature review, we have found that there are many predisposing factors, mechanisms of injury, treatment, and rehab options that are unique to the type of acute ankle sprain sustained. The importance of identifying the type of ankle sprain cannot be stressed enough, as recovery times and return to sport times have been shown to be drastically different. In reviewing the physical and radiographic findings unique to each type of ankle sprain, we hoped to provide a useful guide to identifying and treating ankle sprains appropriately.

After an ALAS, it is important to first exclude the presence of any fractures or concomitant injuries. Subsequently, functional treatment in the form of exercise and functional support (ie, brace or tape) is preferred over immobilization. Still, a short time of immobilization may help diminish complaints of pain and swelling in the case of a lateral ligament injury. In the case of ROM restriction, mobilization therapy may provide help, but a combination with exercise therapy is advised. Surgery should be reserved for patients with lateral ligament ruptures to avoid unnecessary invasive treatment and the risk of complications. In the prevention of ankle sprains, functional support is effective in patients with both first-time and recurrent ALAS, but seems most effective in preventing recurrent sprains. Exercise therapy, however, has only shown a significant preventive effect on recurrent ankle sprains. Overall, there is no clear evidence on the role of other forms of therapy such as (high-fitted and low-fitted and sports) shoe wear, vibration, and electrostimulation therapy in the treatment and prevention of recurrent LAS.

Ankle sprains are very common, and many people sustaining LAS do not seek medical advice. Therefore, the effect of "no intervention" on the outcome after LAS remains unknown. Most of the contradictory results were found in small studies showing both positive and negative effects. Additionally, most studies only included injured patients, whereas there is some conflict in the evidence of certain preventive measures in patients with first-time ALAS. For this, more research is needed to enable adequate comparison between preventive effects based on a history of ankle sprains, preferably within the same study group.

High ankle sprains have been found by reputable high-end athletic organizations like the NFL, NHL, and NCAA to have a significant and variable number of missed games and return to sport times. In addition, high ankle sprains are often missed given the difficulty in detection and diagnosis, resulting in delayed treatment and longer recovery times. While plain radiographs are often helpful in ruling out fractures or other osseous injuries, they often miss high ankle sprains or subtle syndesmotic injuries. MRI scans have a low predictive value for return to sports time, according to studies. It is the recommendation of these authors to obtain MRI scans to definitively identify syndesmotic injuries and elucidate the severity of injury as well as any associated injuries.

Treatment of high ankle sprains may vary depending on the severity of the injury. The prevention of external rotation of the ankle is paramount throughout the treatment and rehabilitation course. While early ROM during ALAS is beneficial, this may be counterproductive for ankle syndesmotic injuries. The implementation of bracing or immobilization is frequently incorporated as the initial treatment for athletes with high ankle sprains without diastasis. Surgical intervention may be required in more severe injuries with diastasis, though. There remains controversy surrounding syndesmotic fixation with screws and/or suture buttons. While correction with screws typically provides a more stable construct, suture buttons have been shown to restore the natural movement of the syndesmosis and have lower rates of additional surgery.

High ankle sprains have demonstrated a longer return to sport recovery period when compared to ALAS, although the rehabilitation process is similar. This recovery time frame can vary greatly depending on the severity of the injury, the athlete's level of play and the type of sport. Incorporating hands-on physical therapy is of utmost importance following high ankle sprains. The use of manual therapy, neuromuscular and proprioceptive training programs has been shown to be beneficial for progressing the athletes' return to play. Gradually, athletes should advance throughout the rehabilitation process to more challenging movements, sport-specific drills, and, ultimately, return to sport.

Universally accepted approaches by both patients and health care professionals in the diagnostic process, treatment, and prevention of ankle sprains have not been elucidated or supported with clear evidence-based medicine related treatment protocols. This is because of a lack of evidence on subjective data, apart from patient satisfaction after undergoing a certain treatment. More evidence on this topic may help identify the best treatment strategy per patient. This article includes procedures and protocols considered and possibly performed by most health care professionals. Further awareness will enable health care providers to follow the state-of-the-art recommendations, which must be raised by means of scientific publication, scientific referral, congresses, and raising awareness among foot and ankle specialists.

DISCLOSURE

The authors have nothing to disclose.

REFERENCES

1. Ivins D. Acute ankle sprain: an update. Am Fam Physician 2006;74(10): 1714–20.
2. Beynnon BD, Renström PA, Alosa DM, et al. Ankle ligament injury risk factors: a prospective study of college athletes. J Orthop Res 2001;19(2):213–20.
3. Woods C, Hawkins R, Hulse M, et al. The Football Association Medical Research Programme: an audit of injuries in professional football: an analysis of ankle sprains. Br J Sports Med 2003;37(3):233–8.
4. Hertel J, Corbett RO. An updated model of chronic ankle instability. J Athl Train 2019;54(6):572–88.
5. Waterman BR, Owens BD, Davey S, et al. The epidemiology of ankle sprains in the United States. J Bone Joint Surg Am 2010;92(13):2279–84.
6. Doherty C, Bleakley C, Delahunt E, et al. Treatment and prevention of acute and recurrent ankle sprain: an overview of systematic reviews with meta-analysis. Br J Sports Med 2017;51(2):113–25.
7. Vuurberg G, Altink N, Rajai M, et al. Weight, BMI and stability are risk factors associated with lateral ankle sprains and chronic ankle instability: a meta-analysis. J ISAKOS 2019;4(6):313–27, published correction appears in J ISAKOS. 2021 Jan;6(1):61.
8. Markolf KL, Jackson SR, McAllister DR. Syndesmosis fixation using dual 3.5 mm and 4.5 mm screws with tricortical and quadricortical purchase: a biomechanical study. Foot Ankle Int 2013;34(5):734–9.
9. Mauntel TC, Wikstrom EA, Roos KG, et al. The epidemiology of high ankle sprains in national collegiate athletic association sports. Am J Sports Med 2017;45(9):2156–63.
10. Tiemstra JD. Update on acute ankle sprains. Am Fam Physician 2012;85(12): 1170–6.
11. Verhagen EA, van Mechelen W, de Vente W. The effect of preventive measures on the incidence of ankle sprains. Clin J Sport Med 2000;10(4):291–6.
12. Anandacoomarasamy A, Barnsley L. Long term outcomes of inversion ankle injuries. Br J Sports Med 2005;39(3):e14.
13. Hiller CE, Nightingale EJ, Raymond J, et al. Prevalence and impact of chronic musculoskeletal ankle disorders in the community. Arch Phys Med Rehabil 2012;93(10):1801–7.
14. Armijo-Olivo S, Fuentes J, da Costa BR, et al. Blinding in physical therapy trials and its association with treatment effects: a meta-epidemiological study. Am J Phys Med Rehabil 2017;96(1):34–44.
15. Malliaropoulos N, Ntessalen M, Papacostas E, et al. Reinjury after acute lateral ankle sprains in elite track and field athletes. Am J Sports Med 2009;37(9): 1755–61.
16. Wagemans J, Bleakley C, Taeymans J, et al. Exercise-based rehabilitation reduces reinjury following acute lateral ankle sprain: a systematic review update with meta-analysis. PLoS One 2022;17(2):e0262023.
17. Sullivan JA, Gross RH, Grana WA, et al. Evaluation of injuries in youth soccer. Am J Sports Med 1980;8(5):325–7.
18. Janda DH, Wojtys EM, Hankin FM, et al. A three-phase analysis of the prevention of recreational softball injuries. Am J Sports Med 1990;18(6):632–5.
19. Larsen E, Angermann P. Association of ankle instability and foot deformity. Acta orthopaedica Scand 1990;61(2):136–9.

20. Strauss JE, Forsberg JA, Lippert FG 3rd. Chronic lateral ankle instability and associated conditions: a rationale for treatment. Foot Ankle Int 2007;28(10): 1041–4.

21. Deben SE, Pomeroy GC. Subtle cavus foot: diagnosis and management. J Am Acad Orthop Surg 2014;22(8):512–20.

22. DeLee JC, Farney WC. Incidence of injury in Texas high school football. Am J Sports Med 1992;20(5):575–80.

23. Wheeler BR. Slow-pitch softball injuries. Am J Sports Med 1984;12(3):237–40.

24. Fordham S, Garbutt G, Lopes P. Epidemiology of injuries in adventure racing athletes. Br J Sports Med 2004;38(3):300–3.

25. Choi WS, Cho JH, Lee DH, et al. Prognostic factors of acute ankle sprain: need for ultrasonography to predict prognosis. J Orthop Sci 2020;25(2):303–9.

26. Chilvers M, Manoli A 2nd. The subtle cavus foot and association with ankle instability and lateral foot overload. Foot Ankle Clin 2008;13(2):315, vii.

27. Coleman SS, Chesnut WJ. A simple test for hindfoot flexibility in the cavovarus foot. Clin Orthopaedics Relat Res 1977;(123):60–2.

28. Mittlmeier T, Rammelt S. Update on subtalar joint instability. Foot Ankle Clin 2018;23(3):397–413.

29. Aynardi M, Pedowitz DI, Raikin SM. Subtalar instability. Foot Ankle Clin 2015; 20(2):243–52.

30. Thermann H, Zwipp H, Tscherne H. Treatment algorithm of chronic ankle and subtalar instability. Foot Ankle Int 1997;18(3):163–9.

31. Keefe DT, Haddad SL. Subtalar instability. Etiology, diagnosis, and management. Foot Ankle Clin 2002;7(3):577–609.

32. Jolman S, Robbins J, Lewis L, et al. Comparison of magnetic resonance imaging and stress radiographs in the evaluation of chronic lateral ankle instability. Foot Ankle Int 2017;38(4):397–404.

33. de César PC, Avila EM, de Abreu MR. Comparison of magnetic resonance imaging to physical examination for syndesmotic injury after lateral ankle sprain. Foot Ankle Int 2011;32(12):1110–4.

34. Prado MP, Mendes AA, Amodio DT, et al. A comparative, prospective, and randomized study of two conservative treatment protocols for first-episode lateral ankle ligament injuries. Foot Ankle Int 2014;35(3):201–6.

35. Bleakley CM, Taylor JB, Dischiavi SL, et al. Rehabilitation exercises reduce re-injury post ankle sprain, but the content and parameters of an optimal exercise program have yet to be established: a systematic review and meta-analysis. Arch Phys Med Rehabil 2019;100(7):1367–75.

36. Blanco-Rivera J, Elizondo-Rodríguez J, Simental-Mendía M, et al. Treatment of lateral ankle sprain with platelet-rich plasma: a randomized clinical study. Foot Ankle Surg 2020;26(7):750–4.

37. Le ADK, Enweze L, DeBaun MR, et al. Current clinical recommendations for use of platelet-rich plasma. Curr Rev Musculoskelet Med 2018;11(4):624–34.

38. Cole BJ, Gilat R, DiFiori J, et al. The 2020 NBA Orthobiologics consensus statement. Orthop J Sports Med 2021;9(5). https://doi.org/10.1177/23259671211002296. 23259671211002296.

39. Jones IA, Togashi RC, Thomas Vangsness C Jr. The economics and regulation of prp in the evolving field of orthopedic biologics. Curr Rev Musculoskelet Med 2018;11(4):558–65.

40. Lamb SE, Marsh JL, Hutton JL, et al. Collaborative ankle support trial (CAST Group). Mechanical supports for acute, severe ankle sprain: a pragmatic, multi-centre, randomised controlled trial. Lancet 2009;373(9663):575–81.

41. Janssen KW, van Mechelen W, Verhagen EA. Bracing superior to neuromuscular training for the prevention of self-reported recurrent ankle sprains: a three-arm randomised controlled trial. Br J Sports Med 2014;48(16):1235–9.
42. Pijnenburg AC, Van Dijk CN, Bossuyt PM, et al. Treatment of ruptures of the lateral ankle ligaments: a meta-analysis. J Bone Joint Surg Am 2000;82(6):761–73.
43. Pihlajamäki H, Hietaniemi K, Paavola M, et al. Surgical versus functional treatment for acute ruptures of the lateral ligament complex of the ankle in young men: a randomized controlled trial. J Bone Joint Surg Am 2010;92(14):2367–74.
44. Cho BK, Kim YM, Kim DS, et al. Comparison between suture anchor and transosseous suture for the modified-Broström procedure. Foot Ankle Int 2012;33(6): 462–8.
45. Ismail MM, Ibrahim MM, Youssef EF, et al. Plyometric training versus resistive exercises after acute lateral ankle sprain. Foot Ankle Int 2010;31(6):523–30.
46. Kim E, Kim T, Kang H, et al. Aquatic versus land-based exercises as early functional rehabilitation for elite athletes with acute lower extremity ligament injury: a pilot study. PM R 2010;2(8):703–12.
47. Prins J, Cutner D. Aquatic therapy in the rehabilitation of athletic injuries. Clin Sports Med 1999;18(2):447, ix.
48. Tenforde AS, Watanabe LM, Moreno TJ, et al. Use of an antigravity treadmill for rehabilitation of a pelvic stress injury. PM R 2012;4(8):629–31.
49. Saxena A, Granot A. Use of an anti-gravity treadmill in the rehabilitation of the operated achilles tendon: a pilot study. J Foot Ankle Surg 2011;50(5):558–61. https://doi.org/10.1053/j.jfas.2011.04.045.
50. Vincent HK, Madsen A, Vincent KR. Role of antigravity training in rehabilitation and return to sport after running injuries. Arthrosc Sports Med Rehabil 2022; 4(1):e141–9.
51. Bassett SF, Prapavessis H. Home-based physical therapy intervention with adherence-enhancing strategies versus clinic-based management for patients with ankle sprains. Phys Ther 2007;87(9):1132–43.
52. Cleland JA, Mintken PE, McDevitt A, et al. Manual physical therapy and exercise versus supervised home exercise in the management of patients with inversion ankle sprain: a multicenter randomized clinical trial. J Orthop Sports Phys Ther 2013;43(7):443–55.
53. Roos KG, Kerr ZY, Mauntel TC, et al. The epidemiology of lateral ligament complex ankle sprains in national collegiate athletic association sports. Am J Sports Med 2017;45(1):201–9.
54. Attenborough AS, Hiller CE, Smith RM, et al. Chronic ankle instability in sporting populations. Sports Med (Auckland, N.Z.) 2014;44(11):1545–56.
55. Herzog MM, Kerr ZY, Marshall SW, et al. Epidemiology of ankle sprains and chronic ankle instability. J Athletic Train 2019;54(6):603–10.
56. Bassett FH 3rd, Gates HS 3rd, Billys JB, et al. Talar impingement by the anteroinferior tibiofibular ligament. A cause of chronic pain in the ankle after inversion sprain. J Bone Joint Surg Am 1990;72(1):55–9.
57. Cannon LB, Hackney RG. Anterior tibiotalar impingement associated with chronic ankle instability. J Foot Ankle Surg 2000;39(6):383–6.
58. Odak S, Ahluwalia R, Shivarathre DG, et al. Arthroscopic evaluation of impingement and osteochondral lesions in chronic lateral ankle instability. Foot Ankle Int 2015;36(9):1045–9.
59. Lavery KP, McHale KJ, Rossy WH, et al. Ankle impingement. J Orthopaedic Surg Res 2016;11(1):97.

60. Robinson P, Bollen SR. Posterior ankle impingement in professional soccer players: effectiveness of sonographically guided therapy. AJR Am J Roentgenol 2006;187(1):W53–8.

61. Jose J, Mirpuri T, Lesniak B, et al. Sonographically guided therapeutic injections in the meniscoid lesion in patients with anteromedial ankle impingement syndrome. Foot & ankle specialist 2014;7(5):409–13.

62. Nery C, Baumfeld D. Anterior and posterior ankle impingement syndromes: arthroscopic and endoscopic anatomy and approaches to treatment. Foot Ankle Clin 2021;26(1):155–72.

63. Yasui Y, Hannon CP, Fraser EJ, et al. Lesion size measured on mri does not accurately reflect arthroscopic measurement in talar osteochondral lesions. Orthopaedic J Sports Med 2019;7(2). 2325967118825261.

64. Georgiannos D, Bisbinas I, Badekas A. Osteochondral transplantation of autologous graft for the treatment of osteochondral lesions of talus: 5- to 7-year follow-up. Knee Surg Sports Traumatol Arthrosc 2016;24(12):3722–9.

65. Yasui Y, Takao M, Miyamoto W, et al. Simultaneous surgery for chronic lateral ankle instability accompanied by only subchondral bone lesion of talus. Arch Orthop Trauma Surg 2014;134(6):821–7.

66. Jiang D, Ao YF, Jiao C, et al. Concurrent arthroscopic osteochondral lesion treatment and lateral ankle ligament repair has no substantial effect on the outcome of chronic lateral ankle instability. Knee Surg Sports Traumatol Arthrosc 2018; 26(10):3129–34.

67. Hunt KJ, Phisitkul P, Pirolo J, et al. High ankle sprains and syndesmotic injuries in athletes. J Am Acad Orthop Surg 2015;23(11):661–73.

68. Gerber JP, Williams GN, Scoville CR, et al. Persistent disability associated with ankle sprains: a prospective examination of an athletic population. Foot Ankle Int 1998;19(10):653–60.

69. Williams GN, Allen EJ. Rehabilitation of syndesmotic (high) ankle sprains. Sports Health 2010;2(6):460–70.

70. Molinari A, Stolley M, Amendola A. High ankle sprains (syndesmotic) in athletes: diagnostic challenges and review of the literature. Iowa Orthop J 2009;29:130–8.

71. Wright RW, Barile RJ, Surprenant DA, et al. Ankle syndesmosis sprains in national hockey league players. Am J Sports Med 2004;32(8):1941–5.

72. Fritschy D. An unusual ankle injury in top skiers. Am J Sports Med 1989;17(2): 282–6.

73. Sikka RS, Fetzer GB, Sugarman E, et al. Correlating MRI findings with disability in syndesmotic sprains of NFL players. Foot Ankle Int 2012;33(5):371–8.

74. Maisonneuve JG. Recherches sur la fracture du perone. Arch Gen Med 1840; 7(165–187):433–73.

75. Stufkens SA, van den Bekerom MP, Doornberg JN, et al. Evidence-based treatment of maisonneuve fractures. J Foot Ankle Surg 2011;50(1):62–7.

76. Savoie FH, Wilkinson MM, Bryan A, et al. Maisonneuve fracture dislocation of the ankle. J Athletic Train 1992;27(3):268–9.

77. Richmond RR, Henebry AD. A maisonneuve fracture in an active duty sailor: a case report. Mil Med 2018;183(5–6):e278–80.

78. Miller BS, Downie BK, Johnson PD, et al. Time to return to play after high ankle sprains in collegiate football players: a prediction model. Sports Health 2012; 4(6):504–9.

79. Chang AL, Mandell JC. Syndesmotic ligaments of the ankle: anatomy, multimodality imaging, and patterns of injury. Curr Probl Diagn Radiol 2020;49(6):452–9.

80. Evans JM, Schucany WG. Radiological evaluation of a high ankle sprain. Proc (Bayl Univ Med Cent) 2006;19(4):402–5.

81. Taweel NR, Raikin SM, Karanjia HN, et al. The proximal fibula should be examined in all patients with ankle injury: a case series of missed maisonneuve fractures. J Emerg Med 2013;44(2):e251–5.

82. Mollon B, Wasserstein D, Murphy GM, et al. High ankle sprains in professional ice hockey players: prognosis and correlation between magnetic resonance imaging patterns of injury and return to play. Orthop J Sports Med 2019;7(9). 2325967119871578.

83. Boyce SH, Quigley MA, Campbell S. Management of ankle sprains: a randomised controlled trial of the treatment of inversion injuries using an elastic support bandage or an Aircast ankle brace. Br J Sports Med 2005;39(2):91–6. https://doi.org/10.1136/bjsm.2003.009233.

84. Zalavras C, Thordarson D. Ankle syndesmotic injury. J Am Acad Orthop Surg 2007;15(6):330–9.

85. Osbahr DC, Drakos MC, O'Loughlin PF, et al. Syndesmosis and lateral ankle sprains in the national football league. Orthopedics 2013;36(11):e1378–84.

86. Laver L, Carmont MR, McConkey MO, et al. Plasma rich in growth factors (PRGF) as a treatment for high ankle sprain in elite athletes: a randomized control trial. Knee Surg Sports Traumatol Arthrosc 2015;23(11):3383–92.

87. Switaj PJ, Mendoza M, Kadakia AR. Acute and chronic injuries to the syndesmosis. Clin Sports Med 2015;34(4):643–77.

88. Huber T, Schmoelz W, Bölderl A. Motion of the fibula relative to the tibia and its alterations with syndesmosis screws: a cadaver study. Foot Ankle Surg 2012; 18(3):203–9.

89. Schepers T, Van Lieshout EM, de Vries MR, et al. Complications of syndesmotic screw removal. Foot Ankle Int 2011;32(11):1040–4.

90. Schepers T, van Zuuren WJ, van den Bekerom MP, et al. The management of acute distal tibio-fibular syndesmotic injuries: results of a nationwide survey. Injury 2012;43(10):1718–23.

91. McKenzie AC, Hesselholt KE, Larsen MS, et al. A systematic review and meta-analysis on treatment of ankle fractures with syndesmotic rupture: suture-button fixation versus cortical screw fixation. J Foot Ankle Surg 2019;58(5):946–53.

92. Klitzman R, Zhao H, Zhang LQ, et al. Suture-button versus screw fixation of the syndesmosis: a biomechanical analysis. Foot Ankle Int 2010;31(1):69–75.

93. Forsythe K, Freedman KB, Stover MD, et al. Comparison of a novel FiberWire-button construct versus metallic screw fixation in a syndesmotic injury model. Foot Ankle Int 2008;29(1):49–54.

94. Boytim MJ, Fischer DA, Neumann L. Syndesmotic ankle sprains. Am J Sports Med 1991;19(3):294–8.

95. Knapik DM, Trem A, Sheehan J, et al. Conservative management for stable high ankle injuries in professional football players. Sports Health 2018;10(1):80–4.

96. DeFroda SF, Bodendorfer BM, Hartnett DA, et al. Defining the contemporary epidemiology and return to play for high ankle sprains in the National Football League. Phys Sportsmed 2021;1–5. https://doi.org/10.1080/00913847.2021. 1924046, published online ahead of print, 2021 May 11.

97. Vancolen SY, Nadeem I, Horner NS, et al. Return to sport after ankle syndesmotic injury: a systematic review. Sports Health 2019;11(2):116–22.

98. Fujii M, Suzuki D, Uchiyama E, et al. Does distal tibiofibular joint mobilization decrease limitation of ankle dorsiflexion? Man Ther 2010;15(1):117–21.

99. Loudon JK, Reiman MP, Sylvain J. The efficacy of manual joint mobilisation/manipulation in treatment of lateral ankle sprains: a systematic review. Br J Sports Med 2014;48(5):365–70.
100. Punt IM, Ziltener JL, Laidet M, et al. Gait and physical impairments in patients with acute ankle sprains who did not receive physical therapy. PM R 2015;7(1):34–41.
101. Feger MA, Goetschius J, Love H, et al. Electrical stimulation as a treatment intervention to improve function, edema or pain following acute lateral ankle sprains: a systematic review. Phys Ther Sport 2015;16(4):361–9.
102. van den Bekerom MP, van der Windt DA, Ter Riet G, et al. Therapeutic ultrasound for acute ankle sprains. Cochrane Database Syst Rev 2011;2011(6):CD001250.
103. Zech A, Hübscher M, Vogt L, et al. Balance training for neuromuscular control and performance enhancement: a systematic review. J Athl Train 2010;45(4):392–403.

Peroneal Pathology in the Athlete

Amelia Mostovoy, DPM[a],*, Thomas Chang, DPM[b]

KEYWORDS

• Peroneal • Lateral ankle • Subluxation • Tendon rupture • Athlete • Sports

INTRODUCTION

The peroneal tendons play a critical role in stabilizing the foot and ankle especially in athletes with high demands on lateral ankle strength. Athletes who run, jump, and frequently perform cutting motions are at increased risk for peroneal injury. Injuries to the peroneal tendons are often misdiagnosed as lateral ankle sprains, and therefore, initial treatment is not targeted to the underlying pathology of the injury. If not promptly diagnosed, peroneal injuries can lead to chronic conditions that are very resistant to conservative treatment and often require invasive or surgical intervention.

There are multiple causes underlying peroneal tendon pathology that can be broken down into intrinsic and extrinsic categories. Intrinsic injury refers to pathology associated with the tendons themselves. Extrinsic pathology refers to injury to the structures surrounding the peroneal tendons such as the tendon sheath and the retinaculum. Peroneal tendon injury can be the result of acute trauma or repetitive chronic trauma in the athlete. Armagan and Shereff further broke down peroneal tendon disorders into 4 categories: peroneal tendinitis/tenosynovitis, tendon tears or ruptures, peroneal subluxation, and painful os peroneum syndrome, all of which are discussed in this article.[1]

Anatomy

The peroneal tendons are extensions of the peroneus longus and peroneus brevis muscles that make up the lateral compartment of the leg. The peroneus longus muscle originates from the lateral tibial condyle as well as the head of the fibula, and the peroneus brevis originates from the middle third of the fibula as well as the intermuscular septum. At the level of the myotendinous junction the tendons share a common synovial sheath and together they course behind the fibula through the retromalleolar groove. In the groove, the peroneus longus is positioned posterior and lateral to the peroneus brevis tendon. The peroneal retinaculum forms the posterolateral boundary

[a] St. Mary's Medical Center, Graduate Medical Office, 450 Stanyan Street, San Francisco, CA 94117, USA; [b] Redwood Orthopedic Surgery Associates, 208 Concourse Boulevard #1, Santa Rosa, CA 95403, USA
* Corresponding author.
E-mail address: ameliajmostovoy@gmail.com

Clin Podiatr Med Surg 40 (2023) 139–155
https://doi.org/10.1016/j.cpm.2022.07.009
0891-8422/23/© 2022 Elsevier Inc. All rights reserved.

of the grove and holds the tendons in place as they slide within the groove, preventing lateral migration and subluxation over the fibula. It originates from the posterolateral distal fibula and forms 2 bands that insert on the lateral calcaneus and lateral Achilles sheath.

As the tendons traverse along the lateral calcaneal wall, they divide into 2 separate sheaths. The peroneus brevis takes a superior course above the peroneal tubercle of the calcaneus and inserts distally on the styloid process of the fifth metatarsal. The peroneus longus takes an inferior course below the peroneal tubercle, travels distally where it wraps around the cuboid in the cuboid groove and inserts on the plantar base of the first metatarsal and medial cuneiform. In addition, the peroneus longus can be in one continuous sheath, or one on the lateral aspect of the ankle and one on the plantar aspect of the foot, where it changes direction under the cuboid.

Both peroneus muscles are innervated by the superficial peroneal nerve, which is a branch of the common fibular nerve and originally stemming from the sciatic nerve. The blood supply for the lateral leg compartment is from the posterior peroneal artery as well as branches of the medial tarsal artery. Although the tendons are encapsulated in a vascular rich paratenon, there is a short area of avascularity where the tendons bend around bony prominences (both tendons in the retromalleolar groove and peroneus longus around the cuboid) (**Fig. 1**).[2]

Biomechanics

The primary biomechanical purpose of the peroneal tendons is to evert the hindfoot (63% of the total work of hindfoot eversion) and keep the first metatarsal purchased to the ground (4% of the total work of ankle plantarflexion). The peroneal tendons balance the forces exerted by the tibialis posterior, flexor hallucis longus, and flexor digitorum longus.[3] In the normal gait cycle, the peroneal tendons contract eccentrically from heel strike to midstance and provide mediolateral stability preventing involuntary inversion at heel strike. From midstance to propulsion, the peroneus longus contracts concentrically to stabilize the first ray and evert the foot during propulsion. The

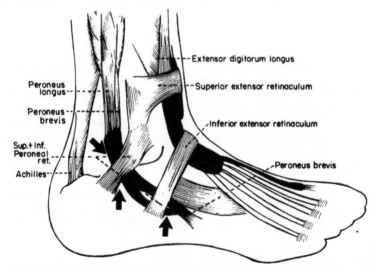

Fig. 1. Anatomy. (*From* L A Gilula, L Oloff, R Caputi, J M Destouet, A Jacobs, and M A Solomon Ankle tenography: a key to unexplained symptomatology. Part II: Diagnosis of chronic tendon disabilities. Radiology 1984 151:3, 581-587.)

peroneus brevis is a stronger evertor of the foot during midstance and an antagonist to the muscles that supinate the subtalar joint.[4]

In athletic movements such as planting and changing direction, the peroneals are essential antagonists to the posterior tibial, flexor hallucis longus, flexor digitorum longus, and anterior tibial tendons to stabilize the lateral ankle and prevent inversion ankle sprains. Weak peroneal tendons are associated with functional ankle instability. Bavdek and colleagues showed that increasing activation of the peroneal tendons such as walking on a medially inclined ramp improves eversion strength, proprioception, and reaction time and could be a suitable exercise for athletes with weak peroneals.[5]

PATHOLOGIES
Peroneal Tendon Tears and Ruptures

Peroneal tendon tears are commonly due to acute inversion ankle injuries or chronic ankle instability. It is more common for the peroneus brevis to tear (about 37% of the population) compared with peroneus longus, and 35% of peroneal tears are asymptomatic.[6] There are 2 proposed pathogenic mechanisms for split lesions of the peroneus brevis. The first mechanism suggests subluxation of the peroneal tendons causing injury from the posterolateral corner of the fibula. The second mechanism suggests split tears during lateral ankle sprain from compression of peroneus brevis between the posterior fibula and the peroneus longus.[7,8]

Physical examination findings of retromalleolar pain with pain on palpation along the course of the peroneal tendons are consistent with peroneal tendon tears. Passively placing the patient in inversion and plantarflexion, applying stress to the lateral ankle, and having the patient both actively evert the hindfoot and dorsiflex the ankle is a reliable test for peroneal pathology if pain is elicited. There is not always loss of eversion strength with peroneal tears, so testing muscle strength is not an accurate examination. Other physical examination findings suggesting peroneal tendon tears are the inability to perform single leg heel raise, given lack of hind foot stability, or inability to balance on one foot with eyes closed, given lack of proprioception.[9]

MRI is crucial in the diagnosis of peroneal tendon tears. The tendons are best evaluated on the axial MR images with the foot in slight plantarflexion. The peroneus brevis is located slightly medial and anterior to the peroneus longus. On MRI, longitudinal tendon split tears seem as multiple tendon slips suggesting separation of the fibers. Another common MRI finding of peroneal tears is severe flattening or a chevron appearance of the peroneus brevis with enveloping of the peroneus longus tendon. As the tendons are followed distally, the separate portions of the brevis tendon reunite below the split tear.[10] Just below the tip of the fibula where the tenon changes directions, it can sometimes mimic the appearance of a tear. This is known as the magic angle phenomenon and is a normal variant.[11] Sobel and colleagues proposed a grading scale for peroneal tendon tears to classify the extent of the tendon splint: grade 1, splayed out tendon; grade 2, partial-thickness split less than 1 cm; grade 3, full-thickness split 1 to 2 cm; and grade 4, full-thickness split greater than 2 cm.[8]

Peroneal tendon injury and tears: surgical considerations

For best operative visualization, the patient is placed in a lateral decubitus position. The incision is classically made parallel to the peroneal tendons behind the lateral malleolus and follows the tendon distally into the foot as far as necessary depending on the presenting pathology; this provides direct dissection onto the peroneal tendon sheath but stays in front of the sural nerve. Once the peroneal sheath is entered, usually a significant amount of hypertrophic synovial inflammation is noted. This sheath is carefully debrided circumferentially around the tendons. Then, it is important to perform a more careful evaluation of the peroneal tendon complex. There is often a distal muscle belly that plays a role in impingement and volume with the peroneal sheath, and this is resected as proximally as possible.

On inspection of the tendons, usually the peroneus brevis is flattened or centrally torn. At times, the central tear within the peroneus brevis tendon corresponds directly to the distal sharp fibular ridge (**Fig. 2**).

All of these areas are evaluated carefully to consider the best repair. Partial tears of up to 50% of the tendon can be treated with debridement of the diseased tendon and tubularization. In the case of acute ruptures or tears of greater than 50% of the tendon, end to end repair, allograft reconstruction, or tendon transfers can be performed. The goal is to attempt a tubularization approach. Usually 3-0 nylon is used, which brings the edges of the tendon together into more of a cylinder or a tube (**Figs. 3** and **4**). The same is done for the peroneus longus tendon, yet this is often not as significantly damaged as the brevis. If greater than 50% of the cross-sectional area of the brevis tendon is damaged, then there could be a consideration of soft tissue graft augmentation or even tenodesis of the peroneus longus to brevis tendon transfer. If there is no subluxation concern, then the peroneal tendon sheath is now closed and the patients are managed with 3 weeks non–weight-bearing.

There are rare situations where both the peroneal tendons are injured and not available for repair or transfer. In these cases, there needs to be consideration of other tendons that can be transferred to replace the damaged peroneal complex. I have used

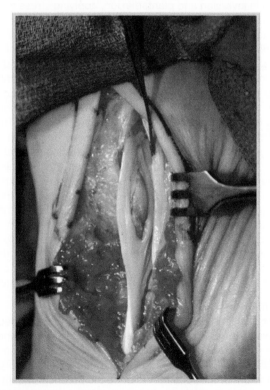

Fig. 2. Brevis tear.

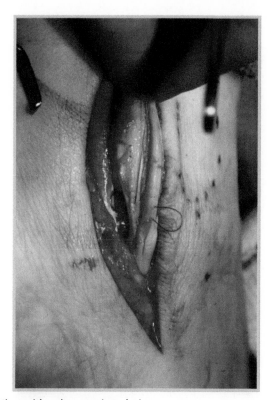

Fig. 3. Tubularization with nylon repair technique.

both the flexor digitorum and flexor hallucis longus tendons, which are taken from the medial side of the foot and ankle (**Fig. 5**).

Care needs to be taken to get adequate length of these tendons so they can travel from the medial to the lateral portion of the ankle, underneath the Achilles tendon, and insert into the styloid process region of the fifth metatarsal base. The flexor digitorum longus (FDL) is often long enough if you can resect this tendon distal to the master knot of Henry. The flexor hallucis longus (FHL) can also be resected there if it is found, but it sits much deeper in the foot and could prove challenging to find. I have also taken the FHL from the planter hallux interphalangeal joint region, and this has been very helpful (**Fig. 6**). The FHL is clearly stronger and more robust than the FDL.

Rehabilitation after peroneal tear or rupture repair is imperative for successful return to sport. Although early literature recommends prolonged cast immobilization of 6 to 12 weeks before any mobilization of the ankle, protocols are being modified to implement earlier range of motion. Van Dijk and colleagues performed a systematic review of 49 rehabilitation protocols after peroneal tendon repair. Although they did not find statistically significant data regarding duration of immobilization or type of surgical repair, they report that there is a trend toward shorter immobilization, most commonly 4 weeks after surgery. Formulated from an evidence-based algorithm, Van Dijk recommends the following treatment of early return to preinjury sport levels: after surgery, lower leg splint for 2 days followed by a non–weight-bearing cast for 12 days and after removal of sutures, weight-bearing in controlled ankle motion boot or walking cast for 4 weeks, followed by 12 weeks of physiotherapy to restore range of motion. Sports-specific training is initiated after completion of 12 weeks of physiotherapy.[12]

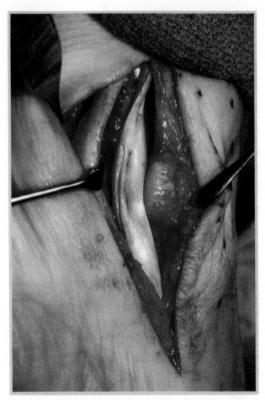

Fig. 4. Tubularization with nylon repair completion.

Peroneal Subluxation

Peroneal subluxation typically occurs secondary to an injury of the superior peroneal retinaculum (SPR), which is the primary ligamentous structure restraining the peroneal tendons. Other causes of subluxation are shallow retromalleolar groove or lateral ankle instability. The most common mechanism of injury occurs during sporting events and occurs from sudden and forceful contraction of the peroneal tendons when the foot is in dorsiflexion. The force generated by the tendons causes an avulsion of the superior peroneal retinaculum from its fibular insertion. Untreated injury to the super peroneal retinaculum will likely cause chronic subluxation of the peroneal tenons.[13]

Eckert and Davis created a classification in 1976 for SPR injuries. Grade 1 injuries involve elevation of the retinaculum creating a pouch into which the tendons can sublux. Grade 2 lesions are when the superior peroneal retinaculum is separated posteriorly from the malleolus and the periosteum. Grade 3 injuries involve separation of the superior peroneal retinaculum from the periosteum with a fibular avulsion.[14] Grade 4, which was added to this classification by Oden, is super peroneal retinaculum's separation from its posterior attachment to the calcaneus and deep fascia of the Achilles. In grade 4, the peroneal tendons are prohibited from relocating because the retinaculum is found deep to the tendons in the retromalleolar sulcus.[15]

Guelfi and colleagues described a new subgroup categorization of peroneal subluxation injuries that did not fit into the aforementioned classification system: intrasheath subluxation characterized by an intact super retinaculum.[16] The peroneus longus and

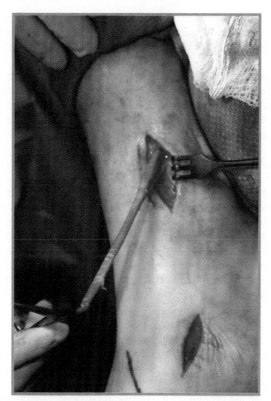

Fig. 5. FDL transfer exposure from medial side leg.

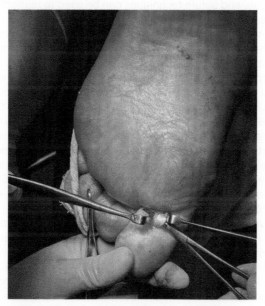

Fig. 6. FHL transfer exposure by harvesting tendon more distally.

peroneus brevis tendons sublux within their tendon sheath in the peroneal groove with an intact superior peroneal retinaculum. The tendons can snap over each other and switch their relative positions or the peroneus longus can sublux through a splint peroneus brevis tear.[17]

On physical examination patients will complain of lateral ankle snapping or popping. Subluxation can be reproduced by isolating and rotating the ankle while stabilizing the lower leg. Occasionally tendons can remain dislocated and will require manual relocation. In the case of intrasheath dislocation, there is no obvious visualized dislocation but patients will experience a clicking or popping sensation in the retromalleolar groove.[13]

Radiographs can be helpful in the diagnosis of chronic subluxing peroneals because it can highlight an avulsion of the lateral malleolus, a sign of a superior peroneal retinaculum rupture. A mortise ankle view allows the best visualization of fleck sign off the lateral malleolus from an SPR avulsion.[18] Ultrasound is a very useful imaging modality for subluxing peroneals, because it allows real-time analysis of the tendons during subluxation; this is especially important in the diagnosis of intrasheath subluxation when the clinical diagnosis is not as obvious. MRI is the gold standard for evaluation of the peroneal tendons as well as the superior peroneal retinaculum. Using MRI, the injury to the superior retinaculum can be classified and the shape of the retromalleolar groove can be evaluated.[13]

Subluxing peroneals: surgical considerations

There are several options when considering repair of a peroneal subluxation. Traditional methods have discussed deepening of the groove and also reattachment of the retinaculum onto the underside of the peroneal ridge, providing tension and tightening of the retinacular compartment (**Fig. 7**). It is usually not beneficial to just use a rotary burr to deepen the groove, as the remaining exposed tissue will be raw cancellous bone and this will usually result in tendon irritation and adhesions. There have been several techniques described where drill holes can be placed on the underside of the peroneal ridge, and suture techniques can be used to reattach the retinaculum to a new attachment location. The technique that has been popularized for many years involves the decancellation of the internal portion of the fibula just anterior to the posterior cortex of the peroneal groove. A guide pin is introduced at the distal tip of the fibula and travels parallel to the posterior surface of the fibula, just a few millimeters anterior to the peroneal groove. A 5-mm cannulated drill is now placed over the guide pin and advanced from the tip of the fibula up 3 to 4 cm into the fibula. Fluoroscopic guidance can also be helpful to assure that the pin and drills are in the right location. Once this is achieved, a sagittal saw can be used to facilitate the process; this attempts to enter the most lateral portion of the circular dill hole created by the cannulated drill and starts just on the medial aspect of the fibular ridge. Once this is done, a bone tamp can be used to collapse the posterior cortical wall of the fibula, resulting in a depression of the groove, therefore deepening the groove effectively (**Fig. 8**). The retinaculum can now be attached through drill holes to the underside of the fibula ridge with nonabsorbable suture.

Another effective way to prevent peroneal tendon subluxation is to combine this with a lateral ligament reconstruction. Often times, lateral ankle instability and peroneal pathology exists in conjunction with each other. Many times I will be performing a double ligament repair, using a drill hole through the fibula with a semitendinosis allograft. A peroneus longus autograft can also be used for the same type of double ligament anatomic reconstruction. The drill hole is placed from the anterior fibula and exits just medial to the fibular ridge, usually close to the origin of the calcaneal fibular

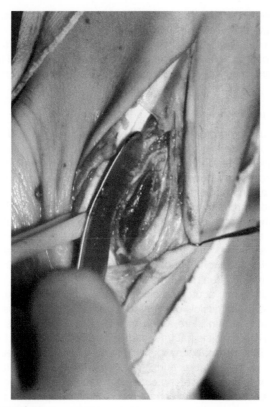

Fig. 7. Groove deepening.

ligament off the distal fibula. When the tendon is passed through the fibular drill hole, the posterior arm is now placed over the 2 peroneal tendons before it is attached to the calcaneal insertion; this will provide a supportive repair of the calcaneal fibular ligament but also prevent future peroneal subluxation from occurring.

In severe cases of subluxation, or in those cases where subluxation has recurred after a repair, there is an option for a fibular osteotomy. A small cortical bone is created

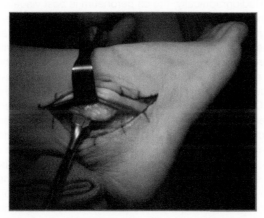

Fig. 8. Tamp groove.

on the lateral malleolar cortex that is rotated posteriorly; this in essence creates an extension of the lateral malleolus posteriorly.[19]

With all of these subluxating peroneal procedures, it is important that the retromalleolar area be prepared to provide more room to accept the perineal tendons. This includes debridement of any low-lying perineal muscle or accessory muscle.

Painful Os Peroneum Syndrome

Painful os peroneum syndrome (POPS), a conditioned named and described by Dr Sobel and colleagues refers to pain caused by trauma to the accessory bone or injury to the peroneus longus tendon from the presence of the accessory bone.[20] The os peroneum is an accessory bone that resides within the peroneus longus tendon at the level of the calcaneocuboid joint. It is ossified and visualized in about 20% of the population and if present, is found bilaterally 60% of the time (**Fig. 9**). This sesamoid bone, as others in the foot, can be inherently bipartite or multipartite.[21] There are 4 soft tissue attachments to the os peroneum sesamoid complex: (1) lateral band of the plantar fascia, (2) band to the base of the fifth metatarsal, (3) band to the peroneus brevis, (4) attachment of the peroneus longus.[19] A painful os peroneum is seen mostly in athletes due to overuse injuries.

POPS has 2 main forms: acute and chronic. The acute form appears as a result of trauma as fractures to the ossicle or injury to an already bipartite ossicle causing diastasis. In the chronic setting there are 4 main causes: (1) diastasis of a multipartite ossicle; (2) healing of an ossicle fracture, causing subsequent callus formation leading to stenosing peroneus longus tenosynovitis; (3) attrition of the peroneus longus tendon distal or proximal to the os peroneum; (4) a hypertrophic peroneal tubercle in the setting of an os peroneum, which can cause entrapment of the tendon and ossicle.

The chronic presentation is more common and mimics a sprained ankle with waxing and waning pain. Common physical examination findings include pain at the os peroneum and along the distal course of the peroneus longus tendon. Patients are especially painful with resisted plantarflexion of the first ray seen with pain during the single heel raise examination. Usually there is near normal strength of the peroneus longus and PB tendons. Occasionally sural nerve dysesthesia/Tinel sign at the lateral calcaneus is experienced.[20]

On imaging, it can be difficult to discern between an ossicle versus a cortical avulsion of the cuboid versus calcification of the peroneus longus or bipartite versus a fractured ossicle. Radiographically, the os peroneum is best visualized on an internal oblique radiograph of the foot. In the case of a multipartite ossicle, the radiographs show multiple fragments with rounded edges and well-defined sclerotic margins. In acute fractures, the ossicle typically appears in multiple fragments with sharp borders. In the case of a stress fracture, the ossicle appears hypertrophic and sclerotic.[21]

The ossicle can also be visualized using an ultrasound with a high-frequency transducer. In the oblique coronal plane, the peroneal tubercle can be seen as a hyperechoic eminence. Once visualized, the peroneal tendon is followed to the cuboid, and if an os peroneum is present, it can be seen at this level as a hyperechoic structure with posterior shadowing. Although the ultrasound is a good tool to visualize the tubercle for local interventional procedures, it typically does not aid in the evaluation of abnormalities of the ossicle.[21] MRI is the gold standard in diagnosis of a painful os peroneal syndrome. Pathologic changes to the bone marrow of the ossicle appear as hypointense on T1 and hyperintense of T2. Computed tomography is the imaging of choice to differentiate a multipartite os peroneum from a nondisplaced fracture when evaluated with submillimeter collimation and sagittal reconstruction.[21]

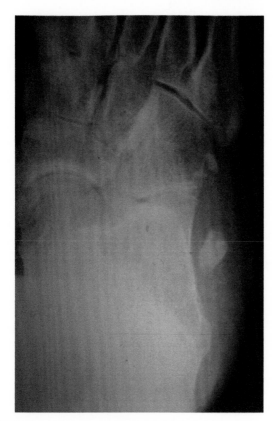

Fig. 9. Os peroneum.

Painful os peroneum surgical considerations

The dissection for an approach to the os perineum is usually along the plantar lateral aspect of the midfoot. The incision is made parallel to the plantar aspect of the calcaneus and cuboid, and this extends out to the styloid process. Usually the sural nerve will be dorsal to the exposure and is not at a risk for damage. The os peroneum is almost always found deep in the cuboid groove and sits much more deeply than expected. The dissection is carried out carefully to preserve the longest fibers in continuity, both proximal and distal to the accessory bone. After this is removed, the remaining portion of the dissected tendon is tubularized as well with 3-0 nylon (**Figs. 10** and **11**). If there is a complete transection of the longus tendon in this area, it is often difficult to repair the 2 ends, as the distal end is so deep within the plantar aspect of the foot. Consideration can be made toward a peroneus longus to a peroneus brevis transfer at this point.

Peroneal Stenosing Tenosynovitis and Tendonitis

Peroneal tendonitis refers to acute inflammation within the peroneal tendon itself, whereas stenosing tenosynovitis refers to inflammation of the synovial sheath of the tendons. Tendons are commonly surrounded by fatty tissue when in an anatomic linear position, but when the direction of a tendon changes about a pully mechanism a sheath usually surrounds the tendon. Ligament and fascia comprise the outer layer of a tendon sheath and a synovial membrane form the inner surface. Between the membrane and the

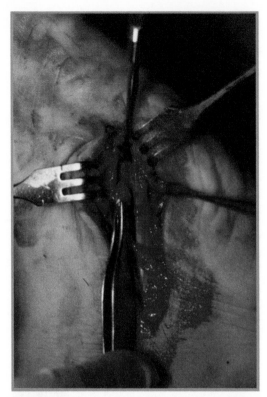

Fig. 10. Os peroneum intra-op.

tendon there is a small amount of synovial fluid.[21] Stenosing tenosynovitis is a more advanced case of tendonitis where scarring has resulted around the tendon, which limits movement of the tendon in its sheath; this typically occurs around the sight of an osseous pulley such as the lateral malleolus for both peroneal tendons and the cuboid for the peroneus longus. With tendon entrapment, the synovial membrane might be hypertrophied due to chronic irritation. In tendonitis, there might be tendon edema or fraying of the tendon as a result of repeated microtrauma from overuse or a single traumatic event.

One of the most prominent causes of peroneal tendonitis and stenosing tenosynovitis is overuse and repetitive mechanical pull on the peroneal tendons commonly seen in athletes.[22] Patients with peroneal tendonitis typically present with gradual onset of posterolateral ankle pain and swelling that worsens with activity and improves with rest. Pain on palpation of the retromalleolar groove with the ankle in eversion and dorsiflexion is considered a positive peroneal compression test, which indicates tendinitis or tenosynovitis.[8] Occasionally redness and swelling are visualized on the posterolateral ankle, along with pain and weak eversion strength.

Clinically it is difficult to differentiate between tendinitis and tenosynovitis, but treatment of the 2 syndromes differ drastically, so it is very important to determine the underlying cause. Although tenosynovitis is amenable to conservative treatments such as antiinflammatories, offloading, physical therapy, and biological regenerative therapy, stenosing synovitis is futile to conservative treatment.[21] MRI and tenogram are the modalities of choice to evaluate tendonitis and tenosynovitis. The pathology is best viewed on a T2 axial MRI, which will show increase signal

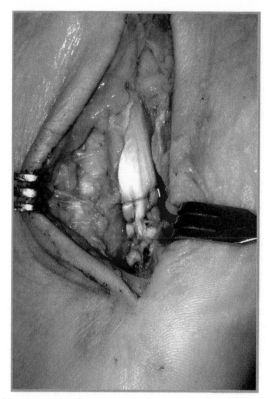

Fig. 11. Peroneus longus repair after removal of os peroneum.

intensity within the tendon and fluid around the tendon. Circumferential fluid within the common peroneal tendon sheath that is wider than 3 mm is a specific finding for tenosynovitis.[11]

Tenogram is not only the gold standard for diagnosing tenosynovitis but can be a treatment modality in and of itself. Tenogram is performed with a 25-gauge needle inserted into the peroneal tendon sheath and injected with a mixture of iothalamate meglumine and 1% lidocaine. The mixture is slowly injected with continuous pressure, and the contrast material is viewed under fluoroscopy as it travels through the tendon sheath (**Fig. 12**). Subsequently the sheath is injected with steroid. The tenogram is then evaluated for areas of stenosis, these being areas where the contrast does not pass through the sheath. In a study performed by Jaffee, it was concluded that 46% of patients who have symptoms of stenosing tenosynovitis had relief after the tenogram due to the dilation of the sheath from the injection of fluid.[23] It is also important to have the patient note relief of pain after tenogram. If patients continue to have pain at the lateral ankle after the sheath was injected with lidocaine, it can be concluded that pain is arising from another location in the lateral ankle that is not the peroneal tendons or sheath.

If stenosing tenosynovitis goes untreated, motion to the peroneal tendons becomes restricted and the foot can develop progressive deformity. When the peroneal tendon becomes immobile the unopposed antagonistic muscle may cause a cavus foot deformity.[24] Surgical intervention includes release of the peroneal tendons from the sheath (**Figs. 13** and **14**).

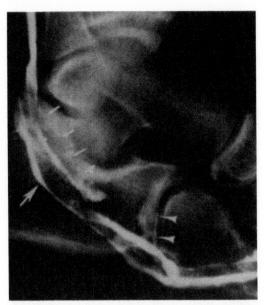

Fig. 12. Stenosing tenosynovitis on tenogram. Lateral view early in the injection shows filling of the left peroneus longus (*large arrow*) and brevis (*small arrows*) tendon sheaths. Contrast material enters the calcaneocuboid joint (*arrowheads*), which indicates capsular tear or defect in the tendon sheath. There is nonfilling of the superior margin of the peroneus brevis, consistent with fibrosis. (*From* L A Gilula, L Oloff, R Caputi, J M Destouet, A Jacobs, and M A Solomon, Ankle tenography: a key to unexplained symptomatology. Part II: Diagnosis of chronic tendon disabilities. Radiology 1984 151:3, 581-587.)

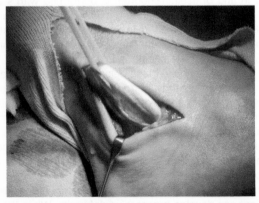

Fig. 13. Tendon stenosis displays abundant fibrosynovial tissue intraoperatively. These restricted band or tissues are easily identified by placing a Penrose drain around proximal healthier tendon and applying tension on the tendon. (*Courtesy of* Lawrence Oloff, DPM, San Francisco, CA.)

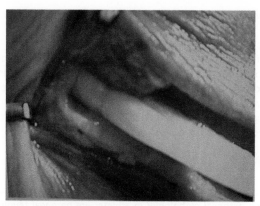

Fig. 14. With tendon stenosis, release of the adhesion may reveal areas of prior tendon stenosis. (*Courtesy of* Lawrence Oloff, DPM, San Francisco, CA.)

SUMMARY

Peroneal tendon tears and ruptures
- The 2 main mechanisms of injury are from tearing due to the sublexation of the peroneal tendons over the sharp posterolateral corner of the fibular or from a lateral ankle sprain due to compression of peroneus brevis between the posterior fibula and the peroneus longus.
- On MRI, longitudinal tendon split tears appear as multiple tendon slips, suggesting separation of the fibers or severe flattening/chevron appearance of the peroneus brevis with enveloping of the peroneus longus tendon.
- Partial tears of up to 50% of the tendon can be treated with debridement of the diseased tendon and tubularization. If greater than 50% of the cross-sectional area of the brevis tendon is damaged, end to end repair, allograft reconstruction, tenodesis, or tendon transfers can be performed.

Peroneal subluxation
- Peroneal subluxation typically occurs secondary to an injury of the superior peroneal retinaculum (SPR), which is the primary ligamentous structure restraining the peroneal tendons. Other causes are shallow retromalleolar groove or lateral ankle instability. A more recently defined category of peroneal subluxation refers to intrasheath sublexation between the 2 peroneal tendons within an intact sheath.
- Radiographs are helpful at diagnosing an avulsion of the lateral malleolus. Ultrasound is useful in analyzing subluxation in real time especially for intrasheath subluxation. MRI is the gold standard for evaluation of the peroneal tendons as well as the superior peroneal retinaculum.
- Surgical intervention includes deepening of the groove, reattachment and reinforcement of the retinaculum as well as combining these procedures with a lateral ligament reconstruction.

Painful os peroneum syndrome
- POPS is defined as pain caused by trauma to the os peroneum accessory bone or injury to the peroneus longus tendon from the presence of the accessory bone.
- On imaging, it can be difficult to discern between an (1) ossicle, (2) a cortical avulsion of the cuboid, (3) a calcification of the peroneus longus, or (4) a bipartite versus a fractured ossicle. MRI is the imaging of choice to evaluate the health of the tendon distal to the accessory ossicle as well as the ossicle itself.

- Surgical intervention includes removal of the os peroneum and repair of the peroneus longus tendon.

Peroneal stenosing synovitis

- Caused by effusion in the tendon sheath where there is a change of direction of the tendon from trauma and mechanical factors such as overuse.
- MRI and tenogram help determine between tendonitis, tenosynovitis, and stenosing tenosynovitis.
- Stenosing tenosynovitis is not amenable to conservative treatment and must be surgically fixed before rigid cavus foot develops

CLINICS CARE POINTS

- The most common peroneal pathologies in athletes are peroneal tendinitis/tenosynovitis, tendon tears or ruptures, peroneal subluxation and dislocation, and painful os peroneum syndrome. Overuse of the peroneal tendon leads to damage to the tendon.

- Accurate diagnosis of peroneal tendon pathology leads to targeted treatment and prevents the development of chronic tendinopathies.

- Proper diagnosis begins with a detailed physical examination followed by targeted imaging. MRI and tenogram are the most helpful modalities of choice, and in some instances tenogram is curative.

- Treatment of athletes with peroneal tendon pain need to be prompt and targeted starting with conservative measures and quickly moving to surgical fixation, if warranted, to prevent chronic damage to the tendon and delay return high function that is required by athletes.

DISCLOSURE

The authors have nothing to disclose.

REFERENCES

1. Armagan O, Shereff MJ, Meyerson. Tendon injury and repair. Foot Ankle Disord 2000;1:942.
2. Lewis OJ. Anatomy of the foot and ankle. Descriptive, topographic, functional. J Anat 1984;138(Pt 2):376.
3. Roukis TS, Scherer PR, Anderson CF. Position of the first ray and motion of the first metatarsophalangeal joint. J Am Podiatr Med Assoc 1996;86(11):538–46.
4. Morgan O, Song J, Hillstrom R, et al. Biomechanics of the peroneal tendons. In: Sobel M, editor. The peroneal tendons: a clinical guide to evaluation and Management. New York: Springer International Publishing; 2020. p. 23–40.
5. Bavdek R, Zdolšek A, Strojnik V, et al. Peroneal muscle activity during different types of walking. J Foot Ankle Res 2018;11:50.
6. Dombek MF, Lamm BM, Saltrick K, et al. Peroneal tendon tears: a retrospective review. J Foot Ankle Surg 2003;42(5):250–8.
7. Munk RL, Davis PH. Longitudinal rupture of the peroneus brevis tendon. J Trauma 1976;16(10):803–6.
8. Sobel M, Geppert MJ, Olson EJ, et al. The dynamics of peroneus brevis tendon splits: a proposed mechanism, technique of diagnosis, and classification of injury. Foot Ankle 1992;13(7):413–22.
9. Banks AS, Downey MS, Martin DE, et al. McGlamry's Comprehensive textbook of foot and ankle surgery (2-volume Set). Foot Ankle Spec 2009;2(4):200.

10. Major NM, Helms CA, Fritz RC, et al. The MR imaging appearance of longitudinal split tears of the peroneus brevis tendon. Foot Ankle Int 2000;21(6):514–9.
11. Erickson SJ, Cox IH, Hyde JS, et al. Effect of tendon orientation on MR imaging signal intensity: a manifestation of the "magic angle" phenomenon. Radiology 1991;181(2):389–92.
12. van Dijk PAD, Lubberts B, Verheul C, et al. Rehabilitation after surgical treatment of peroneal tendon tears and ruptures. Knee Surg Sports Traumatol Arthrosc 2016;24(4):1165–74.
13. Lugo-Pico JG, Kaiser JT, Sanchez RA, et al. Peroneal tendinosis and subluxation. Clin Sports Med 2020;39(4):845–58.
14. Eckert WR, Davis EA. Acute rupture of the peroneal retinaculum. J Bone Joint Surg Am 1976;58(5):670–2.
15. Oden RR. Tendon injuries about the ankle resulting from skiing. Clin Orthop 1987; 216:63–9.
16. Guelfi M, Vega J, Malagelada F, et al. Tendoscopic treatment of peroneal intra-sheath subluxation: a new subgroup with superior peroneal retinaculum injury. Foot Ankle Int 2018;39(5):542–50.
17. Raikin SM, Elias I, Nazarian LN. Intrasheath subluxation of the peroneal tendons. J Bone Joint Surg Am 2008;90(5):992–9.
18. Berquist T. Imaging of the foot and ankle, vol. 3. New York: Wolters Kluwer; 2010.
19. Micheli LJ, Waters PM, Sanders DP. Sliding fibular graft repair for chronic dislocation of the peroneal tendons. Am J Sports Med 1989;17(1):68–71.
20. Sobel M, Pavlov H, Geppert MJ, et al. Painful os peroneum syndrome: a spectrum of conditions responsible for plantar lateral foot pain. Foot Ankle Int 1994; 15(3):112–24.
21. Bianchi S, Bortolotto C, Draghi F. Os peroneum imaging: normal appearance and pathological findings. Insights Imaging 2017;8(1):59–68.
22. Vuillemin V, Guerini H, Bard H, et al. Stenosing tenosynovitis. J Ultrasound 2012; 15(1):20–8.
23. Jaffee NW, Gilula LA, Wissman RD, et al. Diagnostic and therapeutic ankle tenography. Am J Roentgenol 2001;176(2):365–71.
24. Gilula LA, Oloff L, Caputi R, et al. Ankle tenography: a key to unexplained symptomatology. Part II: diagnosis of chronic tendon disabilities. Radiology 1984; 151(3):581–7.

First Metatarsophalangeal Joint Pathology in the Athlete

Emily Khuc, DPM[a], Lawrence M. Oloff, DPM, FACFAS[a,b,*]

KEYWORDS

- First • Great • Toe • Hallux • Metatarsophalangeal • Joint • Athlete • Sports

KEY POINTS

- The most common first metatarsophalangeal joint conditions in athletes are turf toe, sesamoiditis, and hallux rigidus. Extreme movements and contact sports increase the likelihood of damage to the joint.
- The normal function of the joint depends on several key anatomic components, including the sesamoid bones, capsule, tendons, and neurovascular structures.
- Treatment of athletes should involve a care plan which includes options of non-surgical and surgical care and expected recovery timelines for return to sport.
- Athletes can have good surgical outcomes, but procedural decisions should be made to prioritize preservation of the joint in cases where range of motion is essential for sport activity.

INTRODUCTION

The first metatarsophalangeal joint plays an important role in the appropriate function of the foot in normal gait. There are many different anatomic components involved in the structure and function of the first metatarsophalangeal joint and therefore many different places for joint pathologic condition to occur.[1] This is a relatively small-sized joint when compared with the ankle, knee, and hip in the lower extremity but still has all the same basic components of bones, cartilage, tendons, ligaments, and neurovascular structures. Any of these parts of the joint can be injured, and this risk increases with increased demand.

High-level athletic performance in sport is especially dependent on the proper, pain-free functioning of the first metatarsophalangeal joint. Biomechanical studies

[a] Saint Mary's Medical Center San Francisco, Graduate Medical Office, 450 Stanyan Street, San Francisco, CA 94117, USA; [b] Palo Alto Medical Foundation 1501 Trousdale Drive, Ste 115, Burlingame, CA 94010, USA
* Corresponding author. Palo Alto Medical Foundation 1501 Trousdale Drive, Ste 115, Burlingame, CA 94010.
E-mail address: lmop11@comcast.net

Clin Podiatr Med Surg 40 (2023) 157–168
https://doi.org/10.1016/j.cpm.2022.07.010
0891-8422/23/© 2022 Elsevier Inc. All rights reserved.
podiatric.theclinics.com

have shown that peak plantar pressures in the foot occur at the first metatarsophalangeal joint and compound during certain movements including running and jumping, which are common in sport activity.[2] In ballet, correlations have been made between dance participation and loss of first metatarsophalangeal joint cartilage and range of motion.[3,4] In football, there are reports that incidence of turf toe type injuries in professional athletes during their careers can be as high as 45%.[5] First metatarsophalangeal joint injuries are consistently one of the most common injuries seen in collegiate athletes of various sports.[6–8]

The approach to treating the athlete with big toe joint pathologic condition can be a challenge due to the difficulty in offloading this area during an athletic season and the size of the structures involved in injury. Tailoring effective treatment of these athletes requires coming to a specific diagnosis, which starts with an understanding of all of the structures and anatomy involved.

Anatomy

The first metatarsophalangeal joint is made of the articulation between the first metatarsal and the first proximal phalanx. The rounded, convex surface of the metatarsal head meets the concave base of the phalanx to form a ginglymo-arthroidal articulation in areas covered by hyaline cartilage. The sesamoid bones, which track underneath the first metatarsal head within individual grooves, are also covered in cartilage. Variation in the shape of the metatarsal head and the sesamoids can contribute to the development of certain pathologic conditions and lend stability or instability to the complex.[9]

The capsule of the joint supports this structure, the most important portion of which is the plantar plate. Unlike the plantar plates of the lesser metatarsophalangeal joints, which are a simpler singular unidirectional band of ligament, the first metatarsophalangeal joint plantar plate is more of a complex, which consists of several different structures all working in concert to allow proper function of the joint. The proper collateral ligaments, accessory collateral ligaments, intersesamoidal ligament, metatarsalsesamoid ligaments, and sesamoidal phalangeal ligaments, deep intermetatarsal ligament, and fibers from the plantar fascia and the broad extensor hood all encapsulate the joint. The tendons of flexor hallucis brevis, abductor hallucis, and adductor hallucis also contribute to the stability of the joint, with the tendons of the long hallux flexor and extensors responsible for powering plantarflexion and dorsiflexion of the joint.[10]

Finally, the neurovascular structures in this area are vital to the proper functioning of this joint. Four nerves travel along the 4 corners of the base of the toe. The 2 plantar proper digital nerves are supplied by the medial plantar nerve, and the 2 dorsal nerves branch from the superficial peroneal nerve medially and the deep peroneal nerve laterally. The vascular supply of the hallux has more variance and deserves special attention because the plantar blood supply to the sesamoids can predispose patients to certain pathologic conditions and be important for certain surgical considerations. According to anatomic studies done by Rath and colleagues, the first plantar metatarsal artery provides branches to both the tibial and fibular sesamoid bone in most cases; however, the medial plantar artery also contributes to the blood supply of the sesamoid bones in about 18.4% of cases.[11] There is large variation in the size and number of branches of blood flow into the sesamoids, which affects where the areas of ischemia and avascular risk occur.

Evaluation

Clinical evaluation of this joint should begin with inspection and palpation. Palpation of the joint and individual components can determine the presence of osteophytosis, capsulitis, and, most importantly, areas of pain. Evaluation of the alignment of the joint while nonweight-bearing and weight-bearing can reveal triplane structural deformity. A great deal of information can be quickly collected from inspection for overall foot structure and alignment and areas of pain. The next part of evaluation involves thorough observation of the range of motion available in both sagittal and transverse planes. Typically, accepted amount of dorsiflexion in the joint should be 65°, whereas the amount of plantarflexion should be 45°. Crepitus or pain with range of motion may be appreciated. It is additionally important to stress the joint to determine if there is excessive motion dorso-plantar or medial-lateral. Comparison with the opposite side can be useful, except in cases of generalized hypermobility.

Imaging

Plain film radiographs are an important first diagnostic in first metatarsophalangeal joint pathologic condition. Fractures to bones can be seen in settings of trauma. Arthritic changes can be seen once the pathologic condition progresses to involve bone. Weight-bearing radiographs can aid in the evaluation of joint deformity and in the evaluation of overall foot structure and how it is contributing to first metatarsophalangeal pathologic condition. Many pathologic conditions cannot be seen with plain film alone, and other advanced imaging modalities may help diagnose the issue at hand.

For most sports-related first metatarsophalangeal joint complaints, MRI is a helpful next step. MRI can reveal and characterize the extent of osteochondral defects, tendon pathologic condition, ligamentous injury, and more. MRI of the first metatarsophalangeal joint has been shown to correlate well to clinical findings[12] as well as cadaver anatomy.[1,13,14] When ordering MRI for the first metatarsophalangeal joint, it is important to obtain image slices 3 mm thickness maximum and identify the area of complaint so that the planes can be oriented correctly around the joint because this will make a significant difference in the quality and utility of the images.[15]

PATHOLOGIC CONDITIONS
Trauma: Fractures, Sprains, Dislocations, Turf Toe

Athletes are at higher risk to bony trauma to the first metatarsophalangeal joint due to the nature of contact sport and increased demand and cutting, jumping, running, and twisting movements. Avulsion fractures typically indicate injury to collateral ligaments or other portions of the capsule and are treated as such. Fractures of the proximal phalanx or the metatarsal head are typically of consequence if displacement is significant or if the fracture is intra-articular. These fractures should be addressed similarly to any other fractures in that a significant amount of step off in the joint should not be accepted and should be reduced with open reduction and internal fixation, although no studies exist that correlate various levels of first metatarsophalangeal joint involvement to outcome.

Ligament and capsular injuries of the big toe joint can be very disabling, and potentially career ending if neglected. Capsular injuries can be categorized based on cause of injury, specific location of injury, and structures involved. It is therefore important to collect a detailed history of injuries to the joint. There are 2 types to consider that are most commonly encountered: plantar plate and medial collateral. Acute sprains can be immobilized, then rehabilitated with good success. Injuries to the collateral ligaments of the foot typically do well with splinting and immobilization. Acute and more complete plantar plate tears or ruptures tend to require surgical treatment to avoid instability and pain. Chronic instability or capsulitis, regardless of the specific ligamentous or anatomic

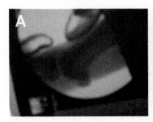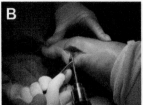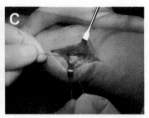

Fig. 1. (*A*) Dorsoplantar stress shows plantar sesamoid-phalangeal ligament tear and resultant instability. (*B*) Anchor being inserted to repair ligament. (*C*) Stability restored by ligament repair.

injury, has a poorer long-term prognosis with conservative care because on either side of the spectrum, these injuries can lead to deformities such as hallux valgus[16,17] or can initiate a cascade down the hallux limitus and rigidus course of joint disease.

Plantar plate tears are the most commonly seen injuries and present as acute injuries caused by forced dorsiflexion.[18] They are described as "Turf Toe," which implies a low morbidity condition, which is not the case. High grade or complete tears of the plantar ligament apparatus of the big toe joint may require surgical repair to best insure a good functional outcome. This surgical repair is best done soon to avoid instability of the joint and joint degeneration. Reattachment of the plantar plate can be approached either through a plantar or medial incision. Anchors help to facilitate the repair (**Fig. 1**A–C). Axial pinning of the toe can help maintain the integrity of the repair. There was interest in the study of this particular injury with the increasing prevalence of artificial turf use, which was linked to increased risk for injury when compared with grass.[19] Fortunately newer artificial turf designs have been modified to reduce this injury risk; however, this is still a commonly encountered injury. Turf toe injuries can be classified in grades of severity, described by Anderson,[20] which have been found to correlate to length of time of return to sport in meta-analysis.[21,22]

Collateral ligament injuries of the big toe joint usually occur when the hallux is restrained on the ground while the body moves internally. This is seen in football and soccer most often. The toe can feel unstable and painful with lateral motion, such as a football player receiver doing a down and out routine. Often, it is helpful to perform stress evaluation under fluoroscopy because these injuries can sometimes seem subtle on clinical examination (**Fig. 2**A, B). They can be treated with

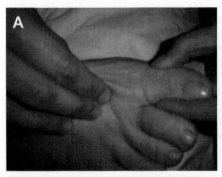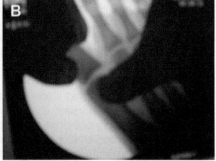

Fig. 2. (*A*) The hallux can be stressed medial to lateral to assess for the integrity of the collateral ligaments. (*B*) Stress of the hallux demonstrating collateral ligament tear and resultant instability.

immobilization, similar to ankle sprains. However, similar to ankle sprains, not all cases resolve with conservative care and instability can occur. Delayed primary repair can be performed successfully, so allowing a trial of conservative care in these cases reasonable.[23]

"Sand Toe" refers to injuries that occur because of extreme plantarflexion of the metatarsophalangeal joint in athletic events typically performed shoeless, such as beach volleyball or certain types of dance.[24] In this case, the dorsal, extensor structures are most commonly injured and these can typically be treated nonoperatively with immobilization.

Another subtype of capsular injury worth mentioning is synovial plicae syndrome. Plica have been well described in knee literature[25,26] but only have one mention in the ankle[27] and one mention in the first metatarsophalangeal joint.[28] Plica are thin, typically transparent folds of capsular synovial tissue that change shape to adapt to joint range of motion. However, when inflamed or injured, plicae can form a thicker fibrotic band within the capsule, which causes impingement. Typically, in the first metatarsophalangeal joint, patients present with history of trauma and a distinct tenderness to palpation to the dorsal joint line without the presence of osteophytosis. There is sometimes loss of range of motion and symptoms may not be reproducible with physical examination. Often, this is a diagnosis of exclusion when all other diagnostic and imaging modalities fail to isolate a specific cause for dorsal metatarsophalangeal joint pain. In the senior author's experience, isolated excision of this structure to be adequate for relief.[28] Active rehabilitation and range of motion following excision is important in avoiding capsular scarring and fibrosis.

Sesamoid Pathologic Conditions

Sesamoids are key components of the plantar plate complex. However, they have their own unique set of intrinsic pathologic conditions that merit a separate discussion. In athletes, the increased axial loading with certain types of motions can cause increased plantar pressure and axial loading on the sesamoids. This can cause repetitive stress injury that pushes the sesamoids down the road of marrow edema, stress fracture,[29,30] and avascular necrosis.[31] It is crucial to recognize and treat sesamoid pathologic conditions early because these injuries are prone to neglect and development into chronic injuries.

Sometimes, sesamoid pathologic condition is easily identifiable clinically with tenderness to palpation directly to the affected sesamoid(s). Other times, patients will describe onset of pain only with activity and have more difficulty with isolating the area of complaint. Plain film radiographs can be helpful in diagnosing acute fracture as long as there is due diligence to rule out bipartite sesamoid.[32] Another helpful modality is MRI, which will rule out other types of first metatarsophalangeal joint pathologic condition and be able to determine the internal structure of the sesamoid to evaluate for avascular necrosis or marrow edema.[33,34] Not all plantar big toe joint pain is sesamoid in origin. In the athlete, one must also consider flexor hallucinations breves tears or tendinopathy, plantar joint chondral injuries, and plantar plate/capsular tears. This can have significant clinical ramifications in an athlete. For example, plantar plate tears may require immediate surgical repair to best insure a good result. Sesamoid injuries do not typically require urgent surgical care.

The mainstays of initial sesamoid pathologic condition treatment are offloading of the area with a dancer's pad, controlled ankle motion boot, cast, any device that aligns with the patient's level of comfort and expected compliance. One issue in conservative treatment of sesamoid stress injuries is that at times the duration of treatment can be long. Even with supplemental modalities such as injections of biologics or bone

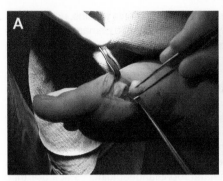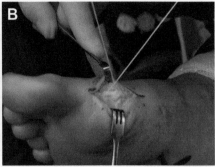

Fig. 3. (*A*) Tibial sesamoid is carefully removed preserving integrity of flexor tendon and all surrounding soft tissue. (*B*) A plicating suture is placed to advance the abductor hallucis to lessen the risk of developing hallux valgus.

stimulation, treatment can often require 3 to 4 months of compliance. The recovery from a sesamoidectomy may be shorter, and this may be favored by the professional athlete whose time span as an elite athlete is relatively short. Sesamoidectomy has been described in athletes as being effective in improving pain and function.[35] This should not be considered a benign procedure, however, because there have been many complications described with sesamoidectomy, including progressive deformity of the first metatarsophalangeal joint and chronic scarring/pain. The senior author prefers to use a medial incision to remove tibial sesamoids and recommends the use of a plicating suture to advance the abductor hallucis to prevent hallux valgus development (**Fig. 3**A, B).

Hallux Valgus

Hallux valgus is the lateral deviation of the hallux at the level of the metatarsophalangeal joint, causing a prominent medial metatarsal head with subluxation of the joint. Hallux valgus has a prevalence of 23% as reported in meta-analysis by Nix and colleagues[36] making it one of the most common foot and ankle issues. Athletic patients will typically complain of medial bump pain with activity in shoes as well as transfer metatarsalgia pain in the lesser metatarsals. Radiographs are essential to evaluate angular deformities present and evaluate foot structures that could be contributing to the development of the hallux valgus.

In athletes, the subluxation of this joint and subsequent loss of appropriate first ray function can become more noticeable with increased demand. In addition, the shoewear required for specific types of sport can exacerbate symptoms caused by hallux valgus. There are examples in the literature of shoewear exacerbating the amount of deformity in rock climbing[37] and wrestling.[38] Injuries to the joint can also lead to traumatic hallux valgus.[17]

There are a multitude of articles that discuss treatment options for hallux valgus in the literature, with options from conservative to surgical based on deformity flexibility and level of angular deformity. The focus of this review is not to review these treatment options in detail but to appreciate that hallux valgus treatment choices in athletes will depend less on these variables and more on what treatments accommodate their desired level and type of sporting activity and time to recovery back to sport.

Osteochondral Injury, Hallux Limitus, and Rigidus

Injury to the first metatarsophalangeal joint surface is common and occurs for a variety of reasons. Acute trauma can cause osteochondral defects but osteochondral injury can also develop because of the accumulation of degenerative changes over time. Although the treatment of osteochondral injury in sports medicine is well described in large joints such as the knee and medium joints such as the ankle, the algorithm in small joints is less clear. These lesions, even if small in metric measurement, can encompass a large percentage of the joint, making treatment challenging. A few studies have reported their experiences with first metatarsophalangeal joint arthroscopy,[39,40] microfracture,[41,42] and cartilage transplant.[43] The motivation for early treatment of these lesions is to prevent further progression of joint disease. Therefore, it is also important to consider the structural contributions to the development of these cartilage defects and treat them accordingly as well.

Hallux limitus is used to describe the limitation of the first metatarsophalangeal joint range of motion for any variety of reasons, which can sometimes progress to even more severe loss of range of motion in the end stage of hallux rigidus.[9,44] In athletes, this can be exacerbated by repetitive strain through jamming types of motions and is known to be more common in certain types of sport, such as basketball[45] and ballet.[3,4] Nonoperative treatments for hallux limitus can delay or prevent the progression of disease to a joint degenerative state. These include forefoot rocker sole shoes and orthotics modifications as well as injections into the joint. However, patients may opt to pursue surgical treatment when there is a definite underlying cause or when symptoms prevent athletic performance. Plain film radiographs and MRI can help determine this.

When considering procedures in athletes, it is less important to consider the grade of disease and more important to consider the patient goals and timeline for treatment and give patients options with estimated recovery times and prognosis. The general approach to the athlete with hallux rigidus is best described as a staged approach, to do the least invasive procedure that returns the athlete to their activities the quickest. Once the athlete retires, definitive reconstruction can then be considered. Cheilectomy with limited cartilage restoration often serves this purpose for athletes. Cheilectomy has been studied in athletes and seen to successfully change peak pressures.[46] In studies of the general population, although many studies report "failure" as reoperation rate or eventual arthrodesis, patient satisfaction with the procedure is high.[47] The authors do not favor Valenti procedures because they may compromise too much geography of the joint, making the late-stage reconstruction after sports career more complicated.

Another excellent procedure choice is the decompressional osteotomy, which has been shown to have favorable patient outcomes in even end-stage joints.[48] Currently available first metatarsophalangeal joint arthroplasty technologies do not provide adequate function and longevity for a high-demand athlete and even have questionable long-term benefit for the low-level recreational athlete,[49,50] also making any future arthrodesis or operation much more technically difficult. Arthrodesis can be appropriate for certain types of sport activity and incompatible with others but has been shown to have high rates of satisfaction.[50] Successful surgical treatment should decrease pain, increase function, and allow for years, if not a lifetime, until any additional procedure.

Joplin's Neuritis/Neuroma

Also known as compression neuropathy or neuritis of the medial plantar digital proper nerve, this condition can be caused by hallux valgus deformity placing increased pressure to this nerve, which tracks along the medial eminence of the first metatarsophalangeal joint.[51–53] Patients will present with typical nerve-type symptoms including burning or tingling in the nerve distribution or sharp pains. There may be a palpable thickening of the nerve on clinical examination. Thickening of the nerve may be seen on MRI. A simple diagnostic block to the nerve can be helpful in isolating the symptoms to this cause.[54] Treatment of any type of peripheral nerve compression syndrome should focus on offloading and decompressing the area externally, as well as any treatment of underlying bony deformities that may be contributing.

DISCUSSION

There are several common first metatarsophalangeal joint pathologic conditions encountered in athletes as reviewed above—turf toe injuries, sesamoid injuries, hallux valgus, hallux limitus/rigidus, and Joplin's neuroma/neuropathy. As in the case with any acute musculoskeletal complaint, anti-inflammatory efforts should be maximized early for both symptom control as well as to prevent the progression of acute inflammation into a chronic state. This can be in the form of cold therapies, compression, oral steroidal, or nonsteroidal anti-inflammatories. The other arms of appropriate treatment are more specific to the severity and accurate diagnosis of the condition.

The first metatarsophalangeal joint is a readily accessible joint to inject with biologics or steroid. There is not yet a large body of evidence for the use of platelet rich plasma (PRP) specifically into the first metatarsophalangeal joint, with one study reporting PRP capsular injections done successfully in ballet dancers to allow return to dance.[55] Other foot and ankle-specific studies on PRP have shown favorable outcomes in reducing the sesamoid injury time to recovery[56] and postponing the time to surgery in ankle osteoarthritis.[57] Concentrated bone marrow aspirate, studied again in sesamoids, may be another option to help get athletes back to preinjury status of performance.[58]

Another important component in the treatment of these issues stems from the fact that often the cause of repetitive strain that leads to these injuries is an essential part of their type of sport. Creative means of offloading the affected area of the joint must be incorporated into the sport activity or the shoewear.[59] Newer shoe technologies that include a full-length carbon fiber shank can help transfer force from heel strike to toe off in the gait cycle more efficiently, placing less strain on the first metatarsophalangeal joint alone. This type of ground reactive force vector modification can also be achieved by way of orthotics and gait training. In athletic sports requiring different types of movement than linear running, taping or bracing of the joint can provide extrinsic support to avoid further damage and aid in joint function.

Surgical interventions in the athlete should always be carefully considered because recovery requires rest and rehabilitation, which is time away from sport. If procedure options are weighed and chosen carefully, this time away from sport can be a worthy investment to gain function and reduce pain during activity. Evidence exists for good postoperative outcomes and high levels of performance in sports after surgical interventions such as sesamoidectomy,[35] bunionectomy, and arthrodesis.[50,60] If surgery is needed, joint sparing procedures such as ligamentous repairs, cheilectomies, or reconstructive osteotomies can be staged until there is no other option but joint destruction. These patients and complaints do not have simple algorithmic approaches. It is important to build a working relationship because they will look to you at multiple disease stages for the management of their great toe pathologic condition.

SUMMARY

Athletes demand higher function from their first metatarsophalangeal joint and therefore experience higher rates of pathologic condition in this joint. At the same time, athletes also seek treatments that minimize time away from sport and maximize function and performance. This can make the treatment of first metatarsophalangeal joint injuries in the athlete a challenging and often prolonged experience through various stages of joint pathologic condition and progression. Orthotics, taping, injections, and shoe modifications can temporize and aid with many of the most common issues, which include turf toe, hallux rigidus, and sesamoiditis. Surgical procedures, if needed, should be chosen to target the specific pathologic condition and should prioritize preservation of the joint, especially when range of motion is important for athletic movement. Fortunately, even in cases where surgery is pursued, athletic patients do have reasonably good outcomes.

CLINICS CARE POINTS

- Accurate diagnosis of the first metatarsophalangeal joint pathologic condition prevents overly aggressive or imprecise treatment in athletes.

- Obtain a complete and accurate history of trauma, both repetitive and acute in nature, and conduct a thorough physical examination with joint anatomy in mind.

- Advanced imaging, such as an MRI with image slices of no more than 3mm, can help narrow a diagnosis. Diagnostic injections can be helpful as well.

- Anti-inflammatory efforts and offloading strategies to decrease repetitive trauma are the mainstays of non-surgical treatment for most conditions.

- If surgical treatment is pursued for hallux rigidus, staged procedures such as a cheilectomy or decompressional osteotomy can reduce pain and maximize sport career performance while delaying or avoiding joint fusion.

DISCLOSURE

The authors have nothing to disclose.

REFERENCES

1. Hallinan JTPD, Statum SM, Huang BK, et al. High-Resolution MRI of the first metatarsophalangeal joint: Gross anatomy and injury Characterization. Radiogr Rev Publ Radiol Soc N Am Inc 2020;40(4):1107–24.
2. Nandikolla VK, Bochen R, Meza S, et al. Experimental gait analysis to study stress distribution of the Human foot. J Med Eng 2017;2017:3432074.
3. van Dijk CN, Lim LS, Poortman A, et al. Degenerative joint disease in female ballet dancers. Am J Sports Med 1995;23(3):295–300.
4. Ambré T, Nilsson BE. Degenerative changes in the first metatarso-phalangeal joint of ballet dancers. Acta Orthop Scand 1978;49(3):317–9.
5. Rodeo SA, O'Brien S, Warren RF, et al. Turf-toe: an analysis of metatarsophalangeal joint sprains in professional football players. Am J Sports Med 1990;18(3):280–5.
6. Hunt KJ, Hurwit D, Robell K, et al. Incidence and Epidemiology of foot and ankle injuries in elite collegiate athletes. Am J Sports Med 2017;45(2):426–33.
7. Lievers WB, Goggins KA, Adamic P. Epidemiology of foot injuries using National collegiate athletic Association Data from the 2009–2010 through 2014–2015 seasons. J Athl Train 2020;55(2):181–7.
8. Chan JJ, Geller JS, Chen KK, et al. Epidemiology of severe foot injuries in US collegiate athletes. Orthop J Sports Med 2021;9(4). 23259671211001132.

9. Zammit GV, Menz HB, Munteanu SE. Structural Factors Associated with hallux limitus/rigidus: a systematic review of case control studies. J Orthop Sports Phys Ther 2009;39(10):733–42.

10. Nery C, Baumfeld D, Umans H, et al. MR imaging of the plantar plate: normal anatomy, turf toe, and other injuries. Magn Reson Imaging Clin N Am 2017; 25(1):127–44.

11. Rath B, Notermans HP, Frank D, et al. Arterial anatomy of the hallucal sesamoids. Clin Anat N Y N 2009;22(6):755–60.

12. Dakkak YJ, Boer AC, Boeters DM, et al. The relation between physical joint examination and MRI-depicted inflammation of metatarsophalangeal joints in early arthritis. Arthritis Res Ther 2020;22(1):67.

13. Wang JE, Bai RJ, Zhan HL, et al. High-resolution 3T magnetic resonance imaging and histological analysis of capsuloligamentous complex of the first metatarsophalangeal joint. J Orthop Surg 2021;16(1):638.

14. De Maeseneer M, Moyson N, Lenchik L, et al. MR imaging-anatomical correlation of the metatarsophalangeal joint of the hallux: ligaments, tendons, and muscles. Eur J Radiol 2018;106:14–9.

15. Crain JM, Phancao JP. Imaging of turf toe. Radiol Clin North Am 2016;54(5): 969–78.

16. Fabeck LG, Zekhnini C, Farrokh D, et al. Traumatic hallux valgus following rupture of the medial collateral ligament of the first metatarsophalangeal joint: a case report. J Foot Ankle Surg Off Publ Am Coll Foot Ankle Surg 2002;41(2):125–8.

17. Covell DJ, Lareau CR, Anderson RB. Operative treatment of traumatic hallux valgus in elite athletes. Foot Ankle Int 2017;38(6):590–5.

18. Aran F, Ponnarasu S, Scott AT. Turf toe. In: StatPearls. StatPearls Publishing; 2022. Available at: http://www.ncbi.nlm.nih.gov/books/NBK507810/. Accessed February 17, 2022.

19. Sivasundaram L, Mengers S, Paliobeis A, et al. Injury risk among athletes on artificial turf: a review of current literature. Curr Orthop Pract 2021;32(5):512–7.

20. Anderson RB. Turf toe injuries of the hallux metatarsophalangeal joint. Tech Foot Ankle Surg 2002;1(2):102–11.

21. Vopat ML, Hassan M, Poppe T, et al. Return to sport after turf toe injuries: a systematic review and meta-analysis. Orthop J Sports Med 2019;7(10). 2325967119875133.

22. McCormick JJ, Anderson RB. Turf toe. Sports Health 2010;2(6):487–94.

23. Walley KC, Muscatelli SR, Singer N, et al. First metatarsophalangeal lateral collateral ligament repair in an athlete: a case report. JBJS Case Connect 2021;11(3). https://doi.org/10.2106/JBJS.CC.20.00901.

24. Frey C, Andersen GD, Feder KS. Plantarflexion injury to the metatarsophalangeal joint ("sand toe"). Foot Ankle Int 1996;17(9):576–81.

25. Casadei K, Kiel J. Plica syndrome. StatPearls Publishing; 2020. Available at: https://www.ncbi.nlm.nih.gov/books/NBK535362/. Accessed February 13, 2021.

26. Lee PYF, Nixion A, Chandratreya A, et al. Synovial plica syndrome of the knee: a commonly Overlooked cause of Anterior knee pain. Surg J 2017;3(1):e9–16.

27. Somorjai N, Jong B, Draijer WF. Intra-articular plica causing ankle impingement in a young handball player: a case report. J Foot Ankle Surg Off Publ Am Coll Foot Ankle Surg 2013;52(6):750–3.

28. By Lawrence M, Oloff DPM. Diagnosing and treating synovial plica syndrome in A patient with first metatarsophalangeal joint pain. Podiatry Today 2021;34(2). Available at: https://www.hmpglobearningnetwork.com/site/podiatry/diagnosing-and-

treating-synovial-plica-syndrome-patient-first-metatarsophalangeal-joint-pain. Accessed February 19, 2022.

29. Hulkko A, Orava S, Pellinen P, et al. Stress fractures of the sesamoid bones of the first metatarsophalangeal joint in athletes. Arch Orthop Trauma Surg Arch Orthopadische Unf-chir 1985;104(2):113–7.

30. Biedert R, Hintermann B. Stress fractures of the medial great toe sesamoids in athletes. Foot Ankle Int 2003;24(2):137–41.

31. Bartosiak K, McCormick JJ. Avascular necrosis of the sesamoids. Foot Ankle Clin 2019;24(1):57–67.

32. Favinger JL, Porrino JA, Richardson ML, et al. Epidemiology and imaging appearance of the normal Bi-/multipartite hallux sesamoid bone. Foot Ankle Int 2015;36(2):197–202.

33. Karasick D, Schweitzer ME. Disorders of the hallux sesamoid complex: MR features. Skeletal Radiol 1998;27(8):411–8.

34. Lombard C, Gillet R, Rauch A, et al. Hallux sesamoid complex imaging: a practical diagnostic approach. Skeletal Radiol 2020;49(12):1889–901.

35. Dean RS, Coetzee JC, McGaver RS, et al. Functional outcome of sesamoid excision in athletes. Am J Sports Med 2020;48(14):3603–9.

36. Nix S, Smith M, Vicenzino B. Prevalence of hallux valgus in the general population: a systematic review and meta-analysis. J Foot Ankle Res 2010;3:21. https://doi.org/10.1186/1757-1146-3-21.

37. Schöffl V, Küpper T. Feet injuries in rock climbers. World J Orthop 2013;4(4):218–28.

38. Yu G, Fan Y, Fan Y, et al. The role of Footwear in the Pathogenesis of hallux valgus: a Proof-of-Concept finite Element analysis in recent Humans and Homo naledi. Front Bioeng Biotechnol 2020;8:648. https://doi.org/10.3389/fbioe.2020.00648.

39. Levaj I, Knežević I, Dimnjaković D, et al. First metatarsophalangeal joint arthroscopy of 36 Consecutive cases. Acta Chir Orthop Traumatol Cech 2021;88(3):211–6.

40. Kuyucu E, Mutlu H, Mutlu S, et al. Arthroscopic treatment of focal osteochondral lesions of the first metatarsophalangeal joint. J Orthop Surg 2017;12(1):68.

41. Bojanić I, Smoljanović T, Kubat O. Osteochondritis dissecans of the first metatarsophalangeal joint: arthroscopy and microfracture technique. J Foot Ankle Surg Off Publ Am Coll Foot Ankle Surg 2011;50(5):623–5.

42. Sherman TI, Kern M, Marcel J, et al. First metatarsophalangeal joint arthroscopy for osteochondral lesions. Arthrosc Tech 2016;5(3):e513–8.

43. Van Dyke B, Berlet GC, Daigre JL, et al. First metatarsal head osteochondral defect treatment with Particulated Juvenile cartilage Allograft Transplantation: a case series. Foot Ankle Int 2018;39(2):236–41.

44. Ho B, Baumhauer J. Hallux rigidus. EFORT Open Rev 2017;2(1):13–20.

45. Trégouët P. An assessment of hallux limitus in university basketball players compared with noncompetitive individuals. J Am Podiatr Med Assoc 2014;104(5):468–72.

46. Mulier T, Steenwerckx A, Thienpont E, et al. Results after cheilectomy in athletes with hallux rigidus. Foot Ankle Int 1999;20(4):232–7.

47. Teoh KH, Tan WT, Atiyah Z, et al. Clinical outcomes following Minimally invasive dorsal cheilectomy for hallux rigidus. Foot Ankle Int 2019;40(2):195–201.

48. Oloff LM, Jhala-Patel G. A retrospective analysis of joint salvage procedures for grades III and IV hallux rigidus. J Foot Ankle Surg Off Publ Am Coll Foot Ankle Surg 2008;47(3):230–6.

49. Daniilidis K, Martinelli N, Marinozzi A, et al. Recreational sport activity after total replacement of the first metatarsophalangeal joint: a prospective study. Int Orthop 2010;34(7):973–9.

50. Da Cunha RJ, MacMahon A, Jones MT, et al. Return to sports and physical activities after first metatarsophalangeal joint arthrodesis in young patients. Foot Ankle Int 2019;40(7):745–52.

51. Melendez MM, Patel A, Dellon AL. The diagnosis and treatment of Joplin's neuroma. J Foot Ankle Surg Off Publ Am Coll Foot Ankle Surg 2016;55(2):320–3.

52. Still GP, Fowler MB. Joplin's neuroma or compression neuropathy of the plantar proper digital nerve to the hallux: clinicopathologic study of three cases. J Foot Ankle Surg Off Publ Am Coll Foot Ankle Surg 1998;37(6):524–30.

53. Merritt GN, Subotnick SI. Medial plantar digital proper nerve syndrome (Joplin's neuroma)–typical presentation. J Foot Surg 1982;21(3):166–9.

54. Burke CJ, Sanchez J, Walter WR, et al. Ultrasound-guided Therapeutic injection and Cryoablation of the medial plantar proper digital nerve (Joplin's Nerve): Sonographic Findings, Technique, and Clinical Outcomes. Acad Radiol 2020; 27(4):518–27.

55. Jain N, Bauman PA, Hamilton WG, et al. Can Elite Dancers Return to Dance After Ultrasound-Guided Platelet-Rich Plasma (PRP) Injections? J Dance Med Sci 2018;22(4):225–32.

56. Le HM, Stracciolini A, Stein CJ, et al. Platelet rich plasma for hallux sesamoid injuries: a case series. Phys Sportsmed 2021;1–4.

57. Repetto I, Biti B, Cerruti P, et al. Conservative Treatment of Ankle Osteoarthritis: Can Platelet-Rich Plasma Effectively Postpone Surgery? J Foot Ankle Surg Off Publ Am Coll Foot Ankle Surg 2017;56(2):362–5.

58. Shimozono Y, Seow D, Kennedy JG. Concentrated Bone Marrow Aspirate Injection for Hallux Sesamoid Disorders. J Foot Ankle Surg Off Publ Am Coll Foot Ankle Surg 2021;S1067-2516(21):00410–5.

59. Colò G, Fusini F, Samaila EM, et al. The efficacy of shoe modifications and foot orthoses in treating patients with hallux rigidus: a comprehensive review of literature. Acta Bio Med Atenei Parm 2020;91(Suppl 14):e2020016.

60. Bouché RT, Adad JM. Arthrodesis of the first metatarsophalangeal joint in active people. Clin Podiatr Med Surg 1996;13(3):461–84.

Orthobiologic Use in Sports Injuries

Lawrence M. Oloff, DPM, FACFAS[a],*, Isaac Wilhelm, DPM[a], Nishit S. Vora, DPM, MPH[b]

KEYWORDS

- Orthobiologics • PRP • BMAC • Tendinopathy • Amniotic • DBM • Sports medicine

KEY POINTS

- Orthobiologics have gained popularity in recent years in the treatment of orthopedic injuries and improving return to activity.
- Platelet-rich plasma, bone marrow aspirate concentrate, amniotic tissue, and demineralized bone matrix have all been found to improve healing in sports-related injuries, although the research is limited.

INTRODUCTION/HISTORY/DEFINITIONS/BACKGROUND

In the past 30 years of medicine, there have been great advances in scientific discovery, improving our understanding of disease pathologic condition and processes, creating a new area of medicine called Orthobiologics. These cell-based therapies are composed of natural growth factors (GF) and cytokines that facilitate cell growth and recruitment, modulate pain receptors and inflammatory mediators, and stimulate blood vessel growth, matrix synthesis, and tissue maturation. Orthobiologics are the biological substances found naturally in the body that are used in regenerative medicine to aid in tissue healing and biological restoration. Orthobiologics have been used in a variety of different areas of medicine, including cardiothoracic surgery, wound healing, ophthalmology, sports medicine, orthopedic surgery, urology, cosmetic surgery, maxillofacial surgery, and dentistry. These therapies used in the field of Sports Medicine have created a paradigm shift in treatment, changing the treatment mindset from temporary symptomatic relief to delaying or preventing onset of disease by modifying the signals within the biologic environment.

The implementation of orthobiologics in treatment therapy has two main benefits. The first benefit is they can reduce the need for surgery, and second benefit is they can increase the effectiveness of current surgical techniques.[1] Orthobiologics come in many different forms to treat soft tissue and bone injuries. These include platelet-

[a] Saint Mary's Medical Center, 450 Stanyan Street, San Francisco, CA 94117, USA; [b] 1501 Trousdale Drive, Suite 115, Burlingame, CA 94010, USA
* Corresponding author. 1501 Trousdale Drive, Suite 115, Burlingame, CA 94010.
E-mail address: lmop11@comcast.net

Clin Podiatr Med Surg 40 (2023) 169–179
https://doi.org/10.1016/j.cpm.2022.07.011
0891-8422/23/© 2022 Elsevier Inc. All rights reserved.

rich plasma (PRP), bone marrow aspirate concentrate (BMAC), amniotic tissue, and demineralized bone matrix (DBM). A recent increase in medical innovation has brought these techniques into mainstream treatment with little clinical evidence. This article provides a current review on the uses of orthobiologics in sports-related injuries.

Platelet-Rich Plasma

PRP is a substance containing a higher concentration of platelets from whole blood, and when administered, will theoretically stimulate a supraphysiologic response. PRP is also known as platelet-enriched plasma, platelet-rich concentrate, and autogenous platelet gel. It initially gained popularity in dentistry and cardiac surgery in the 1980s and 1990s. It was first used by Ferrari and colleagues[2] in 1987 following open heart surgery.

The normal platelet count in a healthy individual is between 150,000 and 450,000/uL, and PRP has a 3- to 5-fold increase in GF concentration. The cytokines in platelets that can contribute to tendon healing include transforming growth factor-β, platelet-derived growth factor, epidermal growth factor, vascular endothelial growth factor, endothelial growth factor, and insulin-like growth factor.[3] The autologous concentrated blood is then mixed with calcium chloride or thrombin to create a more gelatinous substance that can be injected.[4]

There are 2 different types of PRP, and each has their own benefits and limitations. One type is the leukocyte rich (LR-PRP), which is red in color and rich in red blood cells and white blood cells, and the other is leukocyte poor (LP-PRP), which is white blood cell and red blood cell poor. It is widely debated as to which preparation is better for which structures of the musculoskeletal system. LP has been shown to stimulate cartilage better than the LR[5] and found to have more functionality and pain-relieving benefits compared with LR.[6] LR-PRP has been shown to decrease cytokine production and promote tissue regeneration in tenocytes.

PRP has been seen to treat pathologic conditions such as tendinopathy, lumbar radiculopathy, and osteoarthritis.[7] Studies have indicated that the level of concentration matters proportionally with the healing potential.[8] The age of an individual also plays a crucial factor in determining how much blood will be needed to concentrate so as to realize the desired benefits. As a result, older individuals tend to need a higher concentration of PRP in order to start their healing cascade.[9]

PRP therapy has been shown to be an effective method of treating chronic tendinopathy in multiple body areas, including extensor muscles, the Achilles and patellar tendons, and the rotator cuff. Patients treated with PRP therapy reported better functionality and less pain for multiple years after treatment compared with other treatment methods, such as steroid use.

PRP therapy is being heavily looked at as a treatment option for Achilles tendinopathy. Acute Achilles tendinopathy is often treatable with standard practices, such as rest, ice, anti-inflammatories, and so forth. However, chronic Achilles tendinopathy is much more difficult to treat, as the damage is so extensive that there is often a reduction of blood flow and increase in scar tissue. The body is no longer responding to the injured area. The common treatment strategy is to undergo surgery with the intention to increase blood flow and healing in the area. Unfortunately, these surgeries are not often successful.[10] For this reason, PRP therapy is now being tested as a new treatment approach. PRP allows for the direct addition of platelets, which will increase the number of GF.

There have been multiple studies over the effectiveness of PRP with differing results. Filardo and colleagues[11] gave 34 chronic Achilles tendinopathy patients 3 PRP injections over a 6-week period. The patients reported satisfaction with the treatment and would undergo again if necessary. Deans and colleagues[12] treated 28 patients with Achilles tendinopathy. Their treatment was also paired with a standard rehabilitation program of full weightbearing in a pneumatic cast boot for 6 weeks, therapeutic ultrasound treatment, and eccentric exercise program at 2 weeks following injection. They had significant improvement in activities of daily living, quality of life, and ability to perform sports/recreational activities.

Oloff and colleagues[13] were able to study the clinical effects of PRP through imaging. They studied 26 patients, 13 who underwent Achilles tendon debridement with PRP augmentation versus isolated PRP injection for recalcitrant Achilles tendinopathy. MRI was used to image the Achilles tendon preprocedure and postprocedure at an average of 1.8 years apart and was read by one radiologist. Their results showed a statistical significance in the improvement of functional scoring in both groups. Also noted was that there was no difference between the surgical and nonsurgical groups. Whether a standalone PRP injection or combined with surgical debridement, it produced improvement in both clinical outcomes and MRI findings. In some cases, both injection and surgical/injection groups demonstrated almost complete resolution of tendinosis (**Figs. 1** and **2**). Oloff and Lam[14] also studied PRP augmentation with surgery in tibialis posterior tendon tendinosis. They wrote a case study about a soccer player who suffered with this for 2 years and underwent posterior tibial (PT) tendon debridement and intraoperative PRP injection. He returned to activity at 31 weeks with no complication and had an improved tendon appearance at 9 months on MRI and completely normal tendon at 5 years. de Vos and colleagues[15] researched 54 patients in the largest PRP double-blind study. Twenty-seven patients received a PRP injection, whereas the other 27 patients received saline. All participants went through the same postinjection therapy program starting 1 week after injection consisting of 12 weeks of eccentric exercises. They found there was a significant difference in the preinjection and postinjection groups but no difference between the PRP and control group at the 2-, 12-, and 24-week marks. A 1-year follow-up study showed continued improvement in both groups and again no statistical significance between the PRP versus saline injection groups.[16]

PRP is also commonly used in the treatment of osteoarthritis, mainly for the knee and hip,[17] and has been shown to improve functionality and reduce pain, but has not been well documented with the foot and ankle. Patients treated with PRP reported less joint pain and increased joint function compared with a placebo injection in a study conducted by Dai and colleagues.[18] Randomized control trials in which patients with osteoarthritis were stratified suggested that PRP was more effective in

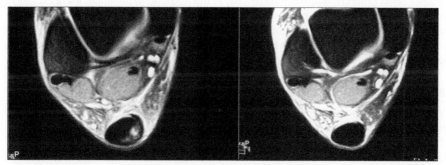

Fig. 1. PRP preinjection and postinjection. (*Courtesy of* Lawrence Oloff, DPM, San Francisco, CA.)

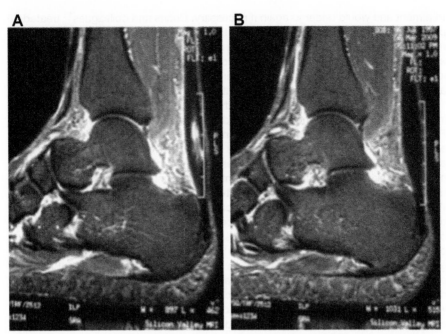

Fig. 2. PRP presurgery and postsurgery. (*From* Oloff L, Elmi E, Nelson J, Crain J. Retrospective Analysis of the Effectiveness of Platelet-Rich Plasma in the Treatment of Achilles Tendinopathy: Pretreatment and Posttreatment Correlation of Magnetic Resonance Imaging and Clinical Assessment. Foot & Ankle Specialist. 2015;8(6):490-497. https://doi.org/10.1177/1938640015599033.)

patients with a lower degree of cartilage degeneration. Careful selection of which patients should receive an intra-articular PRP injection should be considered.[19]

PRP therapy has also been looked into as a treatment of bone healing. Malhotra and colleagues[20] talk about PRP's use in treating fractures. They claim that although PRP contains many GF that have roles throughout the healing process, PRP lacks the necessary scaffolding needed for proper restoration. PRP therapy would be most effective if paired with a cell-supporting matrix.

There has been controversy on the use of PRP and also the best preparation to use its application. There is no standardized PRP treatment protocol, as all of these studies used different treatment regimens. In the authors' experience, immobilization for 3 weeks postinjection has more successful results. After needling the diseased tendon and injecting PRP, the extremity should be immobilized to allow for the PRP to take effect. PRP could be the treatment choice for tendinopathy. It is less invasive, is less chance of complications, and could be an adjunct to surgery.

Bone Marrow Aspirate Concentrate

Various medical procedures have been created with the aim of enhancing regeneration of the cartilage, such as the efforts to deliver reparable agents, the likes of mesenchymal stem cells (MSC) to the defected regions. However, because of the low concentrations that are transported to the defective regions, no method has ever been regarded as optimal when dealing with the regeneration of cartilage.[21] This saw the need for the development of treatment options that could ensure that a high concentration of stem cells was transported to the defected region and enhance the treatment of patients.

One such development is the BMAC. BMAC refers to a concentration of fluid aspirated from bone marrow that is used as an adjunct to encourage GF for bone or cartilage formation. BMAC contains a high number of MSC as well as other osteogenic GF, such as platelet-derived growth factor, transforming growth factor-β, mononuclear cells, and vascular endothelial growth factor. A high concentration of these mononuclear cells have shown the ability to induce osteoblastic growth and differentiation indicating BMAC for a wide variety of procedures, ranging from nonunions, fractures, and osteotomies to revision joint replacement surgery. This material has the ability to produce high amounts of MSC, chondrogenic cells, alongside other cells of the stroma.[22] The amounts of these cells produced by the BMAC even exceed those that are produced by the bone marrow itself and has illustrated that it holds a considerably increased amount of white blood cells as well as platelets.[23]

BMAC can be harvested from the iliac crest, proximal tibia, distal tibia, or calcaneus.[24] The iliac crest is the gold standard for the harvest location with it having the highest concentration of mononuclear cells and lowest associated pain. The bone marrow aspirate is centrifuged to form BMAC, which increases the MSC concentration.[25]

In a study by Murphy and colleagues[26] in 2019, they looked at osteochondral lesions (OLT) of the talus that were treated with microfracture, with and without BMAC. Fifty-two patients were in the microfracture-only group, and 49 patients were in the microfracture plus BMAC group. Both had significant improvement in pain scores, quality-of-life scores, participation in sport, and activities of daily living. Revision rate was 28.8% in the microfracture group and 12.2% microfracture/BMAC group. Lesions were less than 1.5 cm^2 in diameter. They highlighted that the use of BMAC improved outcomes rather than microfracture alone. They also noted that there was no increase in ankle or donor site morbidity in the BMAC group. One study conducted by Pascual-Garrido and colleagues[27] looked at the effectiveness of using ultrasound-guided injection BMAC for patellar tendinitis. The 8 patients were assessed for pain improvement and daily activity scores, quality of life, and functional knee scores (International Knee Documentation Committee) and Knee Injury and Osteoarthritis Outcome Score. Seven of the 8 patients reported back with high scores and said they were satisfied with the treatment.

Although not well supported, BMAC has also been used for prophylactic treatment of nonunions, especially in locations where nonunion is a higher risk. One study by Hunt and Anderson[28] showed that BMAC was an effective treatment option for Jones fractures. Twenty-one elite athletes underwent treatment, with an average return to play of 12.3 weeks and only 1 suffering from refracture. Another study, by Carney and colleagues,[29] looked at 41 athletes across a wide range of sports that had suffered from Jones fractures. They too found that BMAC was effective, as athletes had an average return to play of 11 weeks with no reinjuries.

BMAC can be used as an adjunct to scaffolds to replace bone defects. In a 2011 study by Jäger and colleagues,[30] BMAC was incubated with a collagen scaffold (Col) or hydroxyapatite (HA) before implanting the BMAC into a bone void greater than 1 cm × 1 cm. The Col incubated with BMAC (BMAC-Col) was used in 12 patients and BMAC with HA granules (BMAC-HA) was used in 27 patients. New bone formation was seen in the BMAC-HA group at 6.8 ± 2.7 weeks, which was significantly earlier than the BMAC-Col group at 13.6 ± 13.8 weeks. In 36 of the 39 patients, complete mean time for bone healing for the HA group and Col groups were

17.3 ± 7.8 weeks and 22.4 ± 12.0 weeks, respectively. BMAC used with HA may support a faster recovery time compared with BMAC used with a Col.

The initial studies over BMAC therapy have shown promise to be a treatment option for a wide range of bone, joint, and tendon injuries. The shortcomings in this field are apparent, however. The studies conducted lack standardized, reproducible procedures and are often taken from small sample sizes. There are also a lack of long-term studies to see if there are any long-term physiologic effects. It is also difficult to distinguish the role of BMAC versus other rehabilitation practices often used in conjunction with BMAC. As more studies are conducted, the efficiency and precision of BMAC therapy will likely increase and make a name for itself as a standard rehabilitation option.

Amniotic Tissue

Research into amniotic-derived products has grown in recent years, showing potential therapeutic applications in regenerative orthopedics and sports medicine. The growing interest is primarily because the amniotic tissue is an ethical source and can be easily harvested after cesarean childbirth. They also possess low immunogenicity circumventing the risk of graft-versus-host disease, making them ideal for allogenic use.[31] Furthermore, the amniotic tissue is rich in biofactors that have varied therapeutic applications.

The amniotic tissue makes up the innermost portion of the placenta during pregnancy. It is composed of 2 components: amniotic membrane (AM) and amniotic fluid (AF). The AM is a bilayer with chorion on the outside and amnion on the inside, whereas the AF is surrounded and contained by the amnion. Amniotic tissue has an extracellular matrix comprising collagen, fibronectin, and laminin that provides a natural scaffold for cellular attachment and structural support. In addition, the AF possesses several nutrients, GF, potent antimicrobial agents, antifibrotic factors, and the antiscarring agent hyaluronic acid.[32] Two cell types with stem cell-like characteristics have been identified in AM: human amniotic epithelial cells and human amniotic mesenchymal stromal cells (hAM-MSCs).[33,34]

In vitro and in vivo experiments have demonstrated the beneficial effects of amniotic tissue and tissue-derived products in promoting reepithelialization, decreasing inflammation and fibrosis, and modulating angiogenesis. Amniotic tissue has been shown to inhibit the inflammatory cascade following an adult injury, mediated by anti-inflammatory cytokines secreted by resident dendritic cells, which may benefit healing and scar formation in patients.[35,36] The MSCs in AM implants are capable of homing to injured sites, secreting GF and anti-inflammatory cytokines, and differentiating into osteogenic and chondrogenic lineages.[37,38] The high concentration of epidermal GF in the AF is known to play a role in bone formation,[39] whereas fibroblast GF was shown to restore morphologic and biomechanical properties of injured tendon in animal studies.[40] Thus, transplantation of amniotic tissue at the site of injury can create an environment conducive for repair and regeneration.[32] Furthermore, veterinary and animal studies support the application of AM-derived biologics in healing tendon, ligament, soft tissue, bone, and chondral injuries.[38,41–43]

All these factors combined make human AM-AF a potential therapeutic option for foot and ankle pathologic conditions. Positive results from experimental animal models have paved the way to human trials.[44,45] Preliminary clinical data suggest the administration of hAM-AF as a promising treatment of chronic wounds and pathologic conditions, including plantar fasciitis, Achilles tendinosis, and diabetic ulcers. In this regard, various formulations and modes of applications, such as granulized hAM-AF (gAM-AF) and amniotic suspension allograft, have been tested for safety and optimal efficacy.[46,47]

A study by Werber and colleagues[48] used cryopreserved gAM-AF as an injectable to treat patients with chronic plantar fasciitis and Achilles tendinosis who did not respond to conventional therapies. The injections were directed to the superior surface of the plantar fascia, and along the paratenon starting on the medial aspect in Achilles tendinosis. Interestingly, at 12 weeks posttreatment, all patients reported a significant reduction in pain. Similarly, a randomized clinical trial was conducted to assess the efficacy of 2 doses of micronized dehydrated human amniotic/chorionic membrane injection as a treatment of chronic refractory plantar fasciitis. The research group reported a continued improvement in symptoms and heel function over 8 weeks in the treatment group compared with the control group.[49] Another randomized, controlled, double-blind pilot study showed comparable efficacy outcomes with cryopreserved AM and corticosteroid treatments for plantar fasciitis.[50] Amniotic tissue has also been used for tendon repair. When wrapped around the tendon, the tissue acts as a protective sheath and has benefits that include anti-inflammatory, antiadhesive, and antimicrobial properties. In a study by Liu and colleagues[51] in 2019, they found that freeze-dried AM wrapped around a flexor tendon reduced adhesions and had less complications than poly-DL-lactic acid. The use of gAM-FM was also investigated in treating chronic diabetic foot wounds. In a prospective study, multiple allograft injections to the wounded tissue at 14- to 21-day intervals demonstrated complete wound closure within the 12-week observation period in 90% of the patients.[32] In all the trials, the transplantations were well tolerated with no treatment-related adverse events. However, there are no studies yet that measure long-term safety.

Recent research findings show great promise suggesting amniotic-derived biologics as an adjunct or alternative therapy for tendon, ligament, and bone injuries, including that of foot and ankle pathologic conditions. However, further controlled trials involving more extensive and diverse populations are required to ascertain long-term safety and efficacy outcomes that are statistically significant. Besides, more studies are necessary to standardize the optimal formulation, mode and route of administration, and dosage regimens that can be clinically safe and effective.

Demineralized Bone Matrix

Bone grafting was first reported in 1668 by a Dutch surgeon, Job Van Meerkeren, when he implanted xenograft canine skull into a defect of the skull of a soldier.[52] One of the more popular types of bone grafting, DBM, has become a reliable implant in bone healing during sports-related injuries. Successful bone healing requires 3 major properties: osteoconduction, osteoinduction, and osteogenesis. Osteoconduction aids in bone healing by providing a scaffolding. Examples include bone allograft, bone autograft, DBM, and inert fillers. Osteoinduction aids in providing GF to promote differentiation of host osteoprogenitor cells. Examples include BMPs, PRP, and BMAC. Osteogenesis provides the ability of the graft itself, and its elements, to fabricate new bone. The best example of this is autologous cancellous bone. DBM is a bone allograft that is processed in a way in which its inorganic materials are removed while preserving its organic materials. This allows it to retain both its osteoconductive and its osteoinductive properties through its collagen matrix and BMPs. DBM is another osteobiologic product that can provide favorable outcomes in treating sports injuries and degenerative sequelae in the foot and ankle, as seen in multiple studies.

Yoo studied DBM early on and provided proof that it improved osteoinductivity in skeletally mature rabbits. They implanted different concentrations of DBM with HA and bone marrow aspirate and found that DBM in higher concentrations provided the highest rate of fusion, regardless of the amount of the other compounds added.[52]

Michelson and Curl[53] compared hindfoot fusion augmented with iliac bone graft versus DBM. Fifty-five patients, 11 subtalar joint fusions and 44 triple arthrodesis, were studied. Seven of the 8 subtalar joint fusions that were augmented with DBM went on to fusion with the last having asymptomatic radiographic nonunion. All 29 patients in the triple arthrodesis group with DBM augmentation went on to union. DBM was found to be just as good as iliac bone graft in fusion rates and time to fusion with a decrease in cast and donor site morbidity.

Lareau and colleagues[54] were able to study professional football players from the NFL and quantify their return to work after surgical fixation of their zone 2 and 3 Jones fractures with the supplementation of DBM and BMAC. Twenty-five players were studied with 100% return to work at an average time of 8.7 weeks. Only 3 players suffered refracture and underwent revision surgery for a 12% revision rate. Galli studied the use of DBM in OLT with cystic degeneration. They studied 12 patients with medial cystic OLTs that had failed previous microfracture surgery. The patients underwent medial malleolar osteotomy and DBM grafting and were followed for 2 years. Patients were found to have complete graft incorporation, significant reduction in pain and disability, and no additional complications.

DBM can play an important role in surgical intervention should treatment require surgery. Its innate properties allow for enhanced healing and quicker return to activity. It can be used in conjunction with other osteobiologics to enhance its effects.

SUMMARY

Orthobiologics have gained popularity in recent years. There has not been a robust amount of clinical evidence to support their use yet. In the limited research that has been published, they have been shown to be effective and safe. They can assist in earlier return to activity with the avoidance of surgery. They can also augment current surgical practice to aid in healing and return to sport with almost no complications. With new medical innovation, there is unfortunately a higher cost for these products. The use of orthobiologics will only grow and so will the need for high-level clinical evidence.

CLINICS CARE POINTS

- Platelet-rich plasma and amniotic injections can be used as a last effort before proceeding with surgery. Both are sources of growth factors; however, for older individuals, amnion should be favored because the platelets lose their efficacy for growth factors.
- Patients should be immobilized after platelet-rich plasma injections.
- Demineralized bone matrix can be used in conjunction with BMP or bone marrow aspirate concentrate for improved function.

DISCLOSURE

The authors have nothing to disclose.

REFERENCES

1. Wee J, Thevendran G. The role of orthobiologics in foot and ankle surgery: allogenic bone grafts and bone graft substitutes. EFORT Open Rev 2017;2(6): 272–80.

2. Ferrari M, Zia S, Valbonesi M, et al. A new technique for hemodilution, preparation of autologous platelet-rich plasma and intraoperative blood salvage in cardiac surgery. Int J Artif Organs 1987;10(1):47–50.

3. Foster TE, Puskas PL, Mandelbaum BR, et al. Platelet rich plasma: from basic science to clinical application. Am J Sports Med 2009;37:225916.

4. Toyoda T, Isobe K, et al. Direct activation of platelets by addition of CaCl2 leads coagulation of platelet-rich plasma. Int J Implant dentistry 2018;4(1):23.

5. Cavallo C, Filardo G, Mariani E, et al. Comparison of platelet-rich plasma formulations for cartilage healing: an in vitro study. J Bone Joint Surg Am 2014;96(5):423–9.

6. Riboh JC, Saltzman BM, Yanke AB, et al. Effect of leukocyte concentration on the efficacy of platelet-rich plasma in the treatment of knee osteoarthritis. Am J Sports Med 2016;44(3):792–800.

7. Greer N, Yoon P, Majeski B, et al. Orthobiologics in foot and ankle arthrodesis sites: a systematic review. (US): Department of Veterans Affairs; 2020.

8. Berger DR, Centeno CJ, Steinmetz NJ. Platelet lysates from aged donors promote human tenocyte proliferation and migration in a concentration-dependent manner. Bone Joint Res 2019;8(1):32–40.

9. Roberts TT, Rosenbaum AJ. Bone grafts, bone substitutes and orthobiologics: the bridge between basic science and clinical advancements in fracture healing. Organogenesis 2012;8(4):114–24.

10. Baravarian B. Emerging insights on orthobiologics and Achilles tendon pathology. Podiatry Today 2014;27:11.

11. Filardo G, Kon E, et al. Platelet-rich plasma injections for the treatment of refractory Achilles tendinopathy: results at 4 years. Blood Transfus = Trasfusione Del Sangue 2014;12(4):533–40.

12. Deans VM, Miller A, Ramos J. A prospective series of patients with chronic Achilles tendinopathy treated with autologous-conditioned plasma injections combined with exercise and therapeutic ultrasonography. J Foot Ankle Surg 2012;51:706–10.

13. Oloff L, Elmi E, Nelson J, et al. Retrospective analysis of the effectiveness of platelet-rich plasma in the treatment of Achilles tendinopathy: pretreatment and posttreatment correlation of magnetic resonance imaging and clinical assessment. Foot & Ankle Specialist 2015;8(6):490–7.

14. Oloff L, Lam J. Does PRP have promise for advanced posterior tibial tendinopathy in athletes? Podiatry Today 2017;30:12.

15. de Vos RJ, Adam W, et al. Platelet-rich plasma injection for chronic Achilles tendinopathy: a randomized controlled trial. JAMA 2010;303(2):144–9.

16. de Jonge, Suzan Robert J de Vos, Adam Weir, et al. One-year follow-up of platelet-rich plasma treatment in chronic Achilles tendinopathy: a double-blind randomized placebo-controlled trial. Am J Sports Med 2011;39(8):1623–9.

17. Middleton KK, Barro V, Muller B, et al. Evaluation of the effects of platelet-rich plasma (PRP) therapy involved in the healing of sports-related soft tissue injuries. Iowa orthopaedic J 2012;32:150–63.

18. Dai WL, Zhou AG, Zhang H, et al. Efficacy of platelet-rich plasma in the treatment of knee osteoarthritis: a meta-analysis of randomized controlled trials. Arthroscopy 2017;33(3):659–70.e1.

19. Gato-Calvo L, Magalhaes J, Ruiz-Romero C, et al. Platelet-rich plasma in osteoarthritis treatment: review of current evidence. Ther Adv Chronic Dis 2019;10. 2040622319825567.

20. Malhotra A, Pelletier MH, Yu Y, et al. Can platelet-rich plasma (PRP) improve bone healing? A comparison between the theory and experimental outcomes. Arch Orthop Trauma Surg 2013;133:153–65.
21. Piuzzi NS, Hussain ZB, et al. Variability in the preparation, reporting, and use of bone marrow aspirate concentrate in musculoskeletal disorders: a systematic review of the clinical orthopaedic literature. JBJS 2018;100(6):517–25.
22. Shapiro SA, Kazmerchak, et al. A prospective, single-blind, placebo-controlled trial of bone marrow aspirate concentrate for knee osteoarthritis. Am J Sports Med 2017;45(1):82–90.
23. Chahla J, Mannava S, et al. Bone marrow aspirate concentrate harvesting and processing technique. Arthrosc Tech 2017;6(2):e441–5.
24. Hyer CF, Berlet GC, Bussewitz BW, et al. Quantitative assessment of the yield of osteoblastic connective tissue progenitors in bone marrow aspirate from the iliac crest, tibia, and calcaneus. J Bone Joint Surg Am 2013;95(14):1312–6.
25. Holton J, Imam M, Ward J, et al. The basic science of bone marrow aspirate concentrate in chondral injuries. Orthop Rev 2016;8(3):6659.
26. Murphy EP, et al. A prospective evaluation of bone marrow aspirate concentrate and microfracture in the treatment of osteochondral lesions of the talus. Foot Ankle Surg 2019;25(4):441–8.
27. Pascual-Garrido C, Rolón A, Makino A. Treatment of chronic patellar tendinopathy with autologous bone marrow stem cells: a 5-year-follow up. Stem Cells Int 2012;2012:953510.
28. Hunt KJ, Anderson RB. Treatment of Jones fracture nonunions and refractures in the elite athlete: outcomes of intramedullary screw fixation with bone grafting. Am J Sports Med 2011;39(9):1948–54.
29. Carney D, Chambers MC, Kromka JJ, et al. Jones fracture in the elite athlete: patient reported outcomes following fixation with BMAC. Orthopaedic J Sports Med 2018;6(7_suppl4).
30. Jäger M, Herten M, et al. Bridging the gap: bone marrow aspiration concentrate reduces autologous bone grafting in osseous defects. J Orthop Res 2011;29:173–80.
31. Niknejad H, Peirovi H, Jorjani M, et al. Properties of the amniotic membrane for potential use in tissue engineering. Eur Cell Mater 2008;15:88–99. Published 2008 Apr 29.
32. Werber B, Martin E. A prospective study of 20 foot and ankle wounds treated with cryopreserved amniotic membrane and fluid allograft. J Foot Ankle Surg 2013;52(5):615–21 [published correction appears in J Foot Ankle Surg. 2013 Nov--Dec;52(6):794].
33. Parolini O, Alviano F, et al. Concise review: isolation and characterization of cells from human term placenta: outcome of the first international Workshop on Placenta Derived Stem Cells. Stem cells (Dayton, Ohio) 2008;26(2):300–11.
34. Heckmann N, Auran R, Mirzayan R. Application of amniotic tissue in orthopedic surgery. Am J orthopedics (Belle Mead, N.J.) 2016;45(7):E421–5.
35. Solomon A, Wajngarten M, et al. Suppression of inflammatory and fibrotic responses in allergic inflammation by the amniotic membrane stromal matrix. Clin Exp Allergy : J Br Soc Allergy Clin Immunol 2005;35(7):941–8.
36. Magatti M, De Munari S, Vertua E, et al. Amniotic mesenchymal tissue cells inhibit dendritic cell differentiation of peripheral blood and amnion resident monocytes. Cell Transplant 2009;18(8):899–914.
37. Li J, et al. Human amniotic mesenchymal stem cells promote endogenous bone regeneration. Front Endocrinol (Lausanne) 2020;11:543623.

38. Huddleston HP, Cohn MR, Haunschild ED, et al. Amniotic product treatments: clinical and basic science evidence. Curr Rev Musculoskelet Med 2020;13(2):148–54.
39. Linder M, Hecking M, Glitzner E, et al. EGFR controls bone development by negatively regulating mTOR-signaling during osteoblast differentiation. Cell Death Differ 2018;25(6):1094–106.
40. Moshiri A, Oryan A. Structural and functional modulation of early healing of full-thickness superficial digital flexor tendon rupture in rabbits by repeated subcutaneous administration of exogenous human recombinant basic fibroblast growth factor. J Foot Ankle Surg 2011;50(6):654–62.
41. Ozbölük S, Ozkan Y, Oztürk A, et al. The effects of human amniotic membrane and periosteal autograft on tendon healing: experimental study in rabbits. J Hand Surg Eur 2010;35(4):262–8.
42. Lange-Consiglio A, Tassan S, Corradetti B, et al. Investigating the efficacy of amnion-derived compared with bone marrow-derived mesenchymal stromal cells in equine tendon and ligament injuries. Cytotherapy 2013;15(8):1011–20.
43. Muttini A, Russo V, Rossi E, et al. Pilot experimental study on amniotic epithelial mesenchymal cell transplantation in natural occurring tendinopathy in horses. Ultrasonographic and histological comparison. Muscles Ligaments Tendons J 2015;5(1):5–11 [published correction appears in Muscles Ligaments Tendons J. 2015 Apr-Jun;5(2):1].
44. Coban I, Satoğlu IS, Gültekin A, et al. Effects of human amniotic fluid and membrane in the treatment of Achilles tendon ruptures in locally corticosteroid-induced Achilles tendinosis: an experimental study on rats. Foot Ankle Surg 2009;15(1):22–7.
45. de Girolamo L, Morlin Ambra LF, Perucca Orfei C, et al. Treatment with human amniotic suspension allograft improves tendon healing in a rat model of collagenase-induced tendinopathy. Cells 2019;8(11):1411.
46. Duerr RA, Ackermann J, Gomoll AH. Amniotic-derived treatments and formulations. Clin Sports Med 2019;38(1):45–59.
47. Gomoll AH, Farr J, Cole BJ, et al. Safety and efficacy of an amniotic suspension allograft injection over 12 months in a single-blinded, randomized controlled trial for symptomatic osteoarthritis of the knee. Arthroscopy 2021;37(7):2246–57.
48. Werber B. Amniotic tissues for the treatment of chronic plantar fasciosis and Achilles tendinosis. J Sports Med (Hindawi Publ Corp) 2015;2015:219896.
49. Zelen CM, Poka A, Andrews J. Prospective, randomized, blinded, comparative study of injectable micronized dehydrated amniotic/chorionic membrane allograft for plantar fasciitis–a feasibility study. Foot Ankle Int 2013;34(10):1332–9.
50. Hanselman AE, Tidwell JE, Santrock RD. Cryopreserved human amniotic membrane injection for plantar fasciitis: a randomized, controlled, double-blind pilot study. Foot Ankle Int 2015;36(2):151–8.
51. Liu C, Bai J, et al. Biological amnion prevents flexor tendon adhesion in zone II: a controlled, multicentre clinical trial. Biomed Res Int 2019;2019:2354325.
52. Pacaccio DJ, Stern SF. Demineralized bone matrix: basic science and clinical applications. Clin Podiatr Med Surg 2005;22(4):599–vii.
53. Michelson JD, Curl LA. Use of demineralized bone matrix in hindfoot arthrodesis. Clin Orthop Relat Res 1996;325:203–8.
54. Lareau CR, Hsu AR, Anderson RB. Return to play in national football league players after operative Jones fracture treatment. Foot Ankle Int 2016;37(1):8–16.

Stress Injuries in the Athlete

Eric Shi, DPM[a],*, Lawrence M. Oloff, DPM, FACFAS[b],
Nicholas W. Todd, DPM, FACFAS[c]

KEYWORDS

- Stress fracture • Athlete • Metatarsal • Sports injury • Bone stimulator
- Extracorporeal shockwave therapy • Forteo • Antigravity treadmill training

KEY POINTS

- Stress fractures need to be managed differently based on the level of the athlete.
- A low threshold for advanced imaging is indicated for the diagnosis of stress fractures.
- Evidence to support the use of adjunctive therapy in stress fracture treatment including teriparatide (Forteo), extracorporeal shockwave therapy, and bone stimulators is limited but warrants an increase in judicial use to help improve our understanding of alternative therapy.
- Special conditioning and rehabilitation using techniques such as antigravity treadmill training and deep-water training enable an accelerated return to the high level of play for elite athletes.

INTRODUCTION

Stress injuries are common in athletes due to the repetitive motion in any sport resulting in a gradual buildup of damage to muscles, tendons, bones, and nerves. When a bone is subjected to repeated submaximal stresses, microscopic injuries to the bone cause an imbalance between bone resorption and bone formation, which leads to macro-structural failure and fracture.[1] Lower extremity stress fractures account for 80% to 90% of all stress fractures and affect both recreational as well as high-level athletes alike.[2] In the general population, the incidence of stress fractures ranges from 1% to 15% with long-distance runners most likely affected.[3] They make up 10% of all sports medicine injuries, at a rate of approximately 1.54 per 100,000 athletes.[4] A study looking at stress fractures in division 1 collegiate athletes found an incidence of 1.4%, with the highest rates of fracture in cross-country and track.[5] For professional athletes, stress fractures can be a devastating and career-threatening injury. A study looking at players

[a] Sutter East Bay Medical Foundation, 20101 Lake Chabot Road, Castro Valley, CA 94546, USA;
[b] Sutter Health Palo Alto Medical Foundation, Callan Boulevard, Daly City, CA 94015, USA;
[c] Sutter Health Palo Alto Medical Foundation, 701 East El Camino Real, Mountain View, CA 94040, USA
* Corresponding author.
E-mail address: ericfshi@gmail.com

Clin Podiatr Med Surg 40 (2023) 181–191
https://doi.org/10.1016/j.cpm.2022.07.012
0891-8422/23/© 2022 Elsevier Inc. All rights reserved.

in the National Basketball Association (NBA) found that 30% of players were unable to return to their previous level of play after a stress fracture.[6]

CAUSES AND RISK FACTORS

Athletes at the highest risk of stress fractures are those who abruptly increase the duration, intensity, or frequency of activity without adequate periods of rest. Such injuries are also more likely to occur at the start of the season when the intensity and frequency of activity is just starting to build up.[6] Track and field athletes are known to have higher rates of stress fractures than other sports such as football, basketball, and soccer.[5]

Risk factors for stress fractures include increased age, female sex, poor diet, lower bone mineral density, skeletal malalignment, hormonal imbalance, and poor vascular supply. Of these, a decreased bone mineral density increases stress fracture risk most significantly. The classic "female athlete triad" of amenorrhea, eating disorder, and osteoporosis, describes a combination of conditions that lead to decreased bone mineral density. Care must be taken when treating the female athlete, especially one involved in long-distance running, gymnastics, and figure skating.[7]

CLINICAL PRESENTATION AND EXAMINATION

Typically, athletes who present with a stress fracture describe a progressive and insidious onset of pain and swelling without any obvious traumatic injury. A detailed history regarding the intensity and duration of training, as well as changes in training surface or footwear, is helpful. A thorough medical history including diet, nutrition, as well as any other metabolic deficiencies can be helpful to rule out any underlying risk factors.

DIAGNOSTIC TESTS

Radiographs are routinely used as the first step in working up a potential stress fracture; however, 85% of initial imaging may be negative.[8] At that point, the next steps in diagnostic workup can often depend on the level of clinical suspicion as well as the level of the athlete being treated. For the typical recreational athlete, it may be appropriate to order repeat radiographs in 2 to 3 weeks if symptoms persist, keeping in mind that even up to 50% of follow-up radiographs can still be negative.[8] For higher-level and professional athletes or those with upcoming competitions or events, it may be appropriate to order higher level imaging studies earlier in the workup. An MRI provides the highest sensitivity and specificity in providing a diagnosis and allows the clinician to evaluate for surrounding soft-tissue pathology, which is highly useful in guiding the treatment regimen. Bone scintigraphy, specifically the three-phase bone scan, is highly sensitive in picking up bone stress injuries and was considered the gold standard before the advent of the MRI but can lack in specificity.

TREATMENT

Stress fractures can be categorized into high-risk or low-risk (**Table 1**) based on their ability to heal.[9] Low-risk stress fractures of the foot and ankle include the fibula, calcaneus, and metatarsal can generally be treated nonoperatively with a period of rest and protected weight-bearing with or without immobilization in a walker boot or postoperative shoe. Patients can gradually return to activity when tenderness and swelling have resolved and radiographic evidence of healing is present, which is typically 4 to 6 weeks from the onset of symptoms.[10,11] High-risk stress fractures of the medial

Table 1				
Overview of stress fractures				
Fracture Location	**Mechanism**	**Sport/Risk Factors**	**Risk Level**	**Incidence**
Second and third metatarsal	Plantarflexion at the tarsometatarsal joint	Runners, ballet dancers, and military recruits	Low	Common
Fifth metatarsal	Inversion force	Basketball and cavus foot type	High	Common
Calcaneus	Pull of Achilles during plantar flexion during heel strike	Long-distance running and military recruits	Low	Common
Medial malleolus	Torsional force in ankle	Basketball and running and jumping sports	High	Rare
Navicular	Torsional force in tarsometatarsal joint	Track and field sprinters and jumpers, short first ray and long second ray	High	Uncommon

malleolus, navicular, talus, sesamoid, and proximal fifth metatarsal require a more guarded prognosis and, in many cases, may require surgical management.[9]

STRESS FRACTURE OF THE METATARSAL

Metatarsal stress fractures were often referred to as "march fractures" due to the high incidence in military recruits. These commonly present at the second and third metatarsals and make up to 38% of all stress fractures in athletes.[12] Fractures of the second and third metatarsals are lower risk and heal well with nonoperative treatment. Initial radiographic findings typically show a very subtle periosteal reaction (**Fig. 1**).

Fractures of the fifth metatarsal base are associated with inversion injuries and are a high risk, especially when located proximally at the watershed area metaphyseal diaphyseal junction. For these fractures, primary surgery combined with an autologous bone graft may be a suitable option for athletes wishing to return to sports early. Even with surgical management, up to 43% of players may be unable to return to their prior level of play as found in a study looking at NBA players.[6]

STRESS FRACTURE OF THE CALCANEUS

Stress fractures of the calcaneus are often found in military recruits as well as long-distance runners who present with pain at rest. They are the second most common type of stress fracture, second to metatarsal stress fractures, and can often be misdiagnosed as more routine causes of heel pain such as plantar fasciitis. In cases of suspected fracture, MRI serves as an imaging of choice for early detection (**Fig. 2**). These fractures occur to the posterior tuberosity along the trabecular stress lines.[13] These fractures heal well with a course of rest and protected weight bearing. **Fig. 3**.

STRESS FRACTURE OF THE NAVICULAR

The navicular is known to have a limited blood supply, specifically at a watershed area in the central third portion of the bone creating a physiologically vulnerable area prone to stress fractures and nonunion.[14] Fitch and colleagues[15] proposed that these fractures occur because of the compressive forces between the first and second rays during forefoot loading which create an area of maximal shear force at the central third of the navicular. This makes navicular stress fractures more common in track and field

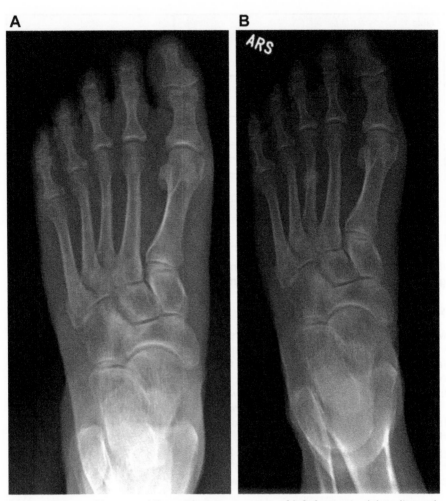

Fig. 1. A 64-year-old woman hiker with an acute onset of left foot pain. (*A*) Radiographs 2 weeks after onset of symptoms show subtle sclerosis mid-shaft of the second metatarsal consistent with stress fracture. (*B*) Radiographs 4 weeks show interval callus formation at prior fracture site, making the diagnosis more apparent. (*Courtesy of* Lawrence Oloff, DPM, San Francisco, CA.)

athletes, specifically sprinters and jumpers, because of the forceful push-off mechanisms required in their sport.

Plain film radiographs have up to a 76% rate of false negatives and higher imaging is indicated when there is a high clinical suspicion. CT scans are particularly useful for navicular stress fractures in providing a detailed image of the fracture pattern as described by the classification system devised by Saxena and colleagues[16] (**Table 2**).

Management of these fractures remains controversial. Nonoperative treatment has been recommended for nondisplaced fractures. For displaced fractures as well as nondisplaced fractures that have failed conservative treatment, operative management can be considered (**Fig. 4**). There remains, however, lack of evidence to support the superiority of operative management over nonoperative management of

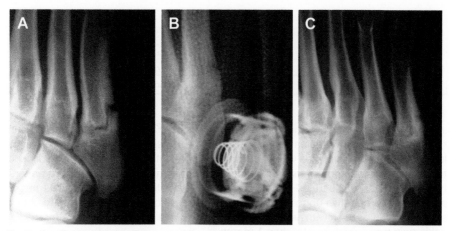

Fig. 2. A collegiate baseball player with a stress fracture that progressed to a fracture of the fifth metatarsal declined surgical intervention. (*A*) Radiographs show fracture at the metaphyseal diaphyseal junction that progressed to the observed nonunion 4 months after the diagnosis. The player again declined surgery and opted for bone stimulation. (*B*) Radiographs taken the cast show overlying bone stimulator and interval osseous bridging. (*C*) Radiographs taken 4 months after starting bone stimulation show healed fracture.

nondisplaced navicular stress fractures. Torg and colleagues[17] found similar outcomes in return to activity and Mallee and colleagues[18] noted a trend toward an earlier return to play with operative treatment, though the difference was not significant.

STRESS FRACTURE OF THE MEDIAL MALLEOLUS

Medial malleolus stress fractures are considered high-risk stress fractures because of their predilection for progressing to a complete fracture, delated union, nonunion, or chronic pain.[19] An accurate diagnosis can often be delayed due to a combination of a clinician's low index of suspicion as well as what can present as mild symptoms,

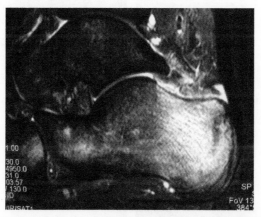

Fig. 3. *Runner presents with heel pain that started 6 weeks ago.* Initial radiographs obtained were negative for fracture. Sagittal STIR MRI shows a posterior calcaneal stress fracture perpendicular to the calcaneal trabecula with surrounding bone marrow edema. (*Courtesy of* Lawrence Oloff, DPM, San Francisco, CA.)

Table 2
Saxena et al classification for navicular stress fracture

Type 1	Dorsal cortical break only
Type 2	Fracture extends into navicular body
Type 3	Bi-cortical fracture

leading athletes to neglect and push through the injury.[20] These fractures are seen in running and jumping athletes and are attributed to torsional forces during repetitive loading.[21] Care is to be taken when examining the patient as symptoms can be difficult to discern from anterior medial ankle impingement symptoms.[9] The fracture pattern typically follows the Lauge-Hansen supination–adduction pattern but initial radiographs can be negative up to 70% of cases.[22,23] It has been recommended to obtain early MRI studies even with negative radiographs to rule out stress fracture for medial ankle pain present for greater than 1 month.[20]

Literature lacks consensus on operative versus nonoperative management of these fractures, except for a systematic review by Irion and colleagues[24] who reported an average of 2.4 weeks to return to play for operative fractures versus 7.6 weeks for nonoperative fractures. Like all other high-risk stress fractures, operative fixation should be considered early for those wishing to return to play quickly and for elite athletes.[21]

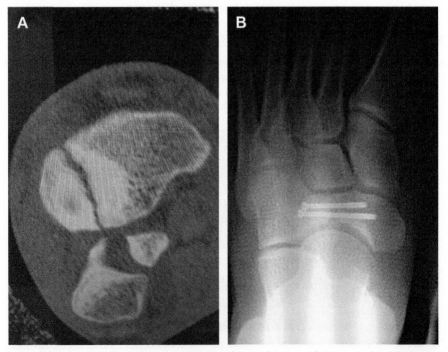

Fig. 4. (*A*) Axial view CT scan shows a bi-cortical stress fracture of the navicular. (*B*) Fixation of the fracture was performed using two partially threaded screws. (*Courtesy of* Lawrence Oloff, DPM, San Francisco, CA.)

AUGMENTED TREATMENT OPTIONS

Care should be taken when treating elite athletes to consider augmented and accelerated treatment options as well as a lower threshold for surgical management. A study looking at players in the NBA found that players who had surgery had significantly better performance at 2 years than those who were managed nonoperatively, regardless of the type of stress fracture.[6]

EXTRACORPOREAL SHOCKWAVE THERAPY

Extracorporeal shockwave therapy (EST) attempts to increase the production of proteins necessary for angiogenesis as well as local growth factors related to bone healing. Studies looking at the use of shockwave therapy in the treatment of stress fractures have been limited to recalcitrant injuries. A study looking at EST in the treatment of tibial stress fractures found a significant reduction in pain and recovery time with one or two sessions of a minimum of 2000 shockwaves of 0.2 mJ/mm.[25] Another study looked at its use in nonunion chronic stress fractures and found an earlier return to sports,[26] though additional high-quality evidence is lacking.

BONE STIMULATORS

Bone stimulators use electrical and ultrasound stimulation to promote angiogenesis and increase growth factor release in the healing of acute fractures. There are few studies that look at the use of bone stimulation for the treatment of stress fractures. Ultrasound bone stimulators have been found effective in stimulating union in up to 98% of delayed and nonunions; however, the use of these has been unclear in acute stress fractures. Studies looking at the use of bone stimulators for tibial stress fractures did not find a significant return to activity when compared with placebo.[27,28]

TERIPARATIDE (FORTEO)

Teriparatide, known under its brand name Forteo, is a synthetic human parathyroid hormone prescription injection used to treat patients with osteoporosis at high risk of fractures. The hormone activates osteoblasts and has been found to increase bone mineral density. Though costly, at $560 for a 1-month supply, studies looking at the medication found it reduced the risk of vertebral fractures as well as shortened the healing time for distal radius fractures in post-menopausal women.[29] Other studies have been limited to the use of Forteo to augment healing in delayed unions[30] or in the treatment of periprosthetic stress fractures.[31] Limited studies looking at the use of Forteo in stress fracture management have been shown to be favorable in the healing of experimentally induced stress fractures[32] as well as an early case report metatarsal stress fractures.[33] A prospective study currently in process during the publication of this article known as the RETURN (Research on Efficacy of Teriparatide Use in the Return of recruits to Normal duty) study, looks at the use of Forteo in treating stress fractures in 136 military recruits[34] and will be one of the first prospective studies to look at outcomes in acute stress fractures.

SPECIAL REHABILITATION

Maintaining conditioning during recovery from a stress fracture is crucial for an athlete's return to sport at a high level. Conditioning activities should be introduced early, as deconditioning can occur in as little as 2 weeks following an injury.[35] Antigravity treadmill training (ATT) or commonly known as AlterG has been reported extensively in physical therapy literature to be used in place of over-ground running to allow runners to return to running at high intensities earlier during recovery with lower bone loading. This can be introduced once the athlete is pain free with walking and with activities of daily living and allows the athlete to maintain fitness while protecting the stress fracture site. An air-filled pressure-controlled chamber surrounds the lower body from the waist down and pressure in the chamber is modulated to offset the runner in increments between 20% and 100% body weight.[35] A study by Saxena and colleagues[36] found that ATT helped Achilles tendon surgery patients return back to running 2 weeks earlier than the control group, but this was not statistically significant. There haven't been any studies that compare the use of ATT versus conventional rehabilitation programs for foot and ankle stress fractures.

Maintenance of physical conditioning during recovery also includes cycling, swimming, and deep-water running (DWR). Deep water running, performed at the deep end of a swimming pool, makes use of the buoyancy of water to provide 100% body weight support while limb movements mimic dry land running to introduce cardiovascular demands close to that of real running.[37,38] Studies looking at DWR training programs in runners found maintenance of VO_2max, anaerobic threshold, land running economy, and leg strength.[39–41] DWR, however, is more useful in maintaining and not increasing conditioning and does not replace the need to progress to dry-land running as part of the rehab process.

PREVENTION

Studies have shown deficiencies in calcium[6] and vitamin D[42] lead to an increase in stress fractures. A randomized controlled trial looking at Navy recruits with suboptimal calcium intake reduced stress fractures by 20% with daily vitamin D and calcium supplementation.[43] Overall, data suggest athletes and high-risk patients should be educated on the benefits of calcium and vitamin D supplementation, and prophylactic supplementation of 2000 IU of vitamin D and 1200 mg calcium daily is recommended.[44–46]

Though not directly applicable to athletes, there is extensive research supporting the use of "shock absorbing" inserts of varying qualities in military training boots and shoes as a preventive measure for stress fractures. In these studies, however, there was no consensus on the best design or type of materials but should be based on the patient's comfort and tolerability.[47] That same study found no benefit from leg muscle stretching during warm-up before exercise as a preventative measure.

Bisphosphonates, a class of drugs that prevent the loss of bone density by inhibiting bone resorption, were looked at as a potential preventative measure for stress fractures. The study found no difference between the experimental and control group in rates of tibial, femoral, metatarsal, or total stress fracture incidence. The study concluded that the use of bisphosphonates to inhibit osteoclast activity would not prevent microcrack repair that leads to stress fractures.[48]

In physical therapy literature, gait retraining has been reported to help runners address underlying biomechanical risk factors that contribute to repeat injuries. Modifying the running program design to reduce bone microdamage formation and its removal can also prevent stress fractures.[35]

SUMMARY

Much thought must be given when treating a stress fracture in an elite athlete. A lower threshold for surgery and an aggressive pursuit for augmented treatment options can accelerate return to play at a higher level than conservative care. Currently, much of the literature looking at augmented treatment options for stress fracture focus on non-unions and less on acute stress fractures. Much more needs to be studied when looking at augmented treatment options to accelerate healing in high-level athletes.

CLINICS CARE POINTS

- The MRI provides the highest sensitivity and specificity in diagnosing stress fracture.
- Surgical repair is the quickest way to manage a non-healing stress fracture in athletes and non-athletes alike.
- Close follow-up with a physical therapist specializing in sports injuries is critical to help an athlete recover from a stress fracture.

DISCLOSURE

The authors have nothing to disclose.

REFERENCES

1. Welck MJ, Hayes T, Pastides P, et al. Stress fractures of the foot and ankle. Injury 2017;48(8):1722–6. Epub 2015 Sep 15.
2. Edwards P, Wright M, Hartman J. A practical approach for the differential diagnosis of chronic leg pain in the athlete. Am J Sports Med 2005;33:1241Y9.
3. Hulkko A, Orava S. Stress fractures in athletes. Int J Sports Med 1987;8(3):221–6.
4. Changstrom BG, Brou L, Khodaee M, et al. Epidemiology of stress fracture injuries among US high school athletes, 2005–2006 through 2012–2013. Am J Sports Med 2015;43:26–33.
5. Hame SL, LaFemina JM, McAllister DR, et al. Fractures in the collegiate athlete. Am J Sports Med 2004;32(2):446–51.
6. Khan Moin, et al. Epidemiology and impact on performance of lower extremity stress injuries in professional basketball players. Sports Health 2018;10(2):169–74.
7. Barrack MT, Gibbs JC, De Souza MJ, et al. Higher incidence of bone stress injuries with increasing female athlete triad-related risk factors: a prospective multisite study of exercising girls and women. Am J Sports Med 2014;42(4):949–58.
8. Spitz DJ, Newberg AH. Imaging of stress fractures in the athlete. Radiol Clin North Am 2002;40(2):313–31.
9. Greaser MC. Foot and ankle stress fractures in athletes. Orthop Clin North Am 2016;47(4):809–22.
10. Gehrmann RM, Renard RL. Current concepts review: stress fractures of the foot. Foot Ankle Int 2006;27(9):750–7.
11. Tangpricha V, Pearce EN, Chen TC, et al. Vitamin D insufficiency among free-living healthy young adults. Am J Med 2002;112(8):659–62.
12. Matheson GO, Clement DB, McKenzie DC, et al. Stress fractures in athletes. A study of 320 cases. Am J Sports Med 1987;15(1):46–58.
13. Leabhart JW. Stress fractures of the calcaneus. J Bone Joint Surg Am 1959;41-A:1285–90.
14. Mann JA, Pedowitz DI. Evaluation and treatment of navicular stress fractures, including nonunions, revision surgery, and persistent pain after treatment. Foot Ankle Clin 2009;14(2):187–204.

15. Fitch KD, Blackwell JB, Gilmour WN. Operation for non-union of stress fracture of the tarsal navicular. J Bone Joint Surg Br 1989;71(1):105–10.
16. Saxena A, Fullem B, Hannaford D. Results of treatment of 22 navicular stress fractures and a new proposed radiographic classification system. J Foot Ankle Surg 2000;39(2):96–103.
17. Torg JS, Moyer J, Gaughan JP, et al. Management of tarsal navicular stress fractures: conservative versus surgical treatment: a meta-analysis. Am J Sports Med 2010;38(5):1048–53.
18. Mallee WH, Weel H, van Dijk CN, et al. Surgical versus conservative treatment for high-risk stress fractures of the lower leg (anterior tibial cortex, navicular and fifth metatarsal base): a systematic review. Br J Sports Med 2015;49(6):370–6.
19. Boden BP, Osbahr DC. High-risk stress fractures: evaluation and treatment. J Am Acad Orthop Surg 2000;8:344–53.
20. Menge TJ, Looney CG. Medial malleolar stress fracture in an adolescent athlete. J Foot Ankle Surg 2015;54(2):242–6.
21. Shelbourne KD, Fisher DA, Rettig AC, et al. Stress fractures of the medial malleolus. Am J Sports Med 1988;16(1):60–3.
22. Lauge-Hansen N. Fractures of the ankle. II. Combined experimental-surgical and experimental roentgenologic investigations. Arch Surg 1950;60(5):957–85.
23. Orava S, Karpakka J, Taimela S, et al. Stress fracture of the medial malleolus. J Bone Joint Surg Am 1995;77(3):362–5.
24. Irion V, Miller TL, Kaeding CC. The treatment and outcomes of medial malleolar stress fractures: a systematic review of the literature. Sports Health 2014;6(6):527–30.
25. Leal C, D'Agostino C, Gomez Garcia S, et al. Current concepts of shockwave therapy in stress fractures. Int J Surg 2015;24:195–200.
26. Furia JP, Rompe JD, Cacchio A, et al. Shock wave therapy as a treatment of non-unions, avascular necrosis, and delayed healing of stress fractures. Foot Ankle Clin 2010;15(4):651–62.
27. Rue JP, Armstrong DW 3rd, Frassica FJ, et al. The effect of pulsed ultrasound in the treatment of tibial stress fractures. Orthopedics 2004;27(11):1192–5.
28. Beck BR, Matheson GO, Bergman G, et al. Do capacitively coupled electric fields accelerate tibial stress fracture healing? A randomized controlled trial. Am J Sports Med 2008;36(3):545–53.
29. Aspenberg P, Genant HK, Johansson T, et al. Teriparatide for acceleration of fracture repair in humans: a prospective, randomized, double-blind study of 102 postmenopausal women with distal radial fractures. J Bone Miner Res 2010;25(2):404–14.
30. Gende A, Thomsen TW, Marcussen B, et al. Delayed-union of acetabular stress fracture in female gymnast: use of teriparatide to augment healing. Clin J Sport Med 2020;30(5):e163–5.
31. Lipof JS, Southgate RD, Tyler WK, et al. Treatment of an acromial stress fracture after reverse total shoulder arthroplasty with teriparatide: a case report. JBJS Case Connect 2020;10(2):e0221.
32. Sloan AV, Martin JR, Li S, et al. Parathyroid hormone and bisphosphonate have opposite effects on stress fracture repair. Bone 2010;47:235–40.
33. Raghavan P, Christofides E. Role of teriparatide in accelerating metatarsal stress fracture healing: a case series and review of literature. Clin Med Insights Endocrinol Diabetes 2012;5(5):39–45.
34. Carswell AT, Eastman KG, Casey A, et al. Teriparatide and stress fracture healing in young adults (RETURN - research on Efficacy of Teriparatide Use in the Return

of recruits to Normal duty): study protocol for a randomised controlled trial. Trials 2021;22(1):580.

35. Warden SJ, Davis IS, Fredericson M. Management and prevention of bone stress injuries in long-distance runners. J Orthop Sports Phys Ther 2014;44(10):749–65.

36. Saxena A, Granot A. Use of an anti-gravity treadmill in the rehabilitation of the operated achilles tendon: a pilot study. J Foot Ankle Surg 2011;50:558Y61.

37. Killgore GL. Deep-water running: a practical review of the literature with an emphasis on biomechanics. Phys Sports Med 2012;40:116–26.

38. Reilly T, Dowzer CN, Cable NT. The physiology of deep-water running. J Sports Sci 2003;21:959–72.

39. Gatti CJ, Young RJ, Glad HL. Effect of water-training in the maintenance of cardiorespiratory endurance of athletes. Br J Sports Med 1979;13:161Y4.

40. Hertler L, Provost-Craig M, Sestili D, et al. Water running and the maintenance of maximum oxygen consumption and leg strength in runners. Med Sci Sports Exerc 1992;24:S23.

41. Wilbur RL, Moffat RJ, Scott BE, et al. Influence of water run training on the maintenance of aerobic performance. Med Sci Sports Exerc 1996;28:1056Y62.

42. Ruohola JP, Laaksi I, Ylikomi T, et al. Association between serum 25(OH)D concentrations and bone stress fractures in Finnish young men. J Bone Miner Res 2006;21:1483–8.

43. Lappe J, Cullen D, Haynatzki G, et al. Calcium and vitamin D supplementation decreases incidence of stress fractures in female Navy recruits. J Bone Miner Res 2008;23:741–9.

44. McCabe MP, Smyth MP, Richardson DR. Current concept review: vitamin D and stress fractures. Foot Ankle Int 2012;33(6):526–33.

45. of Medicine Institute. Dietary reference intakes for calcium and vitamin D. Washington, DC: National Academy of Sciences; 2010.

46. Tenforde AS, Sayres LC, Sainani KL, et al. Evaluating the relationship of calcium and vitamin D in the prevention of stress fracture injuries in the young athlete: a review of the literature. PM R 2010;2(10):945–9. PMID: 20970764.

47. Rome K, Handoll HHG, Ashford RL. Interventions for preventing and treating stress fractures and stress reactions of bone of the lower limbs in young adults. Cochrane Database Syst Rev 2005;Issue 2:CD000450.

48. Milgrom C, Finestone A, Novack V, et al. The effect of prophylactic treatmentwith risedronate on stress fracture incidence among infantry recruits. Bone 2004;35:418–24.

Dance-Related Foot and Ankle Injuries and Pathologies

Varsha Ivanova, DPM[a], Nicholas W. Todd, DPM[b],
Jesse Yurgelon, DPM[b],*

KEYWORDS

• Dance • Ballet • Sesamoiditis • Impingement • Stress fracture

KEY POINTS

• Dancers are highly vulnerable to injuries due to high dynamic overload, extreme positions and motions, and excessive use.
• Most pathologies may be visualized on plain radiographs, stress films, MRI, or computed tomography.
• Primary treatment of most common pathologies includes activity modification with ankle joint immobilization and/or non–weight-bearing.
• Surgical intervention is recommended if return to dance is shorter and complications of conservative treatment can be avoided.

EPIDEMIOLOGY AND CAUSE

Dancers, similar to many athletes, are highly vulnerable to injuries due to high physical demands including dynamic overload, extreme positions and motions, and excessive use. And unlike most athletes, dance is typically performed either barefoot or in shoes that do not aid in shock absorption.[1] The cause of most pedal injuries during dance includes demanding positions, anatomic alignment, lack of good nutrition, and extrinsic factors including poor technique, environmental factors, and inadequate training.[1,2]

Among different forms of dance, ballet is found to have the highest occurrence of injuries.[3] Furthermore, classic ballet is found to have an increased risk of foot and ankle injuries when compared with jazz/contemporary, street, and tap/folk dance.[3] Ballet is a form of performative dance that requires intricate and highly specific body motion and positioning with an emphasis on precise and often elaborate

[a] Kaiser Permanente, 710 Lawrence Expressway, Santa Clara, CA 95051, USA; [b] Palo Alto Medical Foundation Mountain View Center, 701 East EL Camino Real, Mountain View, CA 94040, USA
* Corresponding author.
E-mail address: yurgie16@gmail.com

Clin Podiatr Med Surg 40 (2023) 193–207
https://doi.org/10.1016/j.cpm.2022.07.013
0891-8422/23/© 2022 Elsevier Inc. All rights reserved.

podiatric.theclinics.com

footwork. Various ballet techniques have been developed that put the foot and ankle joints through variable levels of stress. For instance, during *demi releve*, the foot is forced in maximal plantarflexion, and weight-bearing is borne through the dorsiflexed forefoot at the metatarsophalangeal joints; this increases the risk for sesamoid pathology and stress fractures. During *en pointe,* a notably difficult and popularly recognized technique, the dancer is forced to maximally plantarflex the ankle joint and, unlike *demi releve*, bears weight entirely on the distal digits; this predisposes a dancer to posterior ankle impingement and flexor hallucis longus (FHL) tendinopathy, among others. During *demi plie*, bilateral plantigrade feet are forced in complete abduction with the ankle into maximal dorsiflexion, increasing risk for anterior ankle impingement. These positions are not exclusive to ballet, and variations can be found in other dance forms, thus leading to similar patterns of injury.

SESAMOIDITIS
Cause and Diagnosis

With the *demi releve* technique, as well as sudden deceleration after jumps during dance, the sesamoids of the forefoot undergo excessive load and impact. The tibial and fibular sesamoids are embedded within the flexor hallucis brevis tendon and articulate with the plantar first metatarsal proximal to the joint. With repetitive stress and overuse, the sesamoids are thus susceptible to sesamoiditis.[3,4] Sesamoiditis is defined as generalized inflammation to the sesamoids, which may also occur in conjunction with an acute fracture, stress fracture, osteoarthritis, avascular necrosis, or contusion.[5]

Dancers will present with pain at the plantar first metatarsophalangeal joint (MTPJ), with point tenderness at the commonly symptomatic, tibial sesamoid.[5,6] Pain can be reproduced with MTPJ dorsiflexion with and without resistance. Plain radiographs must first be obtained to rule out obvious osseous pathologies. An anteroposterior view of the foot can reveal overall alignment of the sesamoids, whereas the medial and lateral obliques are superior to view the tibial and fibular sesamoids, respectively. A sesamoid-axial radiograph allows direct visualization of the metatarso-sesamoid joint.[5,7] MRI aids will demonstrate diffuse bone marrow edema of the affected sesamoid and surrounding soft tissue (**Fig. 1**). MRI can specifically help diagnose stress or acute fractures, osteonecrosis, and sprains of the sesamoids.[5,6]

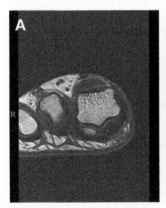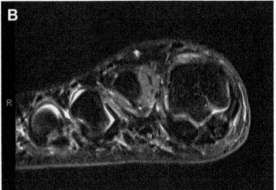

Fig. 1. Coronal MRI view of the distal forefoot of a patient with tibial sesamoiditis. (*A*) T1-weighted image of decreased signal intensity of the medial, tibial sesamoid. (*B*) T2-weighted image demonstrating bone marrow edema of the tibial sesamoid and plantarmedial first MTPJ.

Treatment

Conservative treatment of sesamoiditis includes weight-bearing in a stiff soled shoe, ice, rest, and avoiding the *demi releve* position. Application of a dancers' pad, which allows offloading of the first MTPJ and distributes forces to the rest of the forefoot, can also be helpful.[6] Other conservative treatment options include injection therapy with fluoroscopic guided corticosteroids to help alleviate symptoms. Symptoms may take up to 6 months to resolve; however, in patients with prolonged symptoms, surgical excision of the offending sesamoid is warranted. A tibial sesamoidectomy can be performed with a medial or plantarmedial incision, whereas a fibular sesamoidectomy is performed through the technically demanding dorsal approach or plantar approach. A common complication of complete sesamoidectomy is weakened plantarflexion of the hallux due to the reduced flexion moment arm of the flexor hallucis brevis tendon.[8] Thus, a partial sesamoidectomy can be considered, whereby two-thirds of the sesamoid are removed.

Avoiding such complications is crucial for dancers. Dean and colleagues performed a retrospective study to review functional outcomes of sesamoidectomy in 82 athletes who failed conservative treatment of sesamoiditis. Patients underwent either bilateral sesamoidectomy (n = 10), a tibial sesamoidectomy (n = 54) performed via a medial approach, or fibular sesamoidectomy (n = 18) via a plantar approach. The mean age of all patients was 44.9 years, with 72 females and 10 male patients. Eighty percent of athletes were able to return to sport at a mean of 4.62 months postoperatively.[9]

Robertson and colleagues performed a large systematic review on return to sport following conservative and surgical treatment of stress fractures of the sesamoids.[10] Their review included studies of dance[11–15] as well as a multitude of sports such as figure skating, gymnastics, running, aerobics, and basketball. Out of all papers that specified gender, 54% of patients were women, (with a mean age of 16–36.5 years). Out of the 168 sesamoid fractures, 146 were surgically managed and 22 were conservatively managed. Conservative management included rest, nonsteroidal antiinflammatory drugs, shoe gear modifications (with forefoot rocker-bottom shoes), and custom-made orthotics. Surgical treatment included complete or partial sesamoidectomy, internal fixation (in the event of a complete fracture), and curettage and bone graft. Eighty-six percent of patients who underwent conservative treatment were able to return to sport on average 13.9 weeks, with 64% of patients able to return to their preinjury level. Ninety-five percent of patients who underwent surgical treatment were able to return to sport after 11 weeks, with 88% being able to return to their preinjury level. It was found that a sesamoidectomy offers the quickest return to sport, and internal fixation offers the athlete to return to sport at their preinjury level.[10] The problem with many of these studies is that they lack information specific to dancers. For example, the functional needs of a high-level dancer are not the same as a football player. Hence it is difficult to recommend sesamoidectomy as a safe procedure for dancers. It is generally accepted that it is best to avoid sesamoidectomy in high-level dancers and opt for conservative care management, such as bone stimulators.[16]

POSTERIOR ANKLE IMPINGEMENT
Cause and Diagnosis

En pointe and *demi releve* positions force the ankle in extreme plantarflexion with the dorsum of the foot parallel to the tibia and full weight-bearing at the distal digits. Inability to perform full plantarflexion with pain at the posterior ankle is a common symptom of posterior ankle impingement. Posterior ankle impingement can be separated into soft tissue and osseous or articular, extraarticular, and periarticular causes.[17] Common soft tissue causes of posterior ankle pain and impingement include synovitis or a soft tissue mass. Os trigonum syndrome is the most intraarticular osseous cause of posterior ankle impingement.[18] An os trigonum is the failure of a secondary ossification center at the lateral process of the posterior tubercle of the talus. This secondary ossification center typically presents between the ages of 8 and 10 years in women and 11 and 13 years in men and fuses within the year of visibility.[18,19] In the general population, the prevalence of an os trigonum varies between 7% and 25%, and the prevalence of os trigonum syndrome ranges from 14% to 15%, with an increase in prevalence of 30% in ballet dancers.[19–21] Os trigonum syndrome may also be caused by an acute or stress fracture of the Stieda process, an elongated lateral tubercle of the posterior process of the talus.[19] In addition to limited plantar flexion, posterior ankle impingement and os trigonum syndrome cause stiffness, ankle edema, and chronic pain. On physical examination, pain can be reproduced with passive ankle plantarflexion or palpation of the posterolateral ankle between the Achilles and peroneal tendons. These symptoms often resolve with rest. To compensate for the lack of plantarflexion, dancers may force their ankle in a varus position or "sickling" of the foot.[20]

For diagnosis, it is recommended to obtain plain radiographs of the affected ankle in a lateral view or modified lateral view, whereby the ankle is placed in a forced plantar-flexed position to reveal osseous posterior ankle impingement (**Fig. 2**). A computed tomography (CT) scan can determine the exact position and size of the accessory ossicle.[20] To further assess for any coexisting pathologies, an MRI may also be obtained to rule out soft tissue or cartilaginous abnormalities. An MRI may reveal bone marrow edema to the accessory ossicle and any related FHL tendon pathologies

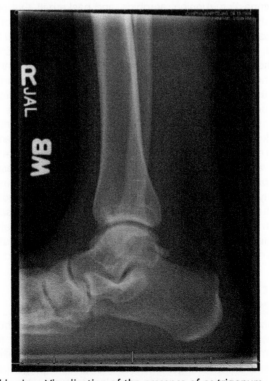

Fig. 2. Lateral ankle view. Visualization of the presence of os trigonum.

(**Fig. 3**).[19] Symptomatic os trigonum syndrome and flexor hallucis longus tendonitis have been found in 63% to 85% of dancers with symptomatic os trigonum.[22]

Treatment

Conservative management is the first line of treatment and includes ice, rest, antiinflammatories, and physical therapy with an emphasis on plantarflexion with the deep posterior muscle compartment. Dancers may also benefit from dance shoe modifications with half or three-quarter shank, allowing decreased compaction of the posterior ankle joint.[1] Mouhsine and colleagues found improvement of symptoms with fluoroscopy-guided local corticosteroid injections.[22] In their case series, Albisetti and colleagues reviewed 12 young trainee ballet dancers who suffered posterior ankle joint pain, both with and without the presence of os trigona. Dancers were treated nonoperatively with decreased activity, antiinflammatories, and physical therapy with increased attention to proprioceptive exercises and strengthen training. Their findings suggest good clinical outcomes with return to dance. Only 3 of 12 dances failed conservative therapies and underwent surgical excision of the os trigonum, with good results.[20]

If consistent conservative treatment for 3 to 6 months fails, then surgical intervention may be considered to resect the accessory ossicle with either endoscopic, arthroscopic, or open approach. Anterior ankle portals can be used to evaluate posterior ankle pathology; however, because of the curvature of the ankle joint, addressing such problems poses a challenge. Thus, van Dijk and colleagues describe a 2-portal endoscopic approach: with the patient in the prone position, the posterolateral mortal is made lateral to the Achilles tendon at the level or slightly more proximal to the lateral malleolus; the posteromedial portal is made medial to the Achilles tendon along the same plane as the posterolateral portal.[23] Both portals can be used to visualize the pathology of posterior process of the talus with or without entering the posterior ankle joint or subtalar joints. However, these joints may also be accessed if necessary for the arthroscopic approach.

An open posterolateral approach avoids the neurovascular bundle, however risks injury to the sural nerve and its branches, whereas a posteromedial approach allows access to address any FHL tendon pathologies.[23] Heyer and Rose performed a retrospective case series of 40 ankles in 38 dancers who failed conservative treatment and

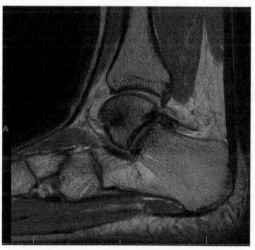

Fig. 3. Sagittal view of ankle. T1-weighted image demonstrated the presence of an os trigonum with surrounding bone marrow edema.

underwent os trigonum excision and FHL tenolysis via an open posteromedial approach. Their study included 39 women with a mean age of 19.2 years, who were primarily ballet dancers (90%). On average, dancers underwent surgery 17.6 months after symptom onset. The open approach was performed at the posterior aspect of the medial malleolus, proceeded by FHL debridement, and excision of the os trigonum using sharp dissection. Dancers returned to full activity 7.9 weeks postoperatively and were pain free after 17.7 months postoperatively, with no reported neurovascular or other major complications.[24]

In their comparative study of open (n = 16) versus endoscopic (n = 25) excision of symptomatic os trigonum that failed conservative treatment, Guo and colleagues found a statistically significant difference in patient satisfaction and complication rate between the 2 groups. There was a higher female-to-male ratio in the open group (37.5%) compared with the endoscopic group (28.0%). Of the open group, 31.5% were dancers and 2% in the endoscopic group; most of the patients in either group were involved in high demanding activities such as soccer, badminton, gymnastics, and basketball. Predictably, the endoscopic excision group had a shorter time to return to activity; there was no statistically significant difference in complication rate. Two complications were observed in the open excision group: 1 patient experienced sensory loss along the sural nerve and another experienced 10-degree loss of dorsiflexion. Only 1 patient in the endoscopic group experienced a complication including sensory loss to the medial heel.[25] Ribbans and colleagues reviewed 47 papers involving open and arthroendoscopic techniques. In the short term, return to activity is faster in the arthroendoscopic group, and long-term outcomes were not able to be assessed due to differing follow-up periods. Their reported complication rates for open medial, open lateral, and arthroendoscopic surgery are 3.9%, 12.7%, and 4.8%, respectively. Of the complications, 4% included neurologic complications (sural and tibial nerve and complex regional pain syndrome) and 2.8% with wound and infection problems.[26]

Thus, regardless of approach used for surgical resection of the os trigonum, meticulous dissection, protection of vital neurovascular structures, and gentle retraction are vital to avoid such complications (**Fig. 4**).

FLEXOR HALLUCIS LONGUS TENDINOPATHY
Cause and Diagnosis

Tendonitis of the FHL has been termed "dancer's tendonitis" and can often be found in conjunction with os trigonum syndrome.[22,27] FHL tendonitis is uncommon in the general population, but is commonly seen in ballet dancers, elicited by the *en pointe* or *demi relevé* positions.[28] The FHL is the largest muscle of the deep posterior compartment and serves to plantarflex both the ankle and hallux. Its tendon travels posteriorly, cradled between the medial and lateral tubercles of the posterior process of the talus, and continues medially, inferior to the sustentaculum tali, and plantarly to its insertion at the hallux distal phalanx. Because of its anatomic course, FHL tenosynovitis (sometimes referred to as dancers' tendinitis) and posterior ankle impingement are often found concurrently and have similar causes. Pain may also be notable at the tarsal tunnel. Entrapment of the tendon may result in stenosing tenosynovitis and the development of microtears or a partial tear.[4] FHL tenosynovitis can be isolated on physical examination with flexion of the hallux eliciting pain at the posterior ankle. Stenosing tenosynovitis of the FHL tendon is due to fusiform thickening of the tendon at the fibro-osseous tunnel at the posterior talus.[2] Crepitus and pain may be palpable with active and passive FHL plantarflexion.[4]

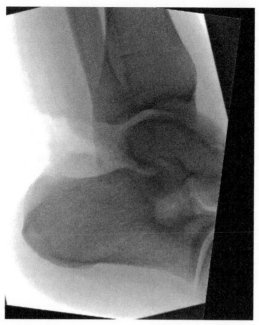

Fig. 4. Fluoroscopic confirmation of Os Trigonum excision

Imaging modalities used to rule out osseous involvement of the os trigonum or posterior ankle joint should initially be performed. To further investigate the integrity of the FHL tendon sheath, a tenogram may be obtained (**Fig. 5**). Foot and ankle tenograms are traditionally performed for the peroneal and posterior tibial tendon due to ease of access. The FHL tendon on the other hand rests in a deeper location along the

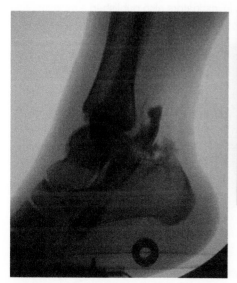
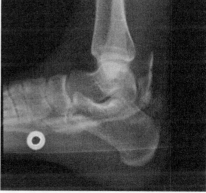

Fig. 5. Flexor hallucis longus tenogram demonstrating contrast confirmation in the sheath of the FHL tendon with stenosis confirmed into the location of the fibro-osseous tunnel.

posteromedial ankle and may pose challenges during needle placement. Na and colleagues describe a technique to locate the tendon more accurately.[29] The patient is laid supine with external rotation of the leg, and the posterior tibial artery is palpated and marked. The skin entry site is marked 1 cm posterior to the artery and 1 cm above the upper border of the calcaneus; this area can be anesthetized using a local anesthetic. The needle is then oriented one-third of the way along the sustentaculum tali in the anteroposterior and superior-inferior direction.[29] Fluoroscopy is used to confirm the orientation before insertion. As the needle advances, it must also be oriented 15 degree off the horizontal to contact the calcaneus rather than the neurovascular bundle. Once the needle is in the correct location, a total of 6 to 8 mL of a mixture of contrast medium—bupivacaine—is injected with multiple spot images obtained. Resistance indicates possible needle insertion into the tendon, whereas localized rounded or irregular shape indicates extravasation; the needle should be reoriented. This examination can demonstrate synovial irregularity or stenoses and fibrous bands. Complications of this procedure includes infection, bleeding, nerve block, tendon injury, and incorrect diagnosis due to improper technique.

MRI continues to remain a useful imaging modality that will demonstrate increased fluid intensity surrounding the tendon in the acute stage and tendon degeneration in the chronic stage (**Fig. 6**).

Treatment

Conservative treatment consists of correction of improper technique, inflammation reduction (with rest, ice, ultrasonography), and physical therapy with reduction or cessation of techniques exacerbating pain such as *en pointe* and *plié*.

Surgical treatment consists of tendon debridement of hypertrophic tendon, repairing tears, and tenolysis and is typically performed with an open approach with a posteromedial incision. In their systematic study, Rietveld and colleagues reviewed 27 papers of endoscopic and open operative treatments for posterior ankle impingement and FHL tendinopathy. Overall surgical outcomes were good to excellent in 89% of cases, with return to dance with an average of 11 weeks for combined and 16 weeks for isolated FHL tendinopathy.[30] In the same year, the investigators also published a retrospective

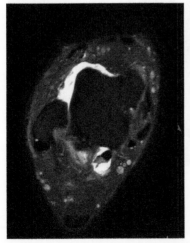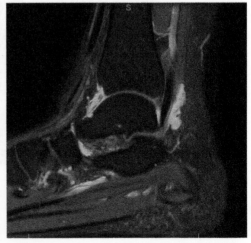

Fig. 6. T2-weighted MRI images. Axial view and sagittal images of the ankle showing anterior ankle joint effusion and FHL tenosynovitis.

study comparing their results of open versus endoscopic operative treatment of posterior ankle impingement syndrome and FHL longus tendinopathy in 32 dancers (39 procedures). Of the procedures, 19 were endoscopic and 20 were open. In the open group, the lateral approach was used in 3 procedures for isolated os trigonum and medial approach used in 17 procedures. Patients were followed-up for an average of 10.2 years for the open and 1.9 years for the endoscopic group. Excellent and good outcomes were noted in 90% of the open group and 79% of the endoscopic group. Both groups were able to return to dance at a mean of 8 weeks. The endoscopic group had a statistically significant increase in complications including hematoma, inflammation, and painful scar formation, thus favoring the open approach.[31]

ANTERIOR ANKLE IMPINGEMENT

In addition to posterior ankle pain, forced plantarflexion causes attenuation of anterior ankle capsular and ligamentous structures. Forced dorsiflexion with external rotation, such as in *demi plié*, can cause impingement of the dorsal talus on the anterior tibial lip. This movement is found to be the most common cause of anterior ankle joint impingement in dancers.[32] Repetitive microtrauma induces bone spur formation at the cartilaginous rim of this articulation (**Fig. 7**).

Anterior ankle impingement can be further divided into anterolateral and anteromedial impingement. Anterolateral gutter impingement usually is due to soft-tissue impingement, particularly the thickening and chronic inflammation of the anterotalofibular ligament. Chronic scarring and hypertrophy of the anterior ankle synovium can lead to mechanical impingement without instability,[33] whereas anteromedial ankle impingement is typically due to osseous impingement of the bone spurs, without joint space narrowing.[1,2] Pain is clinically reproducible with passive ankle dorsiflexion with and without knee flexion. An anterior drawer test and Silfverskiold test should be

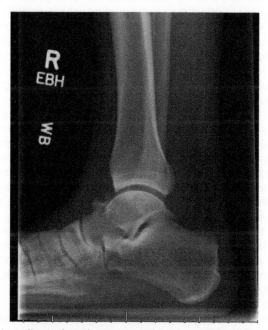

Fig. 7. Lateral plain radiograph with presence of mild osteophytic lipping at the anterior tibia and bone spur formation at the dorsal talus.

performed to rule out presence of lateral ankle instability and equinus contractures, respectively. Radiographs can reveal "kissing exostoses" on the anterior tibia and dorsal talus, with normal ankle joint space.[34] To discern the location of intraarticular osteophytes, an oblique ankle radiograph should be obtained. In his study, van Dijk describes this technique by placing the ankle in neutral, with a 30-degree external rotation of the leg and the x-ray beam 45 degrees craniocaudally from the usual lateral position.[35] Alternatively, a CT scan may also be performed.

Surgical excision of the osteophytes may be performed via open or arthroscopic procedures. Only one study exists in the literature that reviews surgical treatment of anterior ankle impingement. Nihal and colleagues performed a retrospective case series of 11 elite dancers (12 ankles) who underwent arthroscopic treatment of anterior ankle impingement, all who failed conservative treatment. All dancers previously sustained ankle trauma, and anterior ankle exostoses were present in 6 ankles. The arthroscopic approach included the usual anteromedial and anterolateral scope portals for removal of bone spurs, soft tissue impingement, and debridement of synovitis. Patients remained non–weight-bearing for 5 days postoperatively. Nine dancers returned to full activity on an average of 7 weeks postoperatively and one dancer underwent repeat debridement with marked improvement and return to dance performance. One patient was unable to return to dance performance due to other unrelated orthopedic comorbidities.[36] There was no statistically significant difference in recovery between those with osseous or soft tissue impingement.

STRESS FRACTURES IN THE FOOT AND ANKLE
Cause and Diagnosis

With repetitive stress and loading, pedal bones will undergo bone stress reactions. These stress reactions highlight the presence of an imbalance between osteoclastic and osteoblastic activity. Other factors such as metabolic status, nutritional status, menstrual dysfunction, and bone vascularity can further negatively affect this balance. Women form a large proportion of dancers. Female athletes are more susceptible to a constellation of symptoms known as the female athlete triad. In accordance with the updated guidelines, the female athlete triad is described as having reduced energy with or without disordered eating, subclinical menstrual dysfunction, and low bone mineral density.[37,38] These 3 components are thought to be on a spectrum, and all 3 components are not required to be present for diagnosis. Furthermore, low energy availability can influence the release of gonadotropin-releasing hormone, which indirectly disrupts the release of estrogen from the ovaries. Estrogen is an important hormone in regulating bone formation by inhibiting bone remodeling and resorption and enhances bone formation. A decrease in estrogen thus leads to decreased bone mineral density and increase in fragility fractures.[39] A large systematic review by Wentz and colleagues evaluated the incidence of stress fractures in military and athlete populations. The investigators found an increase in incidence of stress fractures in women as compared with men with an incidence of 9.2% and ~3%, respectively. Female athletes with normal weight and bone health are less likely to develop stress fractures.[40] Women with at least one component of the female triad have a higher incidence of stress fractures due to bone remodeling impairment.[41]

Stress fractures typically occur in areas of poorly vascularized bone. Specifically, in the foot and ankle, bones of high-risk stress fractures include the navicular, fifth metatarsal, and anterior tibia.[42] The most common area ballet dancers experience stress fractures are the metatarsals.[43] In a study by Noon and colleagues, 69 Irish dancers with injuries were evaluated for presence of injury types, with one-third found to have stress fractures. These stress fractures were found in the sesamoids (27.7%), metatarsals (23.1%), navicular (12.3%), first proximal phalanx (12.3%), and tibia (9.2%). Similar to ballet dancers, Irish dancers perform the *en pointe* technique, jumps, and *leap over* in which the dancer will jump 2 to 3 feet in the air and land *en pointe*, in a soft tissue "ghille" similar to a ballet slipper.[44]

Clinical symptoms of stress fractures in the lower extremity include nonspecific gradual pain over several weeks. Detailed history should be obtained to assess for the female athlete triad, endocrinopathies, or immune dysfunctions. Workup should include urine and blood tests including complete metabolic panel including serum calcium, albumin, alkaline phosphatase, serum vitamin D levels, and glomerular filtrate rate. Hormonal levels should also be tested for menstrual dysfunction and endocrinopathies. Furthermore, for those with multiple stress fractures or high suspicion for the female athlete triad, a bone density scan should be obtained.[42]

Pain is often reproduced with palpation of the affected bone. Imaging is the most useful for diagnosis and can include plain radiographs, MRI, bone scan, or CT scan. Initially, plain radiographs are obtained and can show subtle radiolucency or ill-defined cortex in stress fractures of cortical bone. Subsequent findings include periosteal reaction and new bone formation.[42] Stress fractures of cancellous bones (such as the calcaneus) show sclerosis oriented perpendicular to the trabecular bone. If radiographs are unremarkable, MRI or bone scan are helpful. MRI shows earlier signs of stress fractures, endosteal marrow edema, periosteal edema, muscle edema, cortical thickening, and hypointensity signal at the fracture site. Technetium-99m–labeled disphosphonate bone scan shows signs of stress fracture before radiographic evidence.[45] Although bone scans are found to be sensitive for any bony remodeling process, such as tumor, infection, acute fracture, and stress fracture, it is not specific for stress fractures.[46] MRI is found to be the same sensitivity and higher specificity as compared with bone scans. In diagnosing stress fractures of superficial bones such as metatarsal fractures, ultrasonography can be used to evaluate the outer surface of the cortex for step-off, a hypoechoic band, periosteal reaction, and hyperechoic callus formation.[47,48]

Treatment

On discovery, stress fractures should initially be treated nonoperatively with a non–weight-bearing (NWB) cast for 6 to 8 weeks with gradual return to activity. Based on clinical, laboratory, and imaging findings, conservative treatment may include a multidisciplinary approach and medications to treat underlying metabolic dysfunction.[42]

With dance positions as *demi relevé*, dancers put increased weight to the second metatarsal, as it bears most of the weight. Radiographically, there may be notable cortical thickening. Fifth metatarsal stress fractures on the other hand are due to lateral column overload or inversion-related fatigue.[49] Stress fractures at the fifth metatarsal are typically located at the metaphyseal-diaphyseal junction, an area of tenuous blood supply. With either stress fracture, initial NWB in a cast is recommended. In their study, Torg and colleagues[50] reported that 93% of 46 athletes with acute fifth metatarsal base fractures healed on an average of 6.5 weeks with an NWB cast. Surgical treatment with intramedullary screw fixation should be considered in those with evidence of delayed union with possible bone grafting.[51] Intramedullary screw fixation can be performed with either an open or a percutaneous approach. DeLee and colleagues reported union of fifth metatarsal stress fractures in 10 athletes on average of 7.5 weeks, with return to sports at 8.5 weeks, without any complications.[52]

The central one-third of the navicular is the zone of maximum shear stress and is devoid of direct blood supply, making it difficult for healing.[53] Because of the tenuous blood supply to this area, aggressive conservative management is the standard of care with non–weight-bearing management until the fractures is healed.[50] Torg and colleagues[51] evaluated 10 patients with navicular stress fractures that underwent conservative management. Patients were immobilized in an NWB cast for 6 to 8 weeks; the average return to activity was found to be 3.8 months.[49] Khan and colleagues[54] evaluated 82 athletes with 86 navicular stress fractures who were treated initially with at least 6 weeks of non–weight-bearing cast (n = 22), at least 6 weeks with weight-bearing of limited activity (n = 24), or less than 6 weeks of conservative treatment (n = 19). Of the patients who underwent initial NWB cast, 86% returned to sports, whereas of the patients who were weight-bearing with limited activity, 26% returned to activity. With patients who failed initial weight-bearing treatment, 86% were successfully treated with NWB cast immobilization, whereas 73% underwent surgical intervention. Their results confirm those of Torg and colleagues that aggressive conservative treatment with NWB cast is important.[51] Surgical management can include either stress fracture fixation percutaneously or fracture exposure based on fracture location. Regardless, postoperative rehabilitation includes a 4-week period of non–weight-bearing for 4 weeks with gradual return to weight-bearing for more than 8 weeks.[42] In a large systematic review and meta-analysis of 315 patients with navicular stress fractures, Attia and colleagues found that operative management provided higher success rate, a lower refracture rate, and a lower nonunion rate compared with conservative management.[55]

SUMMARY

Dancers are subject to many foot and ankle injuries due to high demands, difficult techniques, and repetitive motions. Intrinsic and extrinsic factors can thus lead to sesamoiditis, posterior ankle joint impingement, FHL tendonitis, anterior ankle joint impingement, and stress fractures of various pedal bones. Diagnosis of all pathologies can be made using a focus physical examination, plain radiographs, or MRI if osseous pathologies are not present or obvious. Treatment should initially begin with aggressive conservative treatment with activity cessation, edema control, immobilization, and/or NWB. Surgery should thus be reserved for those who fail conservative treatment. Furthermore, specific treatment options should be tailored to the dancer and should focus on early return to dance.

CLINICS CARE POINTS

- Diagnosis of injuries in dancers should include a detailed physical examination to rule out immunologic, metabolic, or endocrine-related pathologies. Female athlete triad is a known underdiagnosed condition that affects many female athletes and dancers and can lead to several pathologies.

- MRI is helpful in the diagnosis of sesamoiditis, posterior and anterior ankle impingement, flexor hallucis longus tendonitis, and stress fractures if plain radiographs are unremarkable.

- Flexor hallucis longus tenogram is an excellent imaging modality requiring high technical expertise that aids in the diagnosis of flexor hallucis longus tendon pathology.

- Stress fractures are found in areas of bone with decreased vascularity; thus aggressive conservative care should be initially attempted.

DISCLOSURE

The authors have nothing to disclose.

REFERENCES

1. Kadel NJ. Foot and ankle injuries in dance. Phys Med Rehabil Clin N Am 2006; 17(4):813–26, vii.
2. Vosseller JT, Dennis ER, Bronner S. Ankle injuries in dancers. J Am Acad Orthop Surg 2019;27(16):582–9.
3. Campoy FA, Coelho LR, Bastos FN, Netto Júnior J, Vanderlei LC, Monteiro HL, Padovani CR, Pastre CM. Investigation of risk factors and characteristics of dance injuries. Clin J Sport Med 2011;21(6):493–8.
4. Macintyre J, Joy E. Foot and ankle injuries in dance. Clin Sports Med 2000;19(2): 351–68.
5. Sanders TG, Rathur SK. Imaging of painful conditions of the hallucal sesamoid complex and plantar capsular structures of the first metatarsophalangeal joint. Radiol Clin North Am 2008;46(6):1079–92, vii.
6. Prisk VR, O'Loughlin PF, Kennedy JG. Forefoot injuries in dancers. Clin Sports Med 2008;27(2):305–20.
7. Mittlmeier T, Haar P. Sesamoid and toe fractures. Injury 2004;35(Suppl 2). SB87–97.
8. Aper RL, Saltzman CL, Brown TD. The effect of hallux sesamoid excision on the flexor hallucis longus moment arm. Clin Orthop 1996;325:209–17.
9. Dean RS, Coetzee JC, McGaver RS, Fritz JE, Nilsson LJ. Functional outcome of sesamoid excision in athletes. Am J Sports Med 2020;48(14):3603–9.
10. Robertson GAJ, Goffin JS, Wood AM. Return to sport following stress fractures of the great toe sesamoids: a systematic review. Br Med Bull 2017;122(1):135–49.
11. Blundell CM, Nicholson P, Blackney MW. Percutaneous screw fixation for fractures of the sesamoid bones of the hallux. J Bone Joint Surg Br 2002;84:1138–41.
12. Axe MJ, Ray RL. Orthotic treatment of sesamoid pain. Am J Sports Med 1988;16: 411–6.
13. Saxena A, Krisdakumtorn T. Return to activity after sesamoidectomy in athletically active individuals. Foot Ankle Int 2003;24:415–9.
14. Pagenstert GI, Valderrabano V, Hintermann B. Medial sesamoid nonunion combined with hallux valgus in athletes: a report of two cases. Foot Ankle Int 2006; 27:135–40.
15. Pagenstert GI, Hintermann B, Valderrabano V. Percutaneous fixation of hallux sesamoid fractures. Tech Foot Ankle Surg 2008;7:107–14.
16. Bronner S, et al. J Orthop sports Phys ther.: management of a delayed-union sesamoid fracture in a dancer. J Dance Med Sci 2009;13(1):31.
17. Coetzee JC, Seybold JD, Moser BR, Stone RM. Management of posterior impingement in the ankle in athletes and dancers. Foot Ankle Int 2015;36(8): 988–94.
18. Lawson JP. Symptomatic radiographic variants in extremities. Radiology 1985; 157(3):625–31.
19. Nault ML, Kocher MS, Micheli LJ. Os trigonum syndrome. J Am Acad Orthop Surg 2014;22(9):545–53.
20. Albisetti W, Ometti M, Pascale V, De Bartolomeo O. Clinical evaluation and treatment of posterior impingement in dancers. Am J Phys Med Rehabil 2009;88(5): 349–54.

21. Peace KA, Hillier JC, Hulme A, Healy JC. MRI features of posterior ankle impingement syndrome in ballet dancers: a review of 25 cases. Clin Radiol 2004;59(11): 1025–33.

22. Mouhsine E, Crevoisier X, Leyvraz PF, Akiki A, Dutoit M, Garofalo R. Posttraumatic overload or acute syndrome of the os trigonum: a possible cause of posterior ankle impingement. Knee Surg Sports Traumatol Arthrosc 2004;12:250–3.

23. van Dijk CN, Scholten PE, Krips R. A 2-portal endoscopic approach for diagnosis and treatment of posterior ankle pathology. Arthroscopy 2000;16(8):871–6.

24. Heyer JH, Rose DJ. Os trigonum excision in dancers via an open posteromedial approach. Foot Ankle Int 2017;38(1):27–35.

25. Guo QW, Hu YL, Jiao C, Ao YF, Tian DX. Open versus endoscopic excision of a symptomatic os trigonum: a comparative study of 41 cases. Arthroscopy 2010; 26(3):384–90.

26. Ribbans WJ, Ribbans HA, Cruickshank JA, Wood EV. The management of posterior ankle impingement syndrome in sport: a review. Foot Ankle Surg 2015; 21(1):1–10.

27. Hamilton WG. Stenosing tenosynovitis of the flexor hallucis longus tendon and posterior impingement upon the os trigonum in ballet dancers. Foot Ankle 1982;3(2):74–80.

28. Tudisco C, Puddu G. Stenosing tenosynovitis of the flexor hallucis longus tendon in a classical ballet dancer. A case report. Am J Sports Med 1984;12(5):403–4.

29. Na JB, Bergman AG, Oloff LM, Beaulieu CF. The flexor hallucis longus: tenographic technique and correlation of imaging findings with surgery in 39 ankles. Radiology 2005;236(3):974–82.

30. Rietveld ABMB, Hagemans FMT, Haitjema S, Vissers T, Nelissen RGHH. Results of treatment of posterior ankle impingement syndrome and flexor hallucis longus tendinopathy in dancers: a systematic review. J Dance Med Sci 2018;22(1): 19–32.

31. Rietveld ABMB, Hagemans FMT. Operative treatment of posterior ankle impingement syndrome and flexor hallucis longus tendinopathy in dancers open versus endoscopic approach. J Dance Med Sci 2018;22(1):11–8.

32. O'Kane JW, Kadel N. Anterior impingement syndrome in dancers. Curr Rev Musculoskelet Med 2008;1(1):12–6.

33. Laurence Terry. Ankle impingement syndromes. Clin Pract Guidel 2018;290.

34. Talusan PG, Toy J, Perez JL, Milewski MD, Reach JS Jr. Anterior ankle impingement: diagnosis and treatment. J Am Acad Orthop Surg 2014;22(5):333–9.

35. van Dijk CN, Wessel RN, Tol JL, Maas M. Oblique radiograph for the detection of bone spurs in anterior ankle impingement. Skeletal Radiol 2002;31(4):214–21.

36. Nihal A, Rose DJ, Trepman E. Arthroscopic treatment of anterior ankle impingement syndrome in dancers. Foot Ankle Int 2005;26(11):908–12.

37. Frank RM, Romeo AA, Bush-Joseph CA, Bach BR Jr. Injuries to the female athlete in 2017: Part I: general Considerations, Concussions, stress fractures, and the female athlete triad. JBJS Rev 2017;5(10):e4.

38. Nattiv A, Loucks AB, Manore MM, American College of Sports Medicine. American College of Sports Medicine position stand: the female athlete triad. Med Sci Sports Exerc 2007;39(10):1867–82.

39. Syed F, Khosla S. Mechanisms of sex steroid effects on bone. Biochem Biophys Res Commun 2005;328(3):688–96.

40. Wentz L, Liu PY, Haymes E, Ilich JZ. Females have a greater incidence of stress fractures than males in both military and athletic populations: a systemic review. Mil Med 2011;176(4):420–30.

41. Barrack MT, Gibbs JC, De Souza MJ, Williams NI, Nichols JF, Rauh MJ, Nattiv A. Higher incidence of bone stress injuries with increasing female athlete triad-related risk factors: a prospective multisite study of exercising girls and women. Am J Sports Med 2014;42(4):949–58.
42. Shindle MK, Endo Y, Warren RF, Lane JM, Helfet DL, Schwartz EN, Ellis SJ. Stress fractures about the tibia, foot, and ankle. J Am Acad Orthop Surg 2012;20(3): 167–76.
43. Kadel NJ, Teitz CC, Kronmal RA. Stress fractures in ballet dancers. Am J Sports Med 1992;20(4):445–9.
44. Noon M, Hoch AZ, McNamara L, Schimke J. Injury patterns in female Irish dancers. PM R 2010;2(11):1030–4.
45. Roub LW, Gumerman LW, Hanley EN Jr, Clark MW, Goodman M, Herbert DL. Bone stress: a radionuclide imaging perspective. Radiology 1979;132(2):431–8.
46. Gaeta M, Minutoli F, Scribano E, et al. CT and MR imaging findings in athletes with early tibial stress injuries: Comparison with bone scintigraphy findings and emphasis on cortical abnormalities. Radiology 2005;235(2):553–61.
47. Banal F, Gandjbakhch F, Foltz V, et al. Sensitivity and specificity of ultrasonography in early diagnosis of metatarsal bone stress fractures: a pilot study of 37 patients. J Rheumatol 2009;36(8):1715–9.
48. Arni D, Lambert V, Delmi M, Bianchi S. Insufficiency fracture of the calcaneum: Sonographic findings. J Clin Ultrasound 2009;37(7):424–7.
49. Goulart M, O'Malley MJ, Hodgkins CW, Charlton TP. Foot and ankle fractures in dancers. Clin Sports Med 2008;27(2):295–304.
50. Torg JS, Pavlov H, Cooley LH, et al. Stress fractures of the tarsal navicular: a retrospective review of twenty-one cases. J Bone Joint Surg Am 1982;64(5):700–12.
51. Torg JS, Balduini FC, Zelko RR, Pavlov H, Peff TC, Das M. Fractures of the base of the fifth metatarsal distal to the tuberosity. Classification and guidelines for non-surgical and surgical management. J Bone Joint Surg Am 1984;66(2):209–14.
52. DeLee JC, Evans JP, Julian J. Stress fracture of the fifth metatarsal. Am J Sports Med 1983;11(5):349–53.
53. Mann JA, Pedowitz DI. Evaluation and treatment of navicular stress fractures, including nonunions, revision surgery, and persistent pain after treatment. Foot Ankle Clin 2009;14(2):187–204.
54. Khan KM, Fuller PJ, Brukner PD, Kearney C, Burry HC. Outcome of conservative and surgical management of navicular stress fracture in athletes. Eighty-six cases proven with computerized tomography. Am J Sports Med 1992;20(6): 657–66.
55. Attia AK, Mahmoud K, Bariteau J, Labib SA, DiGiovanni CW, D'Hooghe P. Return to sport following navicular stress fracture: a systematic review and meta-analysis of three hundred and fifteen fractures. Int Orthop 2021;45(10):2699–710.

Posterior Ankle Impingement Syndrome

Megan A. Ishibashi, DPM, AACFAS[a], Matthew D. Doyle, DPM, FACFAS[a],*,
Craig E. Krcal Jr, DPM[b]

KEYWORDS

- Posterior ankle impingement • Os trigonum syndrome
- Flexor hallucis longus tenosynovitis • Stieda process

KEY POINTS

- Posterior ankle impingement is typically seen in athletes, primarily dancers and soccer players, secondary to dynamic and repetitive push-off maneuvers and forced hyperplantarflexion.
- Posterior ankle impingement results from chronic, repetitive trauma to the posterior ankle capsule, flexor hallucis longus tendon, and/or os trigonum.
- It is important to perform a thorough workup by isolating and testing the posterior compartment muscles and obtaining proper imaging with radiographs to identify any osseous abnormalities and MRI to evaluate the soft tissue structures.
- Nonsurgical treatment includes activity modification, physical therapy, and steroid injections.
- When conservative treatment fails, surgical treatment should be considered to address either the soft tissue or osseous pathology.

BACKGROUND

Posterior ankle impingement (PAI) is a spectrum of clinical pathologies characterized by posterior ankle pain during plantarflexion. PAI is typically seen in the athletic population, most commonly in dancers, runners, and soccer players. Patients typically experience chronic or recurrent posterior ankle pain after forced or repetitive plantarflexion and push-off maneuvers. PAI is an all-encompassing term that includes not only soft tissue impingement but also bony impingement secondary to the presence of an os trigonum or Stieda process. This condition has been referred to by several names including talar compression syndrome, os trigonum syndrome, hindfoot impingement syndrome, and nutcracker-type impingement.[1]

[a] Silicon Valley Reconstructive Foot and Ankle Fellowship, Palo Alto Medical Foundation, 701 E EL Camino Real, Mountain View, CA 94040, USA; [b] Kaiser San Francisco Bay Area Foot and Ankle Residency Program, 3600 Broadway, Oakland, CA 94611, USA
* Corresponding author.
E-mail address: matthew.doyledpm@gmail.com

Clin Podiatr Med Surg 40 (2023) 209–222
https://doi.org/10.1016/j.cpm.2022.07.014
0891-8422/23/© 2022 Elsevier Inc. All rights reserved.

PATHOANATOMY

The anatomy that comprises the posterior ankle can be divided into osseous and soft tissue structures positioned posterior to the tibiotalar joint, subtalar joint, and calcaneus. The osseous structures responsible for PAI are within the tibiocalcaneal interval including the posterior malleolus, posterolateral talar process (Stieda process), os trigonum, posterior subtalar joint, and the posterior calcaneal tuberosity. The posterior talar process involves the portion of the talus posterior to the articular surface of the joint. This process consists of 2 projections, the posteromedial and posterolateral processes. The posterolateral process is referred to as the trigonal process, and when this process remains a nonfused entity from the talar body, it is referred to as the os trigonum. An os trigonum is an accessory bone that represents failure of the secondary ossification center to fuse with the posterolateral talus. The posterolateral talus typically mineralizes between 7 and 13 years of age and fuses within 1 year; however, in 7% to 14% of adults it remains as a separate accessory bone.[2] When mineralization and fusion is complete, an elongated posterolateral process is called a Stieda process. The overall incidence of os trigonum has been reported to occur in 1.7% to 49% of the population; it is also found to be present bilaterally in about 50% of cases.[3]

Nonosseous posterior ankle joint impingement typically results from anomalous muscle bellies including, most commonly, peroneus quartus or an accessory or low-lying long flexor muscle belly resulting in deep posterior compartment crowding and impingement.[4] The peroneus quartus accessorius has been documented in cadaver dissections in 7% to 22% of the normal population, whereas the presence of other anomalous muscle bellies of the deep posterior compartment is less known.[5] These accessory muscle bellies are typically asymptomatic but have been documented as primary pathologic entities in the posterior ankle.[4] Other causes of nonosseous PAI include soft tissue impingement from native or pathologic hypertrophied synovium or posterior ankle ligaments, particularly the posterior inferior tibiofibular ligament.[6]

The flexor hallucis longus (FHL) tendon originates proximally on the posterior fibula and interosseous membrane and courses distally within its tendon sheath forming a fibro-osseous tunnel in a groove between the posteromedial and posterolateral talar processes. The tendon continues plantarly to the sustentaculum tali of the calcaneus and then forms the "knot of Henry" with the flexor digitorum longus tendon toward its insertion on the base of the distal phalanx of the hallux. The FHL tendon is susceptible to stenosing tenosynovitis, and chronic entrapment of this tendon can occur resulting from either a low-lying muscle belly, impingement from an os trigonum, or incongruity of maximum plantarflexion and dorsiflexion of the ankle and great toe joint, resulting in compression of the tendon.[3,7,8]

CAUSE AND PATHOGENESIS

PAI most commonly presents as a chronic, nonspecific symptom in younger athletes. A high index of suspicion for PAI is vital in timely diagnosis and treatment. The potential causes of PAI are numerous and include soft tissue pathology such as Achilles tendinopathy, retrocalcaneal bursitis, FHL tenosynovitis, and osseous pathology including osteochondral lesions, bony impingement, Haglund deformity, stress fractures, and tarsal coalitions. However, the most common causes of PAI in descending order are os trigonum, large Stieda process, and soft tissue impingement.[9] Dancers, runners, and soccer players encompass the typical patient population presenting with PAI, due to the demands placed on the ankle in the plantarflexed position. In dancers it commonly occurs in the "en pointe" and "demi-pointe" positions.[3] The hyperplantarflexion position causes the posterior talar process to become compressed between the superior calcaneus and posterior distal tibia, causing osseous impingement.

The pathologic processes that lead to pain are either from an acute injury versus chronic repetitive motion. In acute trauma, the Stieda process is compressed between the posterior malleolus and calcaneus, causing a fracture (Shepherd fracture) or injury to the synchondrosis of the os trigonum.[10,11] Impingement may also result from previous fractures or degenerative arthritis, leading to the formation of ankle and subtalar osteophytes. Chronic injury secondary to repetitive plantarflexion results in either soft tissue or osseous impingement. This pathologic process results from the posterior capsule and synovium becoming irritated and consequently inflamed, resulting in pain to the posterior ankle. The posterior ankle ligaments including the posterior talofibular and tibiotalar ligaments can also develop fibrotic and inflammatory changes from the repetitive injury, resulting in ankle stiffness and biomechanical changes.

FHL tendon injuries are one of the more common injuries to the posterior ankle and are similarly seen in athletes performing repetitive push-off maneuvers. This dynamic mechanism results in FHL tenosynovitis or tendinitis, which occurs from compression of the tendon within its sheath. FHL tendon pathology can also result from entrapment secondary to a low-lying FHL muscle belly, friction of the tendon against an os trigonum, or repetitive hyperflexion, resulting in synovial hypertrophy or synovitis.

CLINICAL PRESENTATION

The presentation of PAI is typically characterized by deep posterior ankle pain during maximum plantarflexion, which may be sharp, dull, constant, or positional. The patient may present during an acute exacerbation or trauma or as a chronic irritant from repetitive activity. In the acute setting, pain and inflammation can be expected for 3 to 4 weeks after the initial symptom presentation. More commonly, chronic presentation of PAI presents as a persistent aching during typical activity.[12] It is much less common to encounter posterior ankle pain and impingement in the nonathletic population, and anatomic variation must be considered.

If no obvious structural pathologies can be identified on initial presentation, but posterior ankle joint impingement is suspected, conservative therapy is typically the first-line treatment that may alleviate symptoms including inflammation and pain. Return to activity may result in a recurring cycle of exacerbation and recalcitrant PAI; thus, timely diagnosis and understanding of the causative pathology should be sought out from initial presentation to avoid delayed treatment and to aid in timely return to activity.

DIAGNOSIS

A complete history and physical examination is imperative to successful diagnosis of PAI. Suspicion should be raised when evaluating a younger athlete, particularly dancers, who present with acute on chronic symptoms including pain and limited range of motion during typical activity to the deep, posterior ankle in plantarflexion. PAI is oftentimes a diagnosis of exclusion if no obvious osseous structures can explain the symptoms on plain films, and a thorough evaluation is essential in isolating the pathology.

On examination, the ankle joint should be meticulously examined to rule out other osseous, ligamentous, or tendinous pathologies. Localized tenderness is often not appreciated; however, there may be tenderness to palpation over the posterior medial ankle joint. Active and passive range of motion may or may not elicit symptoms particularly in maximum plantarflexion of the ankle joint or through range of motion of the subtalar joint. Laterally, the peroneal tendons should be carefully examined, and efforts should be taken to isolate and evaluate the posterior tibial tendon, FDL tendon, and FHL tendon. The FHL tendon at the level of the ankle joint should be evaluated by performing active resistance range of motion of the hallux; if this maneuver recreates posterior ankle pain, this may indicate FHL tenosynovitis. It can be difficult to reproduce symptoms for patients with PAI in the clinical setting; however, symptoms are most commonly elicited by weight-bearing "en-pointe," which places an axial load on the posterior ankle reproducing impingement symptoms. This maneuver should be assessed using both manual palpation as well as weight-bearing.[6,12,13]

Imaging and a thorough understanding of the posterior ankle joint anatomy and potential pathologies is essential in appropriate diagnosis and treatment of PAI syndrome. Standard plain film radiographs should be included in all initial evaluations, which may reveal osseous anomalies including os trigonum or Stieda processes (**Fig. 1**). One may also consider ancillary radiographs such as max plantarflexion or "en-pointe" lateral films to assess the posterior ankle joint in the position of pain.[12] A "posterior impingement view" has been described, which involves a nonstandard 25 degree external rotation lateral projection that is described as being more sensitive in diagnosis of osseous posterior ankle joint impingement, as the lateral posterior process is best viewed using this technique.[14] It must also be noted that not all os trigonum and Stieda processes are pathologic, and these anatomic variants can be seen in up to 25% of normal ankle radiographs.[1] For patients with posterior ankle joint pain with nonosseous cause, MRI is more useful in evaluating soft tissue lesions or pathology including capsular or ligamentous impingement or anomalous soft tissue structures such as peroneus quartus and, less commonly, an accessory flexor digitorum accessory muscle.[4] MRI can also be helpful in evaluating any bone marrow edema that may be present within the synchondrosis of the os trigonum, which may indicate a symptomatic os trigonum (**Fig. 2**). Ultrasound-guided posterior ankle joint injections have been found to be quite valuable in treating posterior ankle joint soft tissue impingement and may be used as a diagnostic tool.[15] Other tools described in diagnosing posterior ankle impingement, although less commonly used, involve

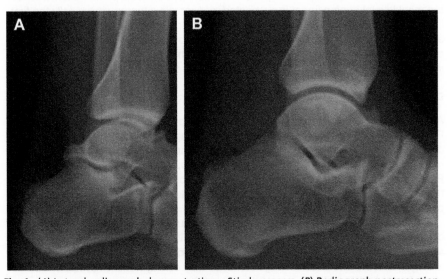

Fig. 1. (*A*) Lateral radiograph demonstrating a Stieda process. (*B*) Radiograph postresection.

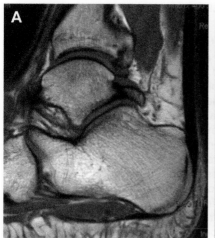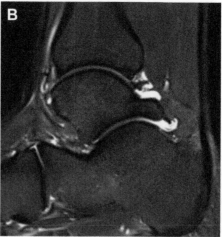

Fig. 2. (*A*) Sagittal T1-weighted MRI of an os trigonum. Note the separation between the posterior talus and os with intact cortical margins of the os fragment. (*B*) Sagittal T2-weighted MRI of a fused Stieda process.

radiographic or MR arthrography, which are typically avoided in the adolescent population. Finally, if plain film radiographs, MRI, and conservative therapy do not identify or manage symptoms consistent with posterior ankle joint impingement, diagnostic and therapeutic posterior ankle joint arthroscopy can be a definitive means of diagnosis and treatment of PAI.

CONSERVATIVE TREATMENT

Treatment of PAI consists of conservative and surgical interventions, where conservative treatments focus on rest, activity modification, physical therapy, and antiinflammatory measures.[12,16] If symptoms do not improve with this first-line therapy, ultrasound-guided injections have been found to be successful especially among high-level athletes.[6] These injections can help athletes either finish their season or can be curative for soft tissue impingement.[15]

Robinson and Bollen[15] treated 10 professional soccer players with PAI with ultrasound-guided injections of 40 mg of triamcinolone acetonide (Kenalog) and 3 mL of 0.5% plain bupivacaine hydrochloride (Marcaine). All players returned to their previous activity level within 3 weeks of the injections. The median follow-up was 26 months (range, 6–42 months). Eight players only had posterolateral synovitis with no os trigonum and did not have any recurrent symptoms on follow-up. The 2 players who had both soft tissue and bony impingement had recurrent symptoms at 4 and 6 months, respectively. These players had a second ultrasound-guided injection and both returned to play within 3 weeks. One player underwent endoscopic resection of the os trigonum and synovitis 4 months after the second injection. Mouhsin and colleagues[10] evaluated 19 recreational and professional athletes with os trigonum syndrome who underwent fluoroscopically guided steroid injections as first-line treatment. Ten athletes required no further treatment, 6 athletes required a second injection, and 3 athletes were recalcitrant to conservative treatment, requiring surgical excision of the os trigonum. Despite the success with the use of local corticosteroid injections, many discourage the routine use of these injections in dancers and high-level athletes because of the potential negative effects on the posterior ankle structures.[17–19]

SURGICAL TREATMENT OF POSTERIOR ANKLE IMPINGEMENT
Open Treatment

Surgical management is indicated for patients if they fail to improve with conservative treatment or if athletic patients want a faster return to play.[12] Surgical options include either an open or an arthroscopic approach. The first cases of surgical treatment of PAI was described in 1982 by Howse and colleagues[20] who performed an open posteromedial approach and Quirk and colleagues[21] who performed an open posterolateral approach to remove an os trigonum in a dancer. The posteromedial approach is well described within the literature as the most common approach for os trigonum resection especially in the dancer population. With this approach, the medial neurovascular bundle is easily identified and protected throughout the procedure. The advantage of this approach is better access to the FHL tendon and sheath, which many dancers and athletes suffer from concomitant FHL tendinitis with PAI.[6] Unlike arthroscopic approaches that resect the joint capsule and os trigonum, the os can be easily dissected from the surrounding soft tissue and capsule allowing for capsular repair, which has shown to decrease postoperative morbidity.[22,23] The posterolateral approach can also be used for os trigonum resection; however, it is not recommended given the potential high rate of sural nerve injury. Some studies have reported up to 20% of permanent or temporary sural nerve sensory loss with a posterolateral approach.[24,25] Abramowitz and colleagues[24] reported good results with open excision of symptomatic os trigonum using a posterior lateral approach in 41 patients; however, 4 patients developed permanent sural nerve sensory loss.

Generally, open debridement has favorable outcomes, with studies reporting approximately 70% to 80% of either good or excellent results at final follow-up.[17,23,24,26–28] This approach has been studied mainly in dancers with an average return to dance in elite dancers from 9 weeks to 20 weeks. Heyer and colleagues[28] used an open posteromedial approach in dancers for os trigonum resection, and the patients had an average return to dance class at an average of 7.9 weeks with full return to prior level of dance at 17.7 weeks. This study is the largest cohort of dancers to undergo excision of an os trigonum with a posteromedial approach.

Several studies have had no permanent injury to the neurovascular bundle or other major complications with the posteromedial approach.[24,28] Labs and colleagues[23] had 1 patient with temporary tibial nerve paralysis and 2 patients with hematomas, 1 of which required reoperation. The several studies on FHL release in dancers via a posteromedial approach have demonstrated no major complications.[29–31] Therefore, the posteromedial approach has been shown to carry a decreased risk of neurovascular injury in comparison to the posterolateral approach. Overall, an open approach for PAI has shown to be safe, reliable, and an effective alternative treatment of arthroscopic treatment of PAI.

Arthroscopic Treatment

Posterior ankle arthroscopy has become an indispensable tool for the treatment of PAI. The widespread use of this approach has provided a better understanding of the anatomy and pathology of the posterior ankle. Arthroscopic treatment of PAI is safer and less invasive with lower rates of complications compared with the standard open approach. The posterior approach was initially described by van Dijk and colleagues[22] using a 2-portal hindfoot approach. The posterolateral portal is created by drawing a straight line from the tip of the lateral malleolus to the Achilles tendon with the portal made just above this line. The posteromedial portal is then located at the same level of the posterolateral portal, just medial to the Achilles tendon (**Figs. 3** and **4**).[22,32] A stab incision is

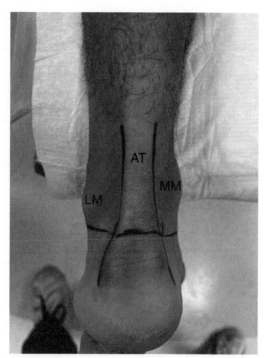

Fig. 3. Before incision placement, the landmarks are marked out including the Achilles tendon (AT), medial malleolus (MM), and lateral malleolus (LM). A horizontal line is made from the inferior aspect of the lateral malleolus.

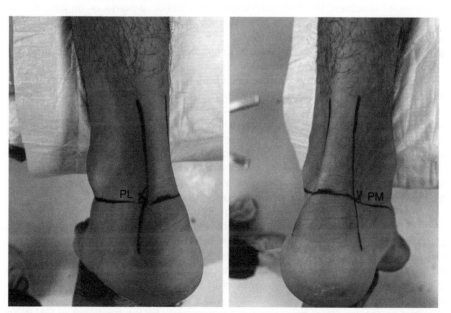

Fig. 4. The posteromedial (PM) and posterolateral (PM) portal sites are marked out about 1 mm anterior to the medial and lateral borders of the Achilles tendon at the level of the horizontal line between the inferior poles of the medial and lateral malleolus.

made over the posterolateral portal, and blunt dissection with a hemostat is carried down to the posterior ankle and subtalar joint. A 4.0- or 2.9-mm arthroscope sleeve with a trocar is advanced via the posterolateral portal to touch the posterior aspect of the talus. After palpating the posterior talus, the trocar can be removed and arthroscope inserted. A spinal or 18-gauge needle can then be used from the posteromedial portal. Once the needle is visualized and confirmed that the level of arthroscopic examination is adequate, a stab incision can be made and an arthroscopic shaver can be inserted. When performing this technique, all instruments should be directed toward the first interdigital web space to prevent iatrogenic neurovascular bundle injury in the hindfoot. Typically, the surgeon will encounter the posterior capsule and/or fibrosis and inflammation that requires debridement for several minutes before adequate visualization of the posterior ankle and talus can be clearly visualized. Once visualization is achieved, finding the FHL tendon is imperative. The FHL becomes the most medial border of the arthroscopic clean up. If the surgeon is not able to adequately visualize the FHL tendon, or debrides medial to the FHL, this can lead to iatrogenic neurovascular injury.

A systematic approach for visualizing all the structures of the posterior ankle and subtalar joints is used by a 4-stage approach with the intermalleolar ligament as the anatomic landmark for defining the quadrants.[12] The superolateral quadrant contains the posterior inferior tibiofibular ligament, transverse ligament, and intermalleolar ligament. During evaluation of each quadrant, the ankle should be passively plantarflexed to check for any impingement. If impingement is noted, the structure is debrided with the shaver. The superomedial quadrant contains the FHL tendon; the neurovascular bundle lies medial to this; therefore, all instruments should stay lateral to the FHL tendon (**Fig. 5**). At this time, anomalous muscles such as a peroneus quartus should be evaluated. Tenosynovitis around the FHL tendon is a common finding, reported up to 65% to 85% in patients with PAI.[26,33] A low-lying FHL muscle belly may also be the source of impingement and should be debrided at this level. Within the inferomedial quadrant, the FHL retinaculum and Stieda process or os trigonum is observed and can be removed with an osteotome, shaver, or burr if causing bony impingement. The investigators typically use a shaver to detach the soft tissues around the os trigonum, then place a burr or small osteotome into the interval between the posterolateral talar process and os trigonum, which is typically a fibrocartilaginous synchondrosis (**Figs. 6** and **7**). The fragment is then removed with a grasper; if the os is too large, it can be broken into 2 or 3 pieces using an osteotome. Alternatively, a spinal needle can be placed percutaneously in the same interval, and the Stieda process or os trigonum can be removed carefully with a burr, starting posterior and debriding anterior until the surgeon reaches the needle. Care should be taken to avoid being overly aggressive and causing damage to the posterior facet of the subtalar joint. Gentle, controlled motion of the burr will prevent this. The inferolateral region contains the posterior talofibular ligament (PTFL) and the calcaneofibular ligament; the PTFL may be thickened and hypertrophied, requiring debridement.

Several clinical studies have reported good clinical outcomes following posterior ankle arthroscopy, with a majority of studies reporting American Orthopedic Foot and Ankle Society (AOFAS) scores greater than 85 at short-term follow-up.[33–42] A recent systematic review by Zwiers and colleagues[18] reported a mean return to full activity was 11.3 weeks (5.9–12.9 weeks) after an arthroscopic approach for PAI. One study evaluated the endoscopic excision of os trigonum in professional dancers and found that the average return to sport was 8 weeks.[43] Sugimoto and colleagues[9] reported on the results of posterior ankle arthroscopy for the treatment of PAI in an athletic population ranging from recreational sports players to professional athletes. There were a total of 59 patients with a mean follow-up of 60 months. The average

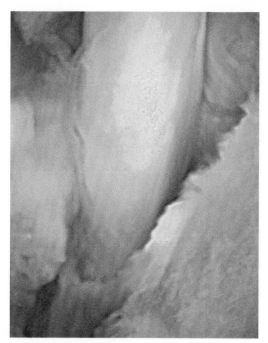

Fig. 5. Arthroscopic image of the superomedial quadrant with fibrosis and stenosis of the FHL tendon.

preoperative AOFAS score improved from 79.6 to 97.6 postoperatively (p < 0.0001). The average time to return to preinjury level was 13.4 weeks. The investigators also reported on the learning curve of performing a posterior ankle arthroscopy and determined that an experience of 26 cases was required to be proficient in this approach.

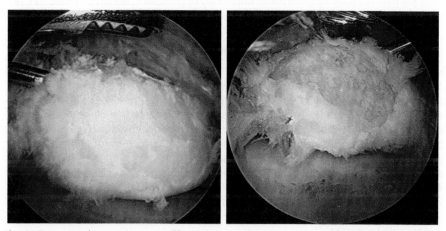

Fig. 6. To resect the os trigonum efficiently, a small osteotome or needle can be placed in the interval between the posterior talus and os trigonum. A burr can then be used to gently resect the os trigonum or Stieda process. Care should be taken to avoid iatrogenic injury to the posterior facet of the subtalar joint.

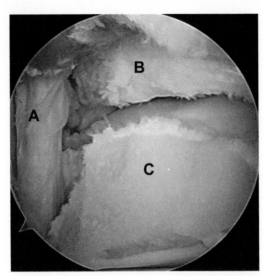

Fig. 7. Arthroscopic image of the posterior ankle joint with the following structures: FHL tendon (A), posterior aspect of the distal tibia (B), and postresection of a Stieda process (C).

Postoperative AOFAS scores between the first and last 10 cases were not statistically different; therefore, despite the learning curve effect, a low volume of experience was not found to affect the results in this study.

Complications in arthroscopic surgery
The most common complication reported is sural nerve injury, reported at a rate of 3.4% to 8.3%.[1] Zwiers and colleagues[18] reported low complication rates after posterior hindfoot arthroscopy, with 1.8% of patients suffering a major complication and 5.4% of patients suffering a minor complication. Major complications consist of deep infection, complex regional pain syndrome, or reoperation, and minor complications are mild nerve symptoms either temporary or persistent, superficial infection, hematoma, persistent leakage, scar issues, or Achilles tightness.[18,44]

Open Versus Arthroscopic/Endoscopic Treatment
Historically, open techniques were used to perform surgery for the resection of osseous or soft tissue PAI with good results. However, since the introduction of endoscopic techniques, advantages attributed to this surgical approach are shorter recovery time, fewer complications, and less pain.[18,45] Georgiannos and Bisbinas[45] conducted a randomized controlled study between endoscopic and open treatment of PAI in an athletic population and reported favorable outcomes for endoscopic surgery regarding lower complication rates and shorter time to return to preinjury level of sports. The mean time to return to training was 9.5 weeks for open treatment and 4.5 weeks for endoscopic treatment ($P < .001$). The time to return to previous sports level was 11.5 weeks for open treatment and 7 weeks for endoscopic treatment ($P < .001$). The overall complication rate was 23% for open treatment and 4% for endoscopic treatment.

A meta-analysis by Zwiers and colleagues[44] compared 32 studies to determine whether endoscopic surgery was superior to open surgery for PAI. There was no difference in postoperative AOFAS scores between open surgery (88.0; 95% confidence interval [CI], 82.1–94.4) and endoscopic surgery (94.4; 95% CI, 93.1–95.7). There was also no difference between patients who rated their overall satisfaction as good or excellent, 0.91 (95% CI, 0.86–0.96) versus 0.86 (95% CI, 0.79–0.94), respectively. No significant difference was found regarding time to return to activity, 10.8 weeks (95% CI, 7.4–15.9 weeks) versus 8.9 weeks (95% CI, 7.6–10.4 weeks), respectively. The proportion of patients with complications for open surgery versus endoscopic surgery was statistically significant, 0.24 (95% CI, 0.14–0.35) versus 0.02 (95% CI, 0.00–0.06), respectively. There was no difference in postoperative AOFAS scores, patient satisfaction, and return to activity between open and endoscopic techniques. The proportion of patients who experienced a complication was significantly lower with an endoscopic approach.

Ahn[46] and colleagues compared anterior ankle/subtalar arthroscopy versus posterior endoscopic excision of symptomatic os trigonum in 28 patients and found that both groups had significant improvement in their VAS and AOFAS scores. There was no difference in outcome scores between the 2 approaches. The average return to sport for the arthroscopic group was 7.5 weeks and 8 weeks for the endoscopic group. The inveastigators concluded that both the anterior and posterior approach were safe and effective in treating PAI; however, the anterior subtalar arthroscopic approach was more technically difficult and should be primarily used if there are any concomitant conditions such as anterior impingement syndrome, sinus tarsi syndrome, or osteochondral lesions of the talus.

POSTOPERATIVE COURSE

Postoperative care depends not only on the surgeon and surgical approach but also the extent of accompanying pathology. If performing an arthroscopic approach for os trigonum excision or to remove FHL adhesions, many patients can bear weight immediately in a boot with a protective dressing. If there is any additional pathology, patients will remain non–weight-bearing until the incisions are healed followed by weight-bearing as tolerated in a boot and gentle ankle range of motion exercises at approximately 2 to 3 weeks to prevent fibrosis and adhesions. For athletes, as soon as the incisions are healed they will begin formal physical therapy to continue to improve strength and range of motion and prevent atrophy during recovery. Many times, for isolated pathology, athletes can return to sport within 1 month.

SUMMARY

PAI is considered a clinical disorder characterized by posterior ankle pain during forced plantarflexion. The most common causes of PAI are pathologic variants of the posterolateral talar process such as either an os trigonum or a Stieda process or soft tissue impingement with or without FHL tendon disorders. PAI can become symptomatic following overuse, ankle trauma, or in athletes such as dancers or runners who are performing repetitive forced plantarflexion of the ankle. Patients typically present with posterior ankle pain, which is exacerbated with plantarflexion. It is important to highlight that patients may have pain with isolated testing of the FHL tendon, which can also be a presenting symptom of PAI. Diagnosis is based on clinical history, physical examination, and imaging. Conservative treatment includes rest, activity modification, physical therapy, and antiinflammatory medications, and steroid injections. Ultrasound-guided injections are useful to help locate the symptomatic lesion and can reduce symptoms to allow a player to finish a season. Therapeutic injections may occasionally cure soft tissue impingement; however, in osseous impingement, symptoms will likely recur requiring surgical excision for symptom resolution. Surgical treatment options include either an open or an arthroscopic approach. Overall, both surgical approaches result in a significant improvement in functional outcomes scores, pain, and a high rate of return to sport or preinjury activity level. Recent studies have found that an arthroscopic approach, despite its technical demands, report a quicker return to sport compared with an open excision. The complication rates between both open and arthroscopic techniques include sural and tibial nerve injury and infection; associated complication rates are similar between the 2 approaches.

CLINICS CARE POINTS

- A thorough clinical exam and history is important in evaluating for posterior ankle impingement.
- Several conservative treatment options are available.
- Surgical treatment is successful in both open and arthroscopic approaches, with arthroscopic approaches leading to quicker return to sport.

DISCLOSURE

The authors have nothing to disclose regarding conflict of interest or commercial relationship related to the content of this work.

REFERENCES

1. Nault M, Kocher MS, Micheli LJ. Os trigonum syndrome. J Am Acad Orthrop Surg 2014;22:545–53.
2. Giannini S, Buda R, Mosca M, et al. Posterior ankle impingement. Foot Ankle Int 2013;34:459–65.
3. Sharpe BD, Steginsky BD, Suhling M, et al. Posterior Ankle Impingement Flexor Hallucis Longus Pathol 2020;39:911–30.
4. Best A, Giza E, Linklater J, et al. Posterior impingement of the ankle caused by anomalous muscles: a report of four cases. J Bone Joint Surg 2005;87:2075–9.
5. Zammit J, Singh D. The peroneus quartus muscle. Anatomy and clinical relevance. J Bone Joint Surg Br 2003;85:1134–7.
6. Roche AJ, Calder JD, Lloyd Williams R. Posterior ankle impingement in dancers and athletes. Foot Ankle Clin 2013;18:301–18.
7. Karasick D, Schweitzer ME. The os trigonum syndrome: imaging features. Am J Roentgenol 1996;166:125–9.
8. Michelson J, Dunn L. Tenosynovitis of the flexor hallucis longus: a clinical study of the spectrum of presentation and treatment. Foot Ankle Int 2005;18:121–5.
9. Sugimoto K, Isomoto S, Samoto N, et al. Arthroscopic treatment of posterior ankle impingement syndrome: mid-term clinical results and a learning curve. Arthrosc Sports Med Rehabil 2021;15:1077–86.
10. Mouhsin E, Djahangiri A, Garofalo R. Fracture of the non fused os trigonum, a rare cause of hindfoot pain. A case report and review of the literature. Chir Organi Mov 2004;89:171–5.
11. Shepherd FJ. A hitherto undescribed fracture of the astragalus. J Anat Physiol 1882;17:79–81.
12. Yasui Y, Hannon CP, Hurley E, et al. Posterior ankle impingement syndrome: a systematic four-stage approach. World J Orthop 2016;7:657–63.

13. Lavery KP, McHale KJ, Rossy WH, et al. Ankle impingement. J Orthop Surg Res 2016;11:97.
14. Wiegerinck JI, Vroemen JC, van Dongen TH, et al. The posterior impingement view: an alternative conventional projection to detect bony posterior ankle impingement. Arthroscopy 2014;30:1311–6.
15. Robinson P, Bollen SR. Posterior ankle impingement in professional soccer players: effectiveness of sonographically guided therapy. Am J Roentgenol 2006;187:53–8.
16. Ribbans WJ, Ribbans HA, Cruickshank JA, et al. The management of posterior ankle impingement syndrome in sport: a review. Foot Ankle Surg 2015;21:1–10.
17. Marotta JJ, Micheli LJ. Os trigonum impingement in dancers. Am J Sports Med 1992;20:533–6.
18. Zwiers R, Wiegerinck JI, Murawski CD, et al. Surgical treatment for posterior ankle impingement. Arthroscopy 2013;29:1263–70.
19. Schulhofer SD, Oloff LM. Flexor hallucis longus dysfunction: an overview. Clin Podiatr Med Surg 2002;19:411–8.
20. Howse AJ. Posterior block of the ankle joint in dancers. Foot Ankle 1982;3:81–4.
21. Quirk R. Talar compression syndrome in dancers. Foot Ankle 1982;3:65–8.
22. Van Dijk CN, Scholten PE, Krips R. A 2-portal endoscopic approach for diagnosis and treatment of posterior ankle pathology. Arthroscopy 2000;16:871–6.
23. Labs K, Leutloff D, Perka C. Posterior ankle impingement syndrome in dancers—a short-term follow-up after operative treatment. Foot Ankle 2002;8:33–9.
24. Abramowitz Y, Wollstein R, Barzilay Y, et al. Outcome of resection of a symptomatic os trigonum. J Bone Joint Surg Am 2003;85:1051–7.
25. Veazey BL, Heckman JD, Galindo MJ, et al. Excision of ununited fractures of the posterior process of the talus: a treatment for chronic posterior ankle pain. Foot Ankle 1992;13:453–7.
26. Hamilton WG, Geppert MJ, Thompson FM. Pain in the posterior aspect of the ankle in dancers. Differential diagnosis and operative treatment. J Bone Joint Surg Am 1996;78:1491–500.
27. Spicer DD, Howse AJ. Posterior block of the ankle: the results of surgical treatment in dancers. Foot Ankle Surg 1999;5:187–90.
28. Heyer JH, Rose DJ. Os trigonum excision in dancers via an open posteromedial approach. Foot Ankle Int 2017;38:27–35.
29. de Landevoisin ES, Jacopin S, Glard Y, et al. Surgical treatment of the symptomatic os trigonum in children. Orthop Traumatol Surg Res 2009;95:159–63.
30. Kolettis GJ, Micheli LJ, Klein JD. Release of the flexor hallucis longus tendon in ballet dancers. J Bone Joint Surg Am 1996;78:1386–90.
31. Rogers J, Dijkstra P, McCourt P, et al. Posterior ankle impingement syndrome: a clinical review with reference to horizontal jump athletes. Acta Orthop Belg 2010;76:572–9.
32. Van Dijk CN, Vuurberg G, Batista J, et al. Posterior ankle arthroscopy: current state of the art. J ISAKOS: Joint Disord Orthopaedic Sports Med 2017;2:269–77.
33. Scholten PE, Sierevelt IN, van Dijk CN. Hindfoot endoscopy for posterior ankle impingement. J Bone Joint Surg Am 2008;90:2665–72.
34. van Dijk CN, de Leeuw PA, Scholten PE. Hindfoot endoscopy for posterior ankle impingement. Surgical technique. J Bone Joint Surg Am 2009;9:287–98.
35. Willits K, Sonneveld H, Amendola A, et al. Outcome of posterior ankle arthroscopy for hindfoot impingement. Arthroscopy 2008;24:196–202.
36. Jerosch J, Fadel M. Endoscopic resection of a symptomatic os trigonum. Knee Surg Sports Traumatol Arthrosc 2006;14:1188–93.

37. Tey M, Monllau JC, Centenera JM, et al. Benefits of arthroscopic tuberculoplasty in posterior ankle impingement syndrome. Knee Surg Sports Traumatol Arthrosc 2007;15:1235–9.

38. Horibe S, Kita K, Natsu-ume T, et al. A novel technique of arthroscopic excision of a symptomatic os trigonum. Arthroscopy 2008;24:121.

39. Galla M, Lobenhoffer P. Technique and results of arthroscopic treatment of posterior ankle impingement. Foot Ankle Surg 2011;17:79–84.

40. Noguchi H, Ishii Y, Takeda M, et al. Arthroscopic excision of posterior ankle bony impingement for early return to the field: short-term results. Foot Ankle Int 2010; 31:398–403.

41. Nickisch F, Barg A, Saltzman CL, et al. Postoperative complications of posterior ankle and hindfoot arthroscopy. J Bone Joint Surg Am 2012;94:439–46.

42. Dinato MC, Luques IU, Freitas Mde F, et al. Endoscopic treatment of the posterior ankle impingement syndrome on amateur and professional athletes. Knee Surg Sports Traumatol Arthrosc 2016;24:1396–401.

43. Morelli F, Mazza D, Serlorenzi P, et al. Endoscopic excision of symptomatic os trigonum in professional dancers. J Foot Ankle Surg 2017;56:22–5.

44. Zwiers R, Miedema T, Wiegerinck JI, et al. Open versus endoscopic surgical treatment of posterior ankle impingement: a meta-analysis. Am J Sports Med 2022;50:563–75.

45. Georgiannos D, Bisbinas I. Endoscopic verus open excision of os trigonum for the treatment of posterior ankle impingement syndrome in an athletic population: a randomized controlled study with 5-year follow-up. Am J Sports Med 2017;45: 1388–94.

46. Ahn JH, Kim YC, Kim HY. Arthroscopic versus posterior endoscopic excision of a symptomatic os trigonum. Am J Sports Med 2013;41:1082–9.

Imaging Tendon Disorders in Athletes

Kanwardeep Singh, MD[a], Nastaran Hosseini, MD[a], Atefe Pooyan, MD, MPH[a],
Firoozeh Shomal Zadeh, MD[a], Majid Chalian, MD[a],*

KEYWORDS

• Tendon • Pathology • Athletes • Injury • Tear • Ultrasound • MRI

KEY POINTS

• Tendon pathology manifests in various forms in athletes including mechanical, degenerative enthesitis, neoplastic, and overuse disease.
• While various modalities are available for imaging tendon pathology, ultrasound and MRI are by far the most common imaging modalities used for this purpose.
• Clinicians need to be familiar with both the normal and pathologic appearance of tendons on ultrasonography and MRI. Common pathologies include tendinosis, tenosynovitis, partial thickness tear, and full thickness tear.
• In addition to the pathologic appearance of tendons, clinicians need to be aware of common normal variants as well as common artifacts encountered on MRI and ultrasound.
• There are various new and emerging imaging techniques for the evaluation of tendon pathologies such as sonoelastography and T2 mapping.

INTRODUCTION

Imaging plays a critical role in evaluating pathology affecting athletes from various fields. Tendon pathology manifests in terms of mechanical, degenerative, enthesitis, neoplastic, and overuse disease.[1] Tendon pathologies in athletes usually involve injuries to commonly injured tendons such as the tendons involving the ankle, elbow, rotator cuff, hip abductors, patellar tendon, and Achilles tendon. For the purposes of this article, the focus will be on the tendons involving the ankle such as the tibialis posterior tendon, peroneal tendons, and achilles tendon. The two most common imaging modalities used for the evaluation of tendons are ultrasound (US) and magnetic resonance imaging (MRI). There are several emerging imaging techniques such as T2 mapping, ultra-short echo time MRI, and sonoelastography.[1] These novel imaging

[a] Department of Radiology, Musculoskeletal Imaging and Intervention, University of Washington, 4245 Roosevelt Way Northeast, Box 354755, Seattle, WA 98105, USA
* Corresponding author.
E-mail address: mchalian@uw.edu
Twitter: @Nas_Hosseini (N.H.); @AtefePooyan (A.P.); @FiroozehShomal (F.S.Z.); @MajidChalian (M.C.)

Clin Podiatr Med Surg 40 (2023) 223–238
https://doi.org/10.1016/j.cpm.2022.07.015
0891-8422/23/© 2022 Elsevier Inc. All rights reserved.

techniques are all in the the research phase and have not been adapted to routine clinical practice.

TENDON ANATOMY

Imaging characteristics of tendons depend on the dense connective tissue and the anatomic relationship between bone and muscle (**Fig. 1**). Tendons are mainly composed of cross-linked triple helices of type 1 collagen which is used to transfer energy from a muscle to bone helping with movement across a joint. Type 1 collagen composes 65% to 80% of the normal tendon by dry weight. The remainder of the collagen structure contains varying degrees of type II, III, IV, and V cartilage among others.[2] Other substances include proteoglycans, glycosaminoglycans, structural glycoproteins, and other inorganic components such as calcium.

These components give rise to the individual collagen fibrils which become organized into collagen fibers. The fascicles are enclosed by an endotendon sheath. The orientation of fibers depends on the location and function of the tendon. In general, collagen fibers are usually arranged parallel to the tendon axis. The force that is applied is directed along the axis. This model becomes more complex when multiple muscles attach to a single tendon as in the Achilles or quadriceps tendon. Schematic **Fig. 2** depicts the normal structure of the tendon.

Some tendons have a synovial sheath while others do not (**Fig. 3**). Typically, synovial sheaths have 2 layers that are in continuity collectively referred to as the mesotenon. The sheath serves to decrease friction wherever a tendon comes in close proximity to bone or fibrous tissue.[3] The mesotenon carries blood vessels into the tendon (**Figs. 4** and **5**). The synovial sheath can become inflamed and result in tenosynovitis with the accumulation of fluid within the tendon sheath. There are several tendons that do not contain a true synovial sheath with the most commonly known example being the Achilles tendon. A paratenon surrounds the Achilles tendon which is separate from the tendon itself. As opposed to the synovial sheath, a paratenon is a single layer of cells composed of adipose tissue which is rich in vascularization.[4] It supplies a significant amount of blood to the underlying tendon. Just like the synovial sheath, the paratenon is also subject to pathology such as paratenonitis resulting in the inflammation of the surrounding adipose tissue.

The ankle anatomy is grossly divided into 3 different tendon compartments. These include the extensor compartment, flexor compartment, and peroneal compartment. The extensor tendons include the tibialis anterior, extensor hallucis longus, and extensor digitorum longus. The flexor compartment includes the tibialis posterior,

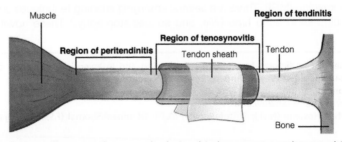

Fig. 1. The diagram illustrates the normal relationship between a tendon attaching muscle to bone with corresponding pathologies affecting various portions of the tendon such as tendinitis, peritendinitis, and tenosynovitis.

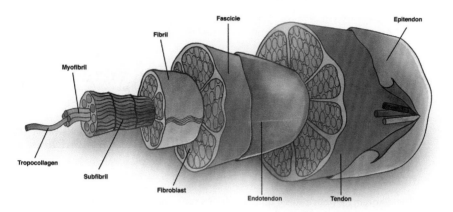

Fig. 2. The diagram illustrates the normal architecture of a tendon. The epitendon surrounds the outer surface with the inner fascicles being surrounded by the endotendon. Each fascicle is made up of multiple fibrils with are further subdivided into subfibril and myofibril. The individual tropocollagen makes up the myofibrils.

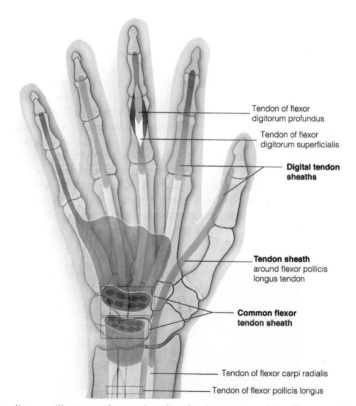

Fig. 3. The diagram illustrates the tendon sheaths that surround the flexor tendons of the digits. More proximally, the tendons of the 2nd–5th digit share a common tendon sheath. Not all parts of the tendons are covered with tendon sheath.

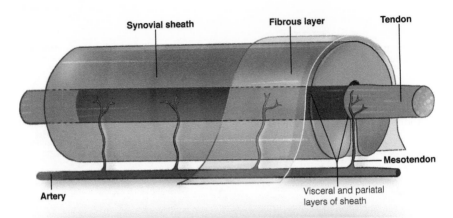

Synovial sheath   Fibrous layer   Tendon

Mesotendon

Artery   Visceral and pariatal
layers of sheath

Fig. 4. The diagram demonstrates a tendon with its surrounding synovial and fibrous layers. The mesotenon can be seen providing blood supply into the tendon.

flexor digitorum longus, and flexor hallucis longus. The peroneal compartment includes the peroneal longus and brevis tendons.

UTILIZATION OF ULTRASOUND AND MAGNETIC RESONANCE IMAGING IN TENDON PATHOLOGY

MRI is one of the most used modalities for the evaluation of tendon pathology. Some of the reasons include the noninvasive nature of the scan and lack of ionizing radiation. Increased utilization of MRI in the medical field has driven forward the inventions of newer MRI-compatible implantable devices. Imaging of tendons relies heavily on microscopic components. The resultant signal is a dark signal void in conventional MRI techniques with the exception of the previously discussed magic angle artifact.

Tendon pathology of athletes on MRI can manifest in various ways such as tendon thickening, partial thickness tear, or full thickness tear. One of the first signs of tendon abnormality is edema resulting from the injury which manifests as an increase in signal intensity on T2 weighted images. Hyperintense signal may also be seen at the site of tendon tear or in the surrounding tissue. Chronic injuries resulting in scarring over time can result in the obscuration of the edema and result in the intermediate signal. Fatty infiltration at the site of injury over time can also occur.[5]

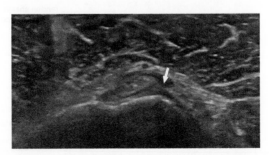

Fig. 5. The ultrasound image of the long head of the biceps tendon on short axis demonstrates fluid surrounding the tendon. Such fluid accumulation can be seen with tenosynovitis. The mesotenon (*arrow*) is seen with fluid on either side.

Ultrasound is another popular modality used as a first-line evaluation for tendon pathology in athletes. Similar to MRI, ionizing radiation is not used in ultrasonography. An important advantage of US is the ability to image tendons in real-time from various angles, weight-bearing positions, and carry out dynamic imaging. However, US is not without limitations. The resolution of the images depends on their ability to penetrate the tissues. The inability to image through bone or gas locules makes visualization and evaluation of deeper tendons difficult. The US appearance of tendons depends on the architectural structure. By using a high-frequency transducer for more superficial tendons like the Achilles, the tendon appears as longitudinal parallel echogenic lines representative of the underlying fascicles. When viewed in a transverse plane, the same linear echogenic parallel lines appear as echogenic points representing each fascicle. The ability to appropriately image a tendon depends on the depth of the structure and availability of transducer frequency.

Tendon pathology disrupts the expected fascicular pattern on ultrasonography. Such pathology includes tendinopathy which results in decreased echogenicity. Hypo echogenicity needs to be differentiated from anisotropy which refers to the artifactual decrease in signal due to the orientation of the imaged tendon. Other pathologic changes include partial thickness tears with resultant increased space between the echogenic fibers. Full thickness tears result in discontinuity of the imaged tendon. Chronic injury can result in thickened appearance on US, similar to MRI. Overuse of tendons in athletes can result in inflammatory enthesitis which may show loss of normal fibrillar pattern, indistinct tendon margins, and irregular fusiform thickening.[6] Chronic injury may also result in calcium deposition which can be visualized as echogenic foci with ultrasonography.

IMAGING APPEARANCE OF NORMAL TENDON

MRI and US are the main diagnostic imaging modalities for the assessment of tendon integrity and pathology. Both techniques do not expose patients to ionizing radiation. In US, tendons appear as fascicular structures visualized as multiple, closely spaced echogenic parallel lines when imaged in a longitudinal plane (**Fig. 6**). In the transverse plane, a tendon seems to have multiple echogenic foci (see **Fig. 5**). On MRI, normal tendons demonstrate low signal intensity on all conventional sequences due to their microstructure and scarcity of internal fluid. When collagen and water molecules are aligned, the dipole interactions shorten the T2 time of normal tendons resulting in loss of signal (**Fig. 7**).

TENDON PATHOLOGIES

There are several different ways to broadly classify tendon pathology in athletes. One such way is to divide it between inflammatory enthesitis and tendinopathy. Inflammatory enthesitis refers to the inflammation of the entheses while the mechanical and

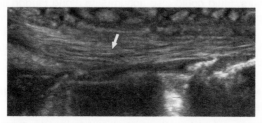

Fig. 6. The longitudinal ultrasound image of extensor tendon at wrist shows the multiple, closely spaced, echogenic, parallel fascicles of the normal tendon architecture (*arrow*).

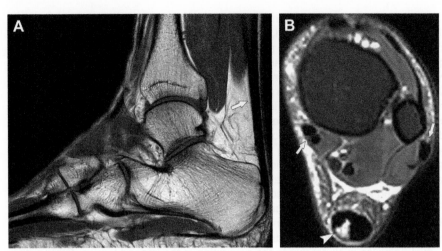

Fig. 7. Normal signal intensity of tendons on MRI. (*A*) The sagittal T1 pulse sequence illustrates the typical hypointense signal of tendons owing to their collagen and water molecule dipole interactions. The normal Achilles tendon is displayed demonstrating diffuse low T1 signal intensity (*arrow*). (*B*) The axial T1 pulse sequence demonstrates the typical hypointense signal of flexor and peroneal tendons within the ankle compartments. Note is made of partial tear of the Achilles tendon (*arrowhead*).

degenerative effects over time culminate in tendinopathy.[7] Inflammation of the attachment sites of tendon, ligament, fascia, or joint capsule to bone is referred to as enthesitis. Imaging features may show edema among other inflammatory markers. On histologic bases, changes such as macrophage-mediated fibrocartilage destruction, lymphocytic infiltration within the bone, lymphocyte paucity at the insertion site, and macrophage infiltration are seen.[8–10]

Tendinopathy refers to mechanical, degenerative, and overuse of the tendon which demonstrates little or no inflammation over time. There is resultant degeneration and disorganization in the structure of tendon fibers which chronically accumulate mucoid, proteoglycan, and water content.[11,12] Macroscopic changes include tendon thickening, loss of mechanical properties, and pain. Age-related changes include structural and compositional changes such as decreased water content and collagenous changes. These changes accumulate over time and predispose to tendinopathy as well as enthesitis. Aging tendons also decrease in vascularity over time which plays a role in tendon imaging.

In addition to the pathologic processes of inflammatory enthesitis and tendinopathy, tendons can undergo tears secondary to trauma, especially in the athletic population. These can be subclassified into partial thickness (see **Fig. 7**B; **Fig. 8**) or full thickness (**Figs. 9** and **10**) tears. Fluid could also accumulate along tendon sheath and cause tenosynovitis, which could be present with tendinopathy or happen in isolation. Tenosynovitis could be secondary to chronic repetitive microtrauma, inflammatory conditions, or infectious etiologies. Discussion on other less common tendon pathologies such as neoplastic lesions is beyond the scope of this article.

COMMON TENDON PATHOLOGIES IN ATHLETES INVOLVING THE ANKLE
Tibialis Posterior Tendon

Tibialis posterior muscle arises from the posterior surface of the tibia beyond the soleal line as well as the fibula. The tendon begins at the lower aspect of the deep posterior

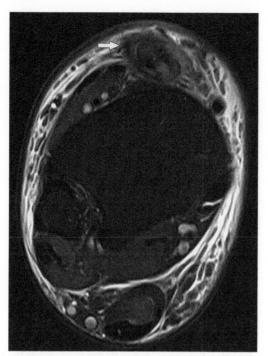

Fig. 8. The axial T2 image illustrates a partial thickness tear of the tibialis anterior tendon (arrow) with thickening of the tendon and fluid signal intensity interspersed in between the fascicles.

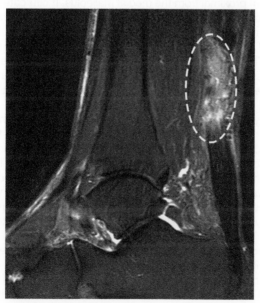

Fig. 9. The sagittal T2 fat-saturated image shows a full thickness tear of the Achilles tendon with fluid filling the tendon gap (dotted oval).

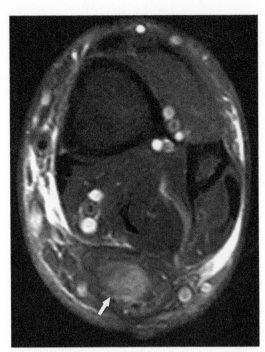

Fig. 10. The axial T2 fat-saturated image demonstrates fluid within the site of a full thickness Achilles tendon tear.

leg compartment running in a fibrous tunnel. There is a synovial sheath that is formed approximately 6 cm proximal from the medial malleolus. It bifurcates into 2 slips after passing inferior to the plantar calcaneonavicular ligament with the superficial slip inserting into the navicular bone or medial cuneiform. The deep slip divides further into slips inserted on the plantar surfaces of the middle cuneiform as well as 2nd–4th metatarsals. The tendon receives its blood supply from the posterior tibial artery and periosteal vessels. There is a segment commencing approximately 15 mm distal to the medial malleolus whereby the tendon's synovial sheath is relatively hypovascular predisposing it to a site of pathology such as a tear.[13]

Ultrasonography is very helpful in imaging tibialis posterior tendon pathologies. For example, ultrasound can depict the degree of fluid surrounding the tendon within the tendon sheath to demonstrate tenosynovitis. Ultrasound can also demonstrate thickening of the tendon which can be seen as long-term sequela of injury in athletes. Disruption of the normal fibrillar pattern can be a result of tendinosis or longitudinal split tears. Hypervascularity can be assessed in real-time secondary to acute inflammatory changes but using Doppler signal. A tear may be visualized as a focal region of hypo echogenicity and discontinuity. Chronic injury can result in tendon thickening and calcification.

Similar to ultrasound, MRI can be very beneficial to demonstrate tibialis posterior pathology. MRI will demonstrate increased signal intensity on fluid-sensitive images secondary to edema with associated tendon thickening.[14] Partial thickness tear will demonstrate fluid signal intensity within the tendon substance with the torn fibers contributing to tendon thinning. Full thickness tears will result in a visible gap typically filled with fluid across the substance of the tendon.[14] Edema may also be seen within the surrounding tissues with both partial and full thickness tears. In addition to the tibialis posterior pathology, MRI can also demonstrate abnormalities of the associated structures which can also be frequently injured in athletes such as spring and deltoid ligament complexes. Its high sensitivity allows for the detection of edema and early intrasubstance tears that may not be appreciated during the physical examination.

Peroneal Tendons

The peroneus longus muscle commences at the proximal aspect of the fibular diaphysis, fibular head, tibiotalar intermuscular septum, and the lateral tibial condyle.[15] The tendon travels distally along the posterior part of the peroneus brevis tendon, inferior to the peroneal tubercle, and medially at the lateral cuboid margin within the cuboid notch toward the first metatarsal. It inserts on the base of the first metatarsal and medial cuneiform. A normal variant os peroneum can be encountered in 5% to 26% of the population.[16] It is a fibrocartilaginous sesamoid bone within the tendon of the peroneus longus. It is fully ossified in 20% of the cases and is usually found whereby the tendon wraps around the cuboid in the cuboid tunnel. Pathology related to this normal variant includes painful os peroneum syndrome. This includes acute or chronic os peroneum fracture, diastasis of the multipartite variant of os peroneum, partial rupture of the peroneus longus tendon, and a prominent peroneal tubercle that can cause entrapment of the peroneus longus or os peroneum.[17] An enlarged prominent tubercle can be seen in up to 29% of specimens.[18]

The peroneus brevis muscle commences at the lower aspect of the fibular diaphysis and intermuscular septum. It travels distally posterior to the lateral malleolus, anterior to the peroneus longus tendon, and superior to the peroneal tubercle of the calcaneus.[15] It has a flattened appearance compared with the peroneus longus and inserts onto the styloid process of the fifth metatarsal base.

Both peroneus longus and brevis share a synovial tendon sheath that begins approximately 2.5 to 3.5 cm proximal to the fibular tip. The synovial sheath then bifurcates with each tendon obtaining its own synovial sheath at the level of the peroneal tubercle. This synovial sheath communicates with the ankle or subtalar joint in 15% of the patients.[19]

Pathology in athletes involving the peroneus tendons includes tenosynovitis, superior peroneal retinaculum (SPR) injury, acute, and chronic tears. One common injury pattern includes traumatic subluxation and dislocation of the peroneal tendons. The displacement occurs from damage to the SPR which is classified into 4 grades. Grade I injuries include lifting the SPR from the fibular periosteum. Grade II injuries include the elevation of the fibrocartilaginous ridge from the fibular. Grade III injuries demonstrate avulsion of the SPR off of the fibula with a small cortical fragment still attached. Grade IV injuries include SPR rupture off of the posterior attachment on the calcaneus and/or Achilles tendon.[20] Callus formation as part of the healing process from an os peroneum fracture can also result in stenosis resulting in tenosynovitis of the peroneus longus tendon.

Both partial and full thickness tears can occur involving the peroneus brevis and longus tendons. These can result from chronic stress, degeneration, and acute inversion injuries involving forced eversion of the supinated foot.[21] Foot malignment such as hindfoot varus and cavovarus can also increase the propensity for injury.[21] Tears of the peroneus brevis can occur at its insertion site near the base of the fifth metatarsal when it is fractured. Peroneus longus tears are less common than peroneus brevis tears. The peroneus longus can be divided into 3 zones: Zone A being from the inferior aspect of the medial malleolus to the peroneal tubercle, Zone B being from the peroneal tubercle to the inferior retinaculum, and Zone C from inferior retinaculum to the cuboid notch. Most of the peroneus longus tears occur in Zone C.[22]

Full thickness tears on US present with focal defects at the site of tendon retraction. Partial thickness tears demonstrate heterogeneity with regions of hypo echogenicity.[23,24] Tendon tears on MRI demonstrated low to intermediate signal on T1 weighted images. Edema represented as increased T2 signal is typically present within the surrounding tissues. Full thickness defects contain a fluid-filled defect at the site of tear. Partial thickness tear could be low grade (less than 50% of tendon thickness) (**Fig. 11**) or high grade (more than 50% of tendon thickness) with residual intact fibers in place.

Tendinopathy manifests as tendon thickening or increased signal intensity on T2 weighted images without tendon thinning or gap (**Fig. 12**). Chronic tendinopathy can result in hypointense calcification or bursitis. Under US, tendinosis can demonstrate heterogenous echogenicity with tendon thickening. Tendon tears may demonstrate thinning or echogenicity. Chronic injury may result in hyperechogenic foci of calcifications. Partial thickness tears demonstrate tendon thinning on T1 weighted MRI images and increased signal on T2 weighted images. Tendon fiber discontinuity associated with increased T2 signal is suggestive of a full thickness tear.[25]

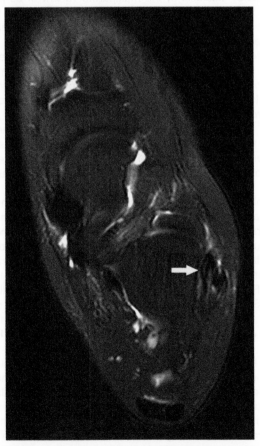

Fig. 11. The axial T2 image demonstrates thinning of the peroneus brevis tendon fibers with surrounding fluid signal consistent and a low-grade partial thickness tear.

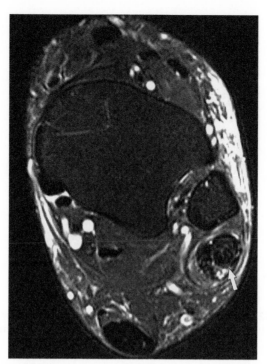

Fig. 12. The sagittal T2 fat-saturated image illustrates fluid signal within the distal aspect of the peroneal tendon with several fibers still in continuity. The findings are consistent with a high-grade partial thickness Achilles tendon.

Achilles Tendon

The Achilles tendon is formed by contributions from the tendons of soleus and both heads of the gastrocnemius on the calcaneus tuberosity. Injuries to the Achilles tendon are often encountered in athletes participating in physical activity such as running. Clinical symptoms accompanying imaging features include swelling, morning stiffness, and pain.[26] The collagen within the connective tissue of the Achilles tendon allows for storage of elastic strain energy and conversion into kinetic energy on recoil.[26] Histologic changes include collagen fiber microstructure disruption, increase in ground substance, neovascularization, and increased fibroblastic activity.[27]

Achilles tendon lacks a true synovial sheath but is instead encased by a paratenon made up of a single layer of cells,[28] which is richly vascularized giving a significant amount of nutrients to the tendon. The most tenuous blood supply is at 2 to 6 cm proximal from the insertion site at the calcaneus.[29] On US, the Achilles tendon seems hypoechoic with typical tightly packed fibrillar tendon structure.[30] On MRI, the tendon demonstrates a low signal intensity across all MRI pulse sequences.[31] During tendinopathy, the Achilles tendon appears thickened with convexity involving the anterior border.[32] Intermediate signal on T1 weighted images maybe seen with high signal surrounding the tendon on the fluid-sensitive sequences. This finding may manifest as retrocalcaneal bursitis or osseous edema. A partial thickness tear results in fluid signal within the tendon fibers resulting in thinning of the overall fibers (see **Fig. 7**; **Fig. 13**). If there is a full thickness tear, hyperintense signal reflecting fluid may fill the gap (see **Figs. 9** and **10**). A Similar gap may be demonstrated using US whereby a hypoechogenicity may separate the typical fibrillar tendon structure.

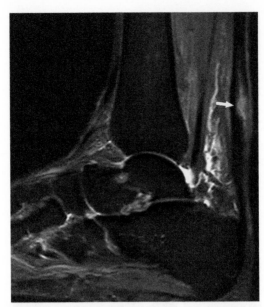

Fig. 13. The axial T2 fat-saturated image illustrates a partial thickness tear involving the peroneus longus and brevis resulting in fluid signal within the tendon fibers.

Pathologies involving extensor tendons are less common and follow the general pattern of peroneal and flexor tendon. Therefore, a detailed description of extensor tendons will not be discussed in this text.

COMMON NORMAL VARIANTS

Common normal variants include accessory anatomic structures especially in the ankle and foot. These include the accessory peroneal muscle such as peroneus quartus.[33] In most cases, it arises from the peroneus brevis muscle and remains medial and posterior to the peroneus brevis and longus (**Fig. 14**). The insertion site can be variable. The accessory soleus muscle is another common variant located in the deep posterior compartment.[33] It arises from the anterior surface of the soleus and remains anterior and medial to the Achilles tendon. It either inserts and contributes to the Achilles tendon or has a direct insertion on the calcaneus.

Examples of normal variants in the shoulder include the aponeurotic expansion of the supraspinatus tendon. In such cases, there is a tendon-like structure localized at the level of the bicipital groove. It is located parallel and anterolateral to the long head of the bicep tendon. It extends from the superficial aspect of the supraspinatus tendon and surrounds the biceps tendon.[34] The assessment and implications of all normal variants are beyond the scope of this text.

COMMON ARTIFACTS ON MAGNETIC RESONANCE IMAGING AND ULTRASOUND

One of the most common artifacts encountered on MRI regarding tendons is the magic angle artifact. If the tendon is aligned at 55° to the bore of the magnet, the signal becomes detectable. This phenomenon is more apparent on short echo time (TE) sequences such as T1, GRE, and PD. Magic angle is mitigated by using long TE

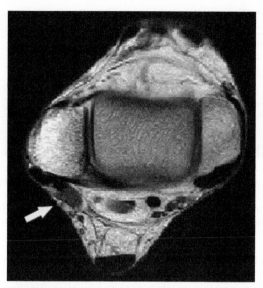

Fig. 14. The axial T2 image at the level of the ankle demonstrates an accessory muscle medial and posterior to the peroneus longus and brevis consistent with a normal variant accessory muscle peroneus quartus.

sequences such as T2. A stronger magnetic field (3T) may also help increase the signal-to-noise ratio and improve image resolution.

A common artifact encountered on US regarding tendon evaluation is anisotropy. It is an artifact generated due to angle created between the US beam and the imaged tendon fibers. It can lead to the preferential reflection of the US beam in one direction. If the imaged structures are not aligned perpendicular to the long axis of the transducer, then the reflection of the beam away from the transducer can result in the artificial reduction in echogenicity referred to as anisotropy (**Fig. 15**).

EMERGING IMAGING TECHNIQUES

While US and MRI are broadly used as the 2 main imaging techniques for the assessment of tendon pathology in athletes, they are not without limitations. US is limited due to its inherent limited field of view and operator dependency. MRI is limited due to the inherent need for homogeneous magnetic field and imaging tissues with a T2 signal that is significantly shorter than 10 microseconds.[7] To overcome the latter, there are possibilities of acquiring images with echo times as low as several microseconds with ultrashort echo time MRI techniques.[35]

Sonoelastography has been implanted in certain medical interpretations within radiology such as liver fibrosis and cirrhosis. The ability to demonstrate the stiffness or softness of tissue by measuring the strain caused on it by tissue compression may be used in tendon pathology as well. Estimation of tissue stiffness is based on the fact that greater tissue displacement occurs with soft tissue rather than hard tissue when external compression is placed.[36,37] This property of tissue can be harnessed to obtain useful information regarding the biochemical properties of a tendon.

T2 mapping can be helpful in the evaluation of biophysical properties of cartilage. It is sensitive to changes in the chemical composition and structure of cartilage. Although traditionally implemented in the evaluation of cartilage, intervertebral discs,

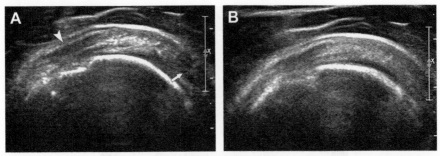

Fig. 15. Anisotropy artifact can lead to artifactual decrease in echogenicity of tendons. (*A*) The ultrasound image illustrates the supraspinatus tendon in long axis with decreased echogenicity at the myotendinous junction. Note is made of high-grade tear at the footprint (*arrow-head*) (*B*) The ultrasound image of the same tendon is obtained after readjusting the probe to demonstrate normal echogenicity of the questionable pathologic region.

and osseous structures, similar biochemical changes in tendon composition such as water content may predispose patients to tendinopathy.

Tenography can be used to evaluate tendons whereby radiopaque contrast medium is injected into a tendon sheath to detect abnormalities of the tendons and their surrounding sheaths. This is typically used when there is suspicion of fibrous adhesions within a tendon sheath.[38] Typically these patients have tendon pain but no evidence on MRI of intrinsic tendon disease. These adhesions can result from acute trauma or mechanical repetitive trauma. With the increasing utilization of US and MRI, the popularity of tenography has since declined. However, tenography can provide valuable complementary diagnostic information as well as potentially provide a therapeutic benefit. Some patients following tenography experience long-term symptoms relief.[38] The most commonly evaluated tendons via tenography are peroneal longus and brevis and posterior tibial.

DISCLOSURE

The authors have nothing to disclose.

REFERENCES

1. Weinreb JH, Sheth C, Apostolakos J, et al. Tendon structure, disease, and imaging. Muscles, ligaments, tendons J 2014;4:1 66–73.
2. Tresoldi I, Oliva F, Benvenuto M, et al. Tendon's ultrastructure. Muscles, ligaments, tendons J 2013;3(1):2–6. https://doi.org/10.11138/mltj/2013.3.1.002.
3. Benjamin M, Kaizer E, Milz S, et al. Structure-function relationships in tendons: a review. J Anat 2008;212(3):211–28. https://doi.org/10.1111/j.1469-7580.2008.00864.
4. Weinfield S. Achilles tendon disorders. Med Clin North Am 2014;98(2):331–8.
5. Goutallier D, Postel J, Bernageau J, et al. Fatty infiltration of disrupted rotator cuff muscles. Rev Rhumengl Ed 1995;62(6):415–22.
6. Kamel M, Eid H, Mansour R. Ultrasound detection of heel enthesitis: a comparison with magnetic resonance imaging. J Rheumatol 2003;30(4):774–8.
7. Hodgson RJ, et al. Tendon and ligament imaging. Br J Radiol 2012;85(1016):1157–72. https://doi.org/10.1259/bjr/34786470.

8. D'Agostino MA, Olivieri I. Enthesitis. Best Pract Res Clin Rheumatol 2006;20(3): 473–86. https://doi.org/10.1016/j.berh.2006.03.007.

9. McGonagle D, et al. Histological assessment of the early enthesitis lesion in spondyloarthropathy. Ann Rheum Dis 2002;61(6):534–7. https://doi.org/10.1136/ard.61.6.534.

10. De Mos M, van El B, DeGroot J, et al. Achilles tendinosis: changes in biochemical composition and collagen turnover rate. Am J Sports Med 2007;35(9):1549–56. https://doi.org/10.1177/0363546507301885. PMID: 17478653.

11. Miller TT, Shapiro MA, Schultz E, et al. Comparison of sonography and MRI for diagnosing epicondylitis. J Clin Ultrasound 2002;30(4):193–202.

12. Kim HM, Dahiya N, Teefey SA, et al. Location and initiation of degenerative rotator cuff TearsAn analysis of three hundred and sixty shoulders. J Bone Joint Surg 2010;92(5):1088–96.

13. Ribbans WJ, Garde A. Tibialis posterior tendon and deltoid and spring ligament injuries in the elite athlete. Foot Ankle Clin 2013;18(2):255–91. https://doi.org/10.1016/j.fcl.2013.02.006.

14. Walz DM, Newman JS, Konin GP, et al. Epicondylitis: Pathogenesis, imaging, and treatment1. Radiographics 2010;30(1):167–84.

15. Altchek DW, DiGiovanni CW, Dines JS, et al. Foot and ankle sports medicine. Philadelphia: LippinCott Williams & Wilkins; 2013.

16. Sammarco VJ, Cuttica DJ, Sammarco GJ. Lasso stitch with peroneal retinaculoplasty for repair of fractured os peroneum: a report of two cases. Clin Orthop Relat Res 2010;468(4):1012–7. https://doi.org/10.1007/s11999-009-0822-x.

17. Sobel M, Pavlov H, Geppert MJ, et al. Painful os peroneum syndrome: a spectrum of conditions responsible for plantar lateral foot pain. Foot Ankle Int 1994; 15(3):112–24.

18. Hyer CF, Dawson JM, Philbin TM, et al. The peroneal tubercle: description, classification, and relevance to peroneus longus tendon pathology. Foot Ankle Int 2005;26(11):947–50.

19. Roster B, Michelier P, Giza E. Peroneal tendon disorders. Clin Sports Med 2015; 34(4):625–41. https://doi.org/10.1016/j.csm.2015.06.003.

20. Oden RR. Tendon injuries about the ankle resulting from skiing. Clin Orthop Relat Res 1987;(216):63–9.

21. Cerrato RA, Myerson MS. Peroneal tendon tears, surgical management and its complications. Foot Ankle Clin 2009;14(2):299–312.

22. Squires N, Myerson MS, Gamba C. Surgical treatment of peroneal tendon tears. Foot Ankle Clin 2007;12(4):675–95, vii.

23. Van Holsbeeck MT, Kolowich PA, Eyler WR, et al. US depiction of partial-thickness tear of the rotator cuff. Radiology 1995;197(2):443–6.

24. De Jesus JO, Parker L, Frangos AJ, et al. Accuracy of MRI, MR arthrography, and ultrasound in the diagnosis of rotator cuff tears: a meta-analysis. Am J Roentgenol 2009;192(6):1701–7.

25. Lequesne M, Djian P, Vuillemin V, et al. Prospective study of refractory greater trochanter pain syndrome. MRI findings of gluteal tendon tears seen at surgery, clinical and MRI results of tendon repair. Joint Bone Spine 2008;75(4):458–64.

26. Child S, Bryant AL, Clark RA, et al. Mechanical properties of the achilles tendon aponeurosis are altered in athletes with achilles tendinopathy. Am J Sports Med 2010;38(9):1885–93. https://doi.org/10.1177/0363546510366234. PMID: 20508077.

27. Khan KM, Cook JL, Bonar F, et al. Histopathology of common tendinopathies: Update and implications for clinical management. Sports Med 1999;27(6):393–408.

28. Schepsis AA, Jones H, Haas AL. Achilles tendon disorders in athletes. Am J Sports Med 2002;30(2):287–305. https://doi.org/10.1177/03635465020300022501. PMID: 11912103.
29. Clain MR, Baxter DE. Achilles tendinitis. Foot Ankle 1992;13(8):482–7. https://doi.org/10.1177/107110079201300810. PMID: 1483611.
30. Maffulli N, Regine R, Angelillo M, et al. Ultra-sound diagnosis of achilles tendon pathology in runners. Br J Sports Med 1987;21(4):158–62.
31. Soila K, Karjalainen PT, Aronen HJ, et al. High-resolution MR imaging of the asymptomatic achilles tendon: new observations. AJR Am J Roentgenol 1999; 173(2):323–8.
32. Calleja M, Connell DA. The Achilles tendon 2010;14(03):307–22.
33. Aparisi Gómez M, Aparisi F, Bartoloni A, et al. Anatomical variation in the ankle and foot: from incidental finding to inductor of pathology. Part I: ankle and hind-foot. Insights Imaging 2019;10:74. https://doi.org/10.1186/s13244-019-0746-2.
34. Moser TP, Cardinal É, Bureau NJ, et al. The aponeurotic expansion of the supra-spinatus tendon: anatomy and prevalence in a series of 150 shoulder MRIs. Skel-etal Radiol 2015;44:223–31. https://doi-org.offcampus.lib.washington.edu/10.1007/s00256-014-1993-4.
35. Tyler DJ, Robson MD, Henkelman RM, et al. Magnetic resonance imaging with ultrashort TE (UTE) PULSE sequences: Technical considerations. J Magn Reson Imaging 2007;25(2):279–89.
36. Hall TJ. AAPM/RSNA physics tutorial for residents: Topics in US beyond the ba-sics: Elasticity imaging with US1. Radiographics 2003;23(6):1657–71.
37. Kulig K, Landel R, Chang N, et al. Patellar tendon morphology in volleyball ath-letes with and without patellar tendinopathy. Scand J Med Sci Sports 2012; 23(2):81–8.
38. Na JB, Bergman AG, Oloff LM, et al. The flexor hallucis longus: tenographic tech-nique and correlation of imaging findings with surgery in 39 ankles. Radiology 2005;236(3):974–82.

Moving?

Make sure your subscription moves with you!

To notify us of your new address, find your **Clinics Account Number** (located on your mailing label above your name), and contact customer service at:

Email: journalscustomerservice-usa@elsevier.com

800-654-2452 (subscribers in the U.S. & Canada)
314-447-8871 (subscribers outside of the U.S. & Canada)

Fax number: 314-447-8029

Elsevier Health Sciences Division
Subscription Customer Service
3251 Riverport Lane
Maryland Heights, MO 63043

*To ensure uninterrupted delivery of your subscription, please notify us at least 4 weeks in advance of move.

ELSEVIER

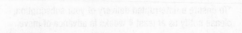

Printed and bound by CPI Group (UK) Ltd, Croydon, CR0 4YY

03/10/2024

01040476-0008